A CULTURAL HISTORY OF THE SENSES

VOLUME 6

A CULTURAL HISTORY
OF THE SENSES

IN THE
MODERN AGE

Edited by David Howes

BLOOMSBURY ACADEMIC
LONDON • NEW YORK • OXFORD • NEW DELHI • SYDNEY

BLOOMSBURY ACADEMIC
Bloomsbury Publishing Plc
50 Bedford Square, London, WC1B 3DP, UK

BLOOMSBURY, BLOOMSBURY ACADEMIC and the Diana logo are trademarks of
Bloomsbury Publishing Plc

First published in Great Britain 2014
This edition published 2019
Reprinted 2019

A catalogue record for this book is available from the British Library.

Library of Congress Cataloging-in-Publication Data.
A cultural history of the senses in the Modern Age, 1920-2000 / edited by David Howes.
pages cm
Includes bibliographical references and index.
ISBN 978-0-85785-344-8 (hardback)
1. Senses and sensation—History—20th century. 2. Perception—History—20th century.
I. Howes, David, 1957–
BF233.C855 2014
152.109'04—dc23
2014005272

ISBN: HB: 978-0-8578-5344-8
       PB: 978-1-3500-7801-7
       ePDF: 978-1-4742-3316-3
       eBook: 978-1-4742-3317-0
       HB Set: 978-0-8578-5338-7
       PB Set: 978-1-3500-7783-6

Series: The Cultural Histories Series

Typeset by RefineCatch Limited, Bungay, Suffolk

To find out more about our authors and books visit www.bloomsbury.com
and sign up for our newsletters.

CONTENTS

     Empowerment of the Patient   149
     Anamaria Iosif Ross

7   The Senses in Literature: From the Modernist Shock of
     Sensation to Postcolonial and Virtual Voices   173
     Ralf Hertel

8   Art and the Senses: The Avant-Garde Challenge to the
     Visual Arts   195
     Hannah B. Higgins

9   Sensory Media: Virtual Worlds and the Training of
     Perception   219
     Michael Bull

     NOTES   243
     BIBLIOGRAPHY   245
     NOTES ON CONTRIBUTORS   269
     INDEX   272

LIST OF ILLUSTRATIONS

INTRODUCTION

CHAPTER ONE

Every effort has been made to trace copyright holders and to obtain their permission for the use of copyright material. The publisher apologizes for any errors or omissions there may be in the credits for the illustrations and would be grateful if notified of any corrections that should be incorporated in future editions of this book.

SERIES PREFACE

GENERAL EDITOR, CONSTANCE CLASSEN

A Cultural History of the Senses is an authoritative six-volume series investigating sensory values and experiences throughout Western history and presenting a vital new way of understanding the past. Each volume follows the same basic structure and begins with an overview of the cultural life of the senses in the period under consideration. Experts examine important aspects of sensory culture under nine major headings: social life, urban sensations, the marketplace, religion, philosophy and science, medicine, literature, art, and media. A single volume can be read to obtain a thorough knowledge of the life of the senses in a given period, or one of the nine themes can be followed through history by reading the relevant chapters of all six volumes, providing a thematic understanding of changes and developments over the long term. The six volumes divide the history of the senses as follows:

Volume 1. A Cultural History of the Senses in Antiquity (500 BCE–500 CE)
Volume 2. A Cultural History of the Senses in the Middle Ages (500–1450)
Volume 3. A Cultural History of the Senses in the Renaissance (1450–1650)
Volume 4. A Cultural History of the Senses in the Age of Enlightenment (1650–1800)
Volume 5. A Cultural History of the Senses in the Age of Empire (1800–1920)
Volume 6. A Cultural History of the Senses in the Modern Age (1920–2000)

EDITOR'S ACKNOWLEDGMENTS

I wish to thank Constance for sharing her vision for *A Cultural History of the Senses* with me and for her untiring work bringing this project to fruition over the last two and a half years. I am grateful to her, in particular, for suggesting the framework for my introductory overview and for her general editorial advice as regards the present volume. I also deeply appreciate having had the opportunity to work with the nine contributors to this volume and I thank them for their participation and their enthusiasm for the project. My editors at Bloomsbury, for their part, have been a constant source of guidance and encouragement.

My own contribution to this volume grows out of an on-going research program in the history and anthropology of the senses funded by the Social Sciences and Humanities Research Council of Canada and the Fonds de recherche du Québec—Société et Culture. I would also like to acknowledge the financial support of the Office of the Vice-President Research and Graduate Studies, Concordia University and the assistance of Dana Samuel and Natalie Doonan. Finally, I would like to thank my family for all the inspiration and advice I received from them during the gestation of this volume and beyond.

Introduction: "Make it New!"— Reforming the Sensory World

DAVID HOWES

The Cold War and hot jazz, the "roaring" twenties and the "swinging" sixties, the silent screen and virtual reality; the dominant sensations of the twentieth century resulted from a mix of technological developments and social and aesthetic changes. Such developments and changes occurred rapidly during the period from 1920 to 2000, and transformed the sensory world so dramatically that it seemed almost a brand-new creation. Indeed, "Make it new!" was the cry of art as of commerce (Armstrong 2005: Ch. 5; Pells 2011).

The twentieth-century world was one in which age-old social distinctions were dissolving, in which the faces seen and the voices heard took on an unprecedented diversity in terms of ethnicity, gender, and class. It was also a world of impossibly tall buildings and incredibly fast vehicles, of soaring aircraft, of moving and talking pictures, of alluring processed foods, and of endlessly malleable synthetic materials. Little wonder that commentators on twentieth-century culture often make prominent reference to Disneyland. For people of previous centuries, the twentieth-century industrial world might have seemed a kind of "Disneyland": fantastical and thrilling, but also, as has often been noted, strangely soulless, a world in which the dominant value seemed to be the pursuit of money in order to achieve a chimeric happiness through the acquisition of material goods. In previous eras, sensory indulgence was often conceptualized as a hindrance to spiritual development. However, in the twentieth century the path to personal fulfillment was increasingly presented as passing through the pleasures of the senses.

In this chapter, characteristic twentieth-century phenomena are coupled in pairs in order to bring out the interplay of different elements of the sensory and social world of the time. The last section briefly examines the late-twentieth-century rise of the "history of the senses" as a field of study which offered a means of investigating the past through material culture, sensory symbols, and lived experience.

THE AUTOMOBILE AND THE AIRPLANE

The twentieth century was quickly identified as an age of speed by modernist writers and artists, and at the center of this whirlwind age was the automobile. The writer F. T. Marinetti declared in the Futurist Manifesto that, due to the automobile, "we believe that this wonderful world has been further enriched by a new beauty, the beauty of speed" (2006: Ch. 2). The sensory impact of the automobile was not limited to the exhilarating sensation of velocity it offered, however, but included a full range of perceptions. As the Dadaist Guillermo de Torre exclaimed in his poem "At the Steering Wheel" (*Al Volante*), "the car is a convex bow that shoots insatiable trajectories . . . the windshield multiplies our eyes . . . and the wind liquefies sounds" (cited by Giucci 2012: 129–30).

The very smell of the automobile symbolized power and freedom for many, as noted by Proust, who found the odor of petrol "delicious" in its evocation of "the joy of speeding over [the countryside]" and "of being on one's way to a longed-for destination" (1984: 48). Automotive odors might also represent progress and success. When the founder of the Honda Motor Company, Soichiro Honda, saw his first car—a Model T Ford—in his Japanese hometown, he knelt to smell its dripping oil and dreamt of one day manufacturing automobiles himself (Ingrassia and White 1994: 236).

A number of modernist artists noted that car windows framed the world as a series of pictures. Henri Matisse brought out this aspect of automobile travel in his painting *The Windshield*, which depicts a car interior with the picturesque nature of the view from the windshield implied by a sketchpad lying on the dashboard (see Danius 2002: 136). The speed of the automobile, however, blurred and scattered the scenes it presented. The perception that the objects seen through car windows were themselves moving was described by Proust in

"Impressions de route en automobile." He imaginatively declared that during his drive, houses "came rushing towards us, clasping to their bosoms vine or rose-bush" while trees "ran in every direction to escape from us" (cited in Danius 2002: 140).

It was not only the view *from* the car, but also the view *of* the car that transformed perception. As a prestige object and a technological wonder, a shiny new automobile attracted admiring looks and desiring touches. The sight of cars hurtling along a road enhanced the impression of living in a whirlwind age. The Futurist Giacomo Balla captured some of this feeling in a series of drawings and paintings which employed abstract representations of spinning wheels, rushing wind, scattered light, and roaring engines to approximate the "thrilling onrush of visual, tactile, and aural sensations" experienced by viewers at an automobile racetrack (Poggi 2008: 29).

At the same time as it dominated the exterior landscape, however, the car isolated its passengers from the environment. This created a sense of alienation from the external world, which, viewed through a windshield, might appear to be little more than a movie projected onto a screen. This tactile isolation was deemed to be a definite advantage by those who decried the indiscriminate contact that might occur among passengers taking public transportation. One early twentieth-century commentator, for example, denounced how, due to the crowding of bodies in Los Angeles trams, "a bishop embraced a stout grandmother" and "a tender girl touched limbs with a city sport" (cited by Bottles 1987: 22). The automobile avoided such blurring of physical and social boundaries by providing each (middle-class) individual and family with a protective and private mode of travel. As a protected and private space, however, the car would also come to function as a central site for intimate encounters and courtship.

The automobile, in fact, not only transformed twentieth-century perceptions, it also fostered new ways of life and new material worlds. With the increase in car ownership, city streets often became more places of passage for automobiles than paths for pedestrians. Highways cut through or bypassed old towns and neighborhoods, spawning their own network of gas stations, diners, motels, and strip malls. Suburbs sprang up in locations once deemed too distant for commuting to urban centers but now seen as only a short drive away. Attached or underground garages enabled drivers to move from car interior to house or building interior without ever stepping outside. As a result, the outdoor world became increasingly foreign to city dwellers—either something one avoided by being in a car, or a place one went to for a change of scene by traveling in a car.

Customs changed, people preferred "driving in the country in the afternoon" to "sitting stiffly in the parlor" (cited by Kihlstedt 1983: 162). Pastors and

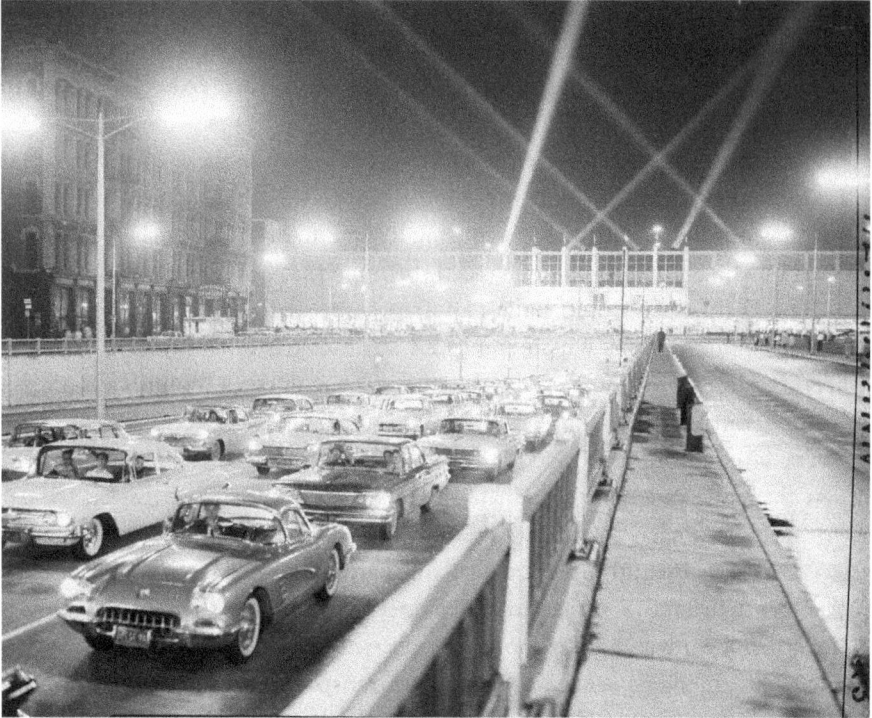

FIGURE I.1: Gleaming automobiles on parade at a Detroit auto show, 1960. Courtesy of Walter P. Reuther Library, Archive of Labor and Urban Affairs, Wayne State University.

priests warned that the new practice of the Sunday family car trip was threatening church attendance (Heitmann 2009: 88). Rushing around in an automobile was said to create a condition of nervousness, a state in which slowing down or stopping were intolerable because they interfered with the pressing impulse to speed ahead. Everything was now required to be speedy and streamlined, including food, work, music, and language itself, which was compressed in both its verbal and literary forms (see, for example, Tichi 1987: 220).

Coupled with the automobile as a marvel of modern transportation, the airplane also transformed people's ways of sensing. Its direct sensory and social impact was not as widespread as that of the automobile. Very few people had private airplanes and, until the latter part of the century, the high cost of flying made it an elite mode of transportation, the prerogative of businessmen, government officials, and the vagabond socialites who came to be known as "the jet set." However, the airplane's impact on the imagination was enormous. "Of all the agencies . . . that made the average man of 1925 intellectually different from [one] of 1900, by far the greatest was the sight of a human being in an airplane," wrote the American journalist Mark Sullivan in 1935 (cited in Bilstein 2003: 16).

Seemingly supernatural in its ability to transport people across the skies, the airplane symbolized the human transcendence of ordinary physical limitations. Numerous people recorded experiencing a sense of spiritual elevation when traveling in or simply watching a plane flying above the earth. In the purity of the sky there was "no ugliness . . . no grasping" and no "mean streets and bickering" (cited in Bilstein 2003: 21).

The airplane freed the human sensorium from earthbound sensations. Blue became the dominant color, the coldness of high altitude the dominant feeling, and the roar of the engine the dominant sound (the onomatopoeic word "zoom" was coined to express the sound and speed of an airplane as it soared into the sky). Flight provided astounding bird's-eye—or God's-eye—views of the world. The Argentine art critic Julio Payró noted in the 1930s that, in contrast to the automobile, with its blurred views and focus on the road, the airplane gave "a cartographic, futurist idea of the landscape" (cited in Giucci 2012: 135). Looking down on earth from a plane made the geographic borders dividing countries seem insignificant—there were no borders in the sky. It was, indeed, hoped by many that "with the new aerial age will come a new internationalism" as people flew from one country to another, dissolving physical and cultural barriers (cited in Bilstein 2003: 20).

Like the automobile, the airplane separated people from the environment; however, in the case of the latter this detachment was total. "Oh! I have slipped the surly bonds of earth," declared aviator John Gillespie Magee in his oft-cited poem "High Flight" (Roberts and Briand 1957: 171). In a very mechanical form of apotheosis, the airplane carried its passengers up into heaven. This pseudo-religious view of air travel was expressed by Apollinaire in his poem "Zone," in which an airplane is likened to Christ and depicted rising into the sky accompanied by angels (1971: 118–19). New, spiritual senses replaced the old, earthly ones. Flying in the "untrespassed sanctity of space" the aviator was able to "put out [his] hand, and touch the face of God" (in Roberts and Briand 1957: 171; see further Corn 1983). That there were, in mundane reality, no gods to be touched and no angels to be seen on the "angel-side of clouds" (Kipling), no "heaven" to be found in the heavens, was discomfiting to many, even though modern science had already put paid to traditional notions of a geographical heaven and hell. The premodern cosmos had been filled with good and evil forces and their sensory manifestations (see Classen 2012: 28). The twentieth-century cosmos seemed chillingly empty. When humans landed on the Moon in 1969, the event aroused a similar range of emotions—awe at what seemed a supernatural feat, and disappointment that, after millennia of myths and stories, that's all there was to the Moon.

It was not only the ability of planes and rockets to leave the earth that riveted the twentieth-century imagination, but also their ability to drop things on earth—in particular, explosives. Many parts of the world experienced the devastation produced by aerial bombing during the twentieth century. The atomic bomb, developed in the United States during the Second World War and "harnessing the basic power of the universe," as President Truman put it (cited by Hein and Selden 1997: 4), vastly intensified the destructive power of aerial bombing. The sudden transformation of the city of Hiroshima into a pile of formless rubble after an atomic bomb had been dropped on it by one single airplane made it clear that the god-like power of modern technology could destroy as well as enhance life. The picture of the giant mushroom cloud produced by the detonation of an atomic bomb became one of the most powerful and disturbing images of the latter part of the century. The purely visual nature of the picture made it all the eerier because its silence seemed to convey a silencing of voices and an annihilation of listeners.

The wartime use of the airplane tarnished its image as an agent for spiritual and social transformation. The final blow to the notion of the airplane elevating its passengers above worldly cares and conflicts came not in the twentieth century, however, but in 2001, when four American passenger planes were hijacked by terrorists and used as weapons of mass destruction. The era of the airplane as otherworldly was over.

THE SKYSCRAPER AND THE BUNGALOW

The same desire to rise above the ground which produced the airplane manifested itself architecturally in the skyscraper. Made possible by advances in engineering and the invention of the elevator, skyscrapers were erected in major cities around the world from the 1930s on. In city centers where land was limited and expensive, it made sense to build upwards rather than outwards, to house people in the sky, rather than on the ground. However, skyscrapers were not only monuments to efficiency, they were also emblems of corporate and urban might, and even sublimity—for their great height aroused the feelings of awe evoked in previous centuries by soaring cathedral spires. The majesty of the skyscraper did not point to the power of God, however, but rather to human ingenuity.

> . . . Who made the skyscrapers?
> Man made 'em, the little, two-legged joker, Man.
> Out of his head, out of his dreaming, scheming skypiece . . .
>
> Sandburg 2003: 320

Standing up straight and tall like giants, skyscrapers were figurative men, proudly displaying themselves as conquerors of the landscape.

The sensory impact of skyscrapers was experienced corporeally through their looming presence on city streets and the upward movement of their elevators, but it was their visual effects, the views of and from skyscrapers, that were most often remarked. Seen from a distance, a skyline of skyscrapers presented the city as a site of power and wonder. And while "close up there are things that are not very comforting: littered streets, corner drug deals, broken down tenements" (Douglas 1996: 2), by keeping eyes looking upwards, skyscrapers diverted the senses from the often far less attractive scenario of the ground environment. The view *from* the skyscraper, in turn, minimized the significance of the sensory experiences of life on the ground as it maximized the power of sight to encompass and survey.

It was not just its height which gave the skyscraper its particular visual potency, but also its lack of ornamentation. The sleek, often reflective, facade of the skyscraper seemed to transform the building into pure presence. Making no allusions, affording no distractions, it was simply, mammothly, *there*. The smooth, clean surfaces of the skyscraper matched the smoothness and cleanliness of pavement, and the smoothness of automobile travel, to offer an illusion of urban life as similarly smooth and clean; ordered and controlled by modern technology.

The skyscraper's lack of ornamentation also suggested that the work undertaken in such a building would be highly functional, and even ruthless, with no deviations from the prescribed course. The main use of the skyscraper was as a corporate office building and therefore its design mimicked the supposedly no-nonsense office work which took place inside, and which ideally resulted in a commercial dominance equivalent to the architectural dominance of the building. Furthermore, just as the skyscraper's facade lacked distinguishing features, so, one might assume, did the lives of workers toiling inside: each individual simply contributed to the monumental effect of the whole. As skyscrapers were the most prominent buildings in the big city, the big city itself became a symbol of faceless corporate power and functionalism.

The aesthetic and symbolic values of the skyscraper were mirrored in many of the artistic productions of the century. While the prosaic, commercial

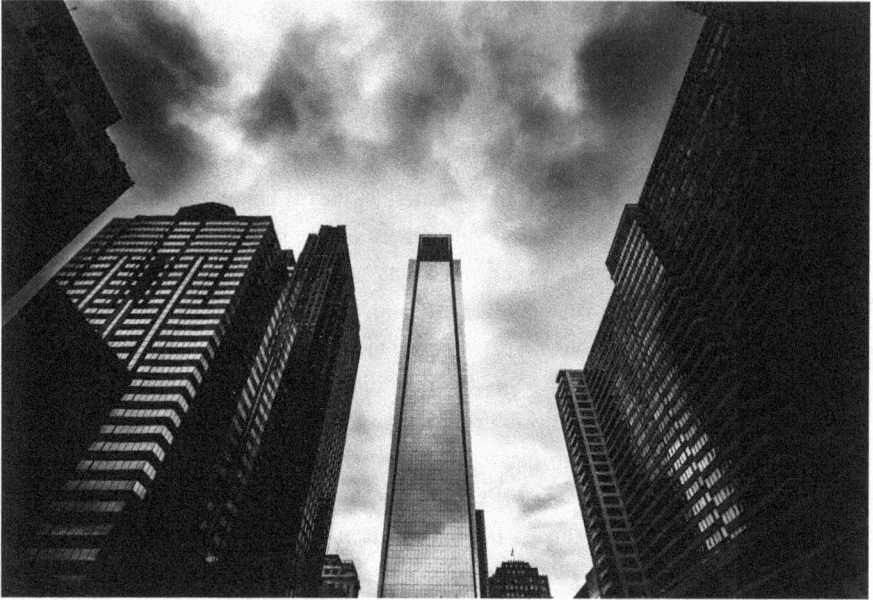

FIGURE I.2: Looming skyscrapers in Philadelphia. Photograph by andrearoad. Getty Images.

functions of the skyscraper might not appeal to the artistic imagination, its clean, functional lines, soaring height, and display of technological mastery did. Depicting a skyscraper in a painting became a sign of an artist who was confronting the realities of modern life. Painters such as Joseph Stella (*Skyscrapers*) and Georgia O'Keefe (*Manhattan*, 1932), depicted the buildings as stark geometrical patterns of light and dark rising into the sky. The Brazilian composer Hector Villa-Lobos traced a picture of the New York City skyline onto a musical staff and used it as the basis for an orchestral suite. The term "Skyscraper moderne" was coined to refer to furniture and housewares inspired by the forms of skyscrapers. In 1934 Malcolm Cowley proclaimed that "the writers of our generation . . . had one privilege: to write a poem in which all was but order and beauty, a poem rising like a clean tower" (cited in Tichi 1987: 289).

The counterpart to the urban skyscraper was the suburban bungalow. Imported from India and redesigned by the British in the early century, the low-profile, open-layout bungalow went on to gain popularity in cities around the world (King 1984). That its airy design was particularly suited for hot climates made no difference, as modern heating systems could take care of any chilling effects of open spaces and large windows in colder climates.

The growth of bungalow-filled suburbs was made possible by the spread of the family automobile. In the nineteenth century, the suburbs had often been regarded as undesirable places to live. Most people who could afford it wished to live within convenient walking distance of work and amenities. The urban outskirts were frequently considered unhealthy, poor, and criminal, emitting a "great variety of fetid and disgusting smells" (Bottles 1987: 6). In the twentieth century, the greater mobility provided by the automobile transformed the outskirts of cities into places of respite from the "concrete jungle" of the city center—places where inexpensive housing, green spaces, and fresh air abounded (see Howes 2010).

The bungalow captured the spirit of the time by offering a more informal space for family living that was suggestive of the easier-going social relations of the new century. The low profile and large windows of the bungalow and its mid-twentieth century variation, the ranch house, allowed it to be filled with the sunshine which was absent from downtown streets perpetually shaded by office towers. The lawn that stretched out in front of the house and the roomy yard behind added a relaxing, natural aspect, and the possibility of outdoor cooking—even swimming in a pool if the budget allowed—which contributed to the bungalow's "vacation home" atmosphere and its cultural value as an antidote to the pressures and formalities of city life.

For many, making the switch from renting an urban apartment to owning a suburban bungalow—however humble and undistinguished—was also an important step up the social ladder. In England, bungalow-ownership was even said to be accompanied by a new style of speech to go along with the new social status it conferred: the so-called "bay window" accent (McKibbin 1998: 79).

However, some viewed the expanding tracts of bungalows with dismay. The social historian Lewis Mumford condemned such suburbs as:

> a multitude of uniform, unidentifiable houses, lined up inflexibly, at uniform distances, on uniform roads, in a treeless communal waste, inhabited by people of the same class, the same income, the same age group, witnessing the same television programs, eating the same tasteless pre-fabricated foods, from the same freezers, conforming in every outward and inward respect to a common mold.
>
> Cited in Clark 1986: 227

Bestselling books, such as *The Organization Man* by William H. White, *The Man in the Gray Flannel Suit* by Sloan Wilson, and *The Crack in the Picture*

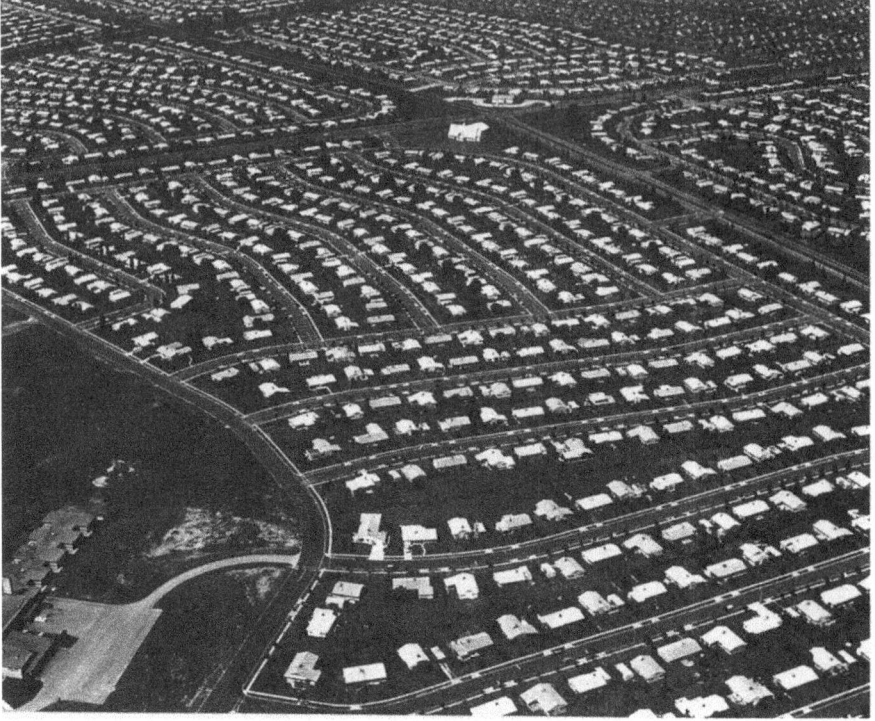

FIGURE I.3: The sensory monotony of suburbia: Levittown, USA. Public domain.

Window by John Keats, warned that the suburbs united with the corporate world in offering stifling monotony and imposing mindless conformity. A song called "Little Boxes," sung by Pete Seeger, refers to bungalows as "little boxes made of ticky tacky . . . little boxes all the same," which produced families "all the same." If people escaped to the suburbs hoping to find more scope for individuality and more sensory diversity than in their downtown office buildings, it seems they were out of luck (see Baxandall and Ewen 2000; Creadick 2010).

The reputed dullness of the suburbs, in fact, gave a new prominence to the city center as a hub of activity. This was particularly the case at night when the suburbs lay dark and silent and the city scintillated with light and movement. In her catchy hit song of 1964, "Downtown," Petula Clark urged people to go downtown and "listen to the music of the traffic in the city," look at the "pretty" neon lights, and dance the night away. During the day, the city center might be a cold and hard-edged arena for business transactions, but at night it became a fantasy land of sensuous pleasures. However, such pleasures were assumed to be for the most part off-limits to the family men and women who inhabited the suburbs.

As the century progressed, women, in their role as housewives, especially came to be seen as the "victims" of suburban monotony. While suburban men drove off every weekday to their jobs in the city, women remained ensconced in the family bungalow. Indeed, the bungalow itself—low-profile, close to "nature," and the center of family life—conveyed notions of femininity in contrast to the masculine associations of the vertical, business-centered, skyscraper. New labor-saving devices such as vacuum cleaners and washing machines meant that the women left at home had more free time but, stuck in the suburbs as they were, limited possibilities for creative action or mental stimulation. In 1963 Betty Friedan's *The Feminine Mystique* detailed the plight of the "trapped" housewife in terms of her supposedly drab sensory life: "Each suburban wife struggled with her [dissatisfaction] alone. As she made the beds, shopped for groceries, made slipcover material, ate peanut butter sandwiches with her children, chauffeured Cub Scouts and Brownies, lay beside her husband at night—she was afraid to ask even of herself the silent question—'Is this all?'" (1963: 15). The bungalow, which had once represented freedom, now seemed to be a prison. The time, it seemed, had come for women's liberation.

By the last decades of the century, the bungalow had lost much of its appeal. Rather than appearing fresh and stimulating it looked tired and boring. In 1946, the authors of *Tomorrow's House* had claimed that "even a poor architect has a hard time making a spreading, one-story house unattractive" (Clark 1986: 177). In the 1980s the generation that had grown up in such houses appeared to think just the opposite, that even a *good* architect would have a hard time making a spreading, one-story house attractive.

The desire for home comforts that the bungalow awakened, however, had not disappeared, the "dream house" had simply taken another, and grander, form. It had two stories instead of one, two (if not more) bathrooms and two garages—for the liberated woman of the house needed her own car now. If anything, the home was regarded as even more of an oasis from the stress of city living than before, due to innovations in home media technologies and the trend towards "cocooning" or retreating into the home. Nor had the drive for conformity epitomized by the uniformity of suburbia disappeared. Instead it had become masked by the seeming diversity of options offered by such things as customized interior fittings, cable television, multiple flavors of ice cream, and assorted varieties of toothpaste. These might all simply be choices from a limited menu (Archer 2005: 337), however, they provided a pleasant sense of individuality while ensuring that life in the little (though increasingly bigger) boxes of suburbia carried on.

THE CAMERA AND THE SCREEN

The twentieth century was marked by an increasing proliferation of visual imagery. Photography, once the domain of professionals, became a hobby that almost anyone could practice with the aid of an inexpensive compact camera and a photo-developing service. Every middle-class family could have albums filled with snapshots (first black-and-white and then color) of family celebrations and vacations. As a key means of embodying personal history, the family photo album transformed the past into a series of visual images. If Proust had lived a few decades later, perhaps it might have been a photo album, and not a madeleine dipped in tea, that awakened his recollections of the past.

Home photography supplemented the multiplicity of photographs in magazines, newspapers, and books. The realistic quality of these images added to their impact. Unlike illustrations, they appeared to offer unmediated visual access to the people and scenes they represented and thus transform their viewers into eyewitnesses. Susan Sontag observed that photographs "have virtually unlimited authority in a modern society" due to the fact that they are not perceived merely as representations of reality, but as "something directly stencilled off the real," a skimming, as it were, of actual visual surfaces (1973: 154). By the end of the century, the photograph had in some ways become more "real" than the real thing, as photographs and films posted on the internet began to acquire a life and value of their own (see Howes and Classen 2014: 89–92).

The relatively effortless process of taking a photograph, compared to drawing a picture, placed the sensory emphasis on the visual end result, rather than on the manual craft. As Walter Benjamin wrote in 1936: "photography freed the hand of the most important artistic functions which henceforth devolved only upon the eye looking into a lens" (1969: 219). The photograph itself, by eliminating all sensory information but the visual, gave an added value to visual appearance. If the visual was all that this wondrous new technology of reproduction could depict, then it was essential to make the most of visuality. This emphasis on "looking good" in contemporary culture was enhanced by pervasive advertising imagery which promoted products and the people pictured with them in terms of their visual appeal (Ewen 1988).

The function of the camera in modern society, however, was not only to record significant people and places, to capture "slice-of-life" moments, or to showcase desirable merchandise. It was also to survey. First World War cameras, carried aloft on airplanes, were put to the service of military reconnaissance. Over the course of the century the camera became essential to peacetime surveillance as well. Introduced in the 1970s, video surveillance of public spaces as a form of social control was widespread by the century's close: "Today, the ubiquitous video 'security' camera stares blankly at us in apartment buildings, department and convenience stores, gas stations, libraries, parking garages, automated banking outlets, buses, and elevators. No matter where you live you are likely to encounter cameras; some places simply bristle with them" (Staples 2000: 59). Even in the sky, cameras mounted on satellites circled the Earth, capturing images which were viewed down on the ground. The world had never been so watched. "Has the camera replaced the eye of God?" asked John Berger (1991: 57).

This constant monitoring elicited less public concern than one might have expected. Perhaps its social benefits seemed greater than its intrusiveness. Perhaps the visualism of twentieth-century culture had accustomed people to being looked at. However, it did raise questions about the loss of privacy in contemporary society and spawn a thriving academic sub-field called Surveillance Studies (i.e. Lyon 2007).

Turning from the camera to the screen, cinema, the most popular form of entertainment in the first half of the century, further contributed to the optical orientation of the age. Viewing a film was not an exclusively visual experience, of course. After sound came to the "silent screen" in the late 1920s, movies engaged the ears as well as the eyes. Even the early cinematic experience could, in fact, be quite synaesthetic. The more elaborate cinemas showcased sumptuous architectural fittings, featured a live orchestra, and had elegant cafés (Richards 2010). The movie theater also served as a site for familial or romantic handholding and cuddling. Nonetheless, it was the visual effects of the films shown there that drew the most attention.

Cinema seemingly magnified the power of sight by presenting larger-than-life images. At the same time, techniques of filming and editing—close-ups, slow motion, camera angles, abrupt changes of scene—trained movie audiences in radically new ways of seeing and gave a whole new interest to being a spectator. The fact that movies were shown in a dark theater—or "picture palace"—in which people sat motionless and (ideally) silent, enhanced their sensorial power. While the fantasy fare of cinema provided an "escape" from the tedium and restrictions of everyday life, it also taught people to seek release only though their eyes, ears, and imaginations, while not moving an inch. The cinema audience seemed like a collection of eyes all fixed on one point.

With the invention of television in the mid-twentieth century, however, a new form of leisure viewing emerged. Television shows had many of the same traits as the movies shown at the cinema, but they appeared on a small screen and were intended for private viewing in the home. Watching television was not something one went out to do, but something one stayed in to do. In 1938, the Anglo-Irish novelist Elizabeth Bowen gave as one of her reasons for enjoying the cinema: "I like sitting in a packed crowd in the dark, among hundreds riveted on the same thing" (cited by Richards 2010: 23). Millions of television viewers might all be "riveted on the same thing" but they were no longer sitting together in a packed crowd. Twentieth-century spectatorship changed from being communal to being largely familial or individualist.

As watching a television show was as easy as pressing a button and setting the channel, and as there was no need to leave one's home to do it, television also vastly increased the amount of time people spent passively viewing a screen. Instead of being a once-a-week activity, as cinema was in its heyday, television became a daily activity. A good part of people's lives in the second half of the century, therefore, was spent passively watching images flickering on a screen.

The declining cost of television ownership resulted in it becoming a fixture in virtually all homes in the developed world. In his dystopic novel of 1956 about life in the suburbs, *The Crack in the Picture Window*, John Keats (1957: 79) described the sensory uniformity created by mass television viewing in the days when there were few channels:

> Every house . . . was dark . . . but within every shuttered living room there gleamed a feeble phosphorescence, a tiny picture flickering in that glow. Over the bewitched community there swelled a common sound. Sometimes it was the fanfare, introducing a commercial. Sometimes it was the thin, jubilant cry of the studio audience in New York . . . Sometimes it was the dumb-de-dumb-dumb musical signature of a period crime piece. But whatever the sound, it was a common sound, rising above the darkened houses, for everyone watched the same shows.

Watching shows at home did allow viewers to participate in a variety of activities not possible in a movie theater, such as eating a meal. However, it also significantly shaped activities within the home. For example, many families began eating meals in front of a TV set instead of around a table. This new custom of clustering around the television led to its being considered the modern successor to the hearth (Spigel 1992). Whereas sitting around a hearth had left people free to converse and look at each other, however, the television interfered with familial interaction through its demands for visual and auditory attention. At the same time, the mass diffusion of television programs and advertising created a widely-shared visual and sonic pool of information and tropes which helped to dissolve differences of class, gender, and ethnicity.

This emphasis on seeing at the expense of other, more traditional, forms of sensory engagement was disturbing to many. Parents worried that their children were spending too much time watching television and not enough playing outside. Social critics feared that the twentieth century's obsession with visual surfaces signaled an ailing and alienated society. American educator Neil Postman warned that we were "amusing ourselves to death" with the facile "visual delight" of television (1985). "From television to newspapers, from advertising to all sorts of mercantile epiphanies, our society is characterized by a cancerous growth of vision, measuring everything by its ability to show or be shown, and transmuting communication into a visual journey," proclaimed the French philosopher Michel de Certeau (1983: 18). And then came the personal computer and the internet, which turned even greater numbers of people into "hypervisualists," constantly scanning images and texts on a screen. However, the fact that images and texts could be created and transmitted, as well as viewed on the internet, meant that the new medium of the computer did not simply continue the sensory trajectory of the cinema and television, but rather fostered a new sensory dynamic which would await the next century to disclose its social effects.

PLASTIC AND POLLUTION

The substance that characterized the physical world of the twentieth century, and provided a material base for much of its cultural expression, was plastic. The term "plastic," in fact, covers a variety of synthetic or semi-synthetic substances, from the celluloid used in film and cheap jewelry to the vinyls employed in records, raincoats, and exterior siding. However, plastic became the umbrella term for all these creations of the chemical industry. Technical advances resulted in plastics that were amazingly durable, as well as low cost. "Plastic is forever" touted one industry pioneer, "and a lot cheaper than diamonds" (cited in Meikle 1995: 9).

Over the course of the century the material became a familiar component of ordinary life. A family celebrating Christmas in the United States in the 1970s, for example, might have a plastic Christmas tree decorated with plastic ornaments and plastic Barbie dolls and Lego blocks as presents. In a famous line from the 1967 movie *The Graduate*, a recent college graduate who is uncertain about his future is told by his businessman father: "I want to say one word to you. Just one word . . . There's a great future in plastics. Think about it" (cited in Meikle 1995: 3).

Like its material uses, the sensory properties of plastic were multiple. Easy to shape, color, and texture, plastic might approximate anything. It could be made to look like wood or it could be made to look like glass, it could resemble flowers or it could mimic gemstones. Nonetheless, on close inspection, it always retained something "plasticky" in its look and feel. Plastic itself had no imitators, for who would imitate such a cheap and indeterminate substance?

Due to its mutability, plastic engendered a notion of the malleability of the material world. The French philosopher Roland Barthes wrote of plastic in the 1950s that it embodied "the very idea of . . . infinite transformation" (1972: 79). Plastic's mutability coincided with twentieth-century desires to reshape not only the physical environment, but also society, and even the human body through cosmetic and surgical procedures. Limits set by nature or by custom no longer seemed to hold in a plastic world. Anything could take on a new form.

While plastic was embraced by the twentieth century for its malleability and low cost, however, it was despised (at least by the educated classes) for its "inauthenticity." Over the course of the century, in fact, the word plastic came

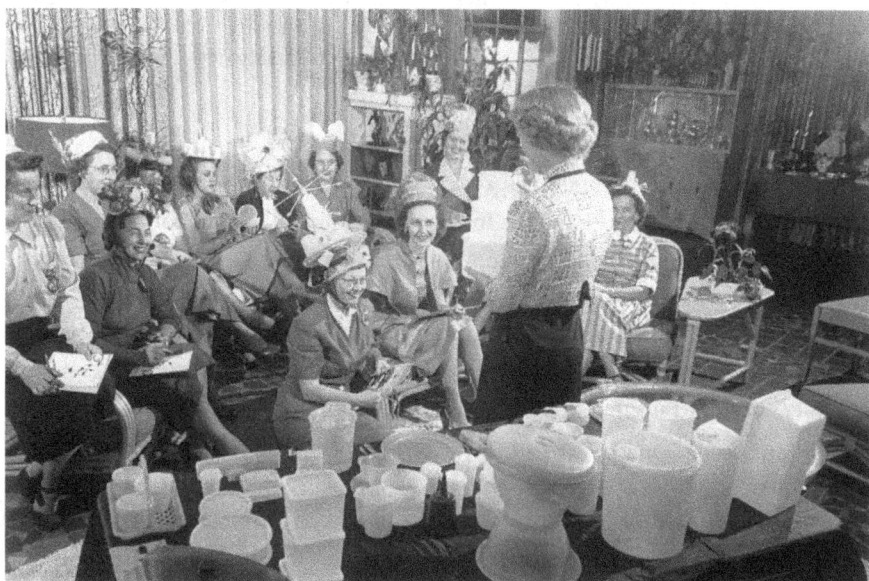

FIGURE I.4: The look and feel of plastic: a Tupperware party. Getty Images.

to be a synonym for fake. Social critics saw plastic as sign and symptom of a society in which simulations had a greater appeal than reality. When the businessman in *The Graduate* affirmed that there was a great future in plastics, the line was not intended to serve as an indicator of commercial acumen, but as an indictment of the superficiality and materialism of Western culture.

It was not only the look and feel of the twentieth-century industrialized world that breathed artificiality, however, but also the taste. Convenience foods—from the quick meals served up by fast food restaurants to the prepared foods stocked at the supermarket (such as the frozen "TV dinners" made to be warmed and eaten while watching television)—became increasingly popular during the century. The new processed foods also had new artificial flavors and colors, many of them derived from petrochemicals, just like most plastics (see Classen *et al.* 1994: 187–200). In their song of 1972, "Plastic Man," The Kinks sung disparagingly of a "plastic man" who "eats plastic food with a plastic knife and fork." Many processed foods, of course, were packaged in plastic, if not canned or boxed. The contents of the supermarket thus seemed, from one perspective, to represent one more triumph of modern technology, and, from another, one more of the shams of contemporary life.

Within the context of a material culture that seemed increasingly artificial, the natural world acquired a new value as a place and source of authenticity, where one could experience the "real" thing. The sights, sounds, and scents of nature were extolled as both physically and spiritually refreshing. This desire for natural experiences was bolstered by the dramatic growth in urban populations during the century. Trips to the countryside and camping became popular ways for urbanites to replenish their senses and spirits through immersion in natural settings, especially after workers won the right to paid vacation time in many countries (Aron 1999).

At the same time as the pure air and green vistas of the wilderness were acquiring a new value for city dwellers, however, an awareness developed of how the natural world was being depleted and polluted by industrialization and technological development (Barr 1970; Parr 2010). The lumber industry was devastating forests, factory smoke and automobile exhausts were poisoning the air, chemical waste was contaminating rivers, nuclear power created radioactive byproducts, and mass production was resulting in mass garbage. All the wondrous inventions and sensations of modernity, it seemed, had negative counterparts in environmental degradation and sensory malaise. In return for the thrill of speeding in an automobile one breathed air tainted with smog. One "paid" for the spectacle of electric light by giving up the view of the night sky. That plastic lasted "forever" no longer seemed such a good thing when that plastic was piling up in landfills and creating vast "garbage patches" in the ocean.

Discussing the "sensory shock" occasioned by this new awareness of environmental pollution, Constance Classen wrote: "Even the clean look of the modern city with its subterranean sewers, its electrical energy, its sleek buildings, its shiny cars and its synthetic products has turned out to simply be a mask for immense waste. We are dismayed to learn that, in the end, dirt is 'cleaner' than plastic" (2013: 177). Nor was the issue only a matter of aesthetics; human health and the wellbeing of the whole ecological system were adversely affected. Rachel Carson began her pioneering work on environmentalism, *Silent Spring* by contrasting the sensory experience of a country town before and after intensive use of pesticides. The "before" description spoke of "green fields" and "white clouds of bloom," of "barking foxes" and "clear, cold streams." In the "after" description, animals and children have sickened and died, the apple trees bear no fruit, the vegetation is brown and withered, and "on the mornings that had once throbbed with the dawn chorus of robins, catbirds, doves, jays, wrens, and scores of other bird voices there was now no sound; only silence lay over the fields and woods and marsh" (1962: 1–2).

In Carson's account, aesthetic blight accompanies and testifies to environmental blight. Even pleasant sensations, however, might warn of environmental disaster. A late twentieth-century counterpart to Carson's book, for example, might have been titled *Warm Winter* and detailed how, due to the effects of global warming, an unusually warm winter could no longer be regarded as a pleasant break from the customary cold weather of the season, but rather now served as one more ominous sensory sign of an ailing world.

The natural world had once been conceptualized as immensely powerful, with limitless resources, but by the last decades of the century this view was seriously challenged. It was not only accounts and experiences of the proliferation of garbage, smog, oil-spills, and deforestation which led to a change in attitude, however. The view from above provided by airplanes and, more dramatically, space ships, contributed greatly to the perception of the Earth as bounded and frail. Astronaut Russell Schweickhart, who spent ten days in orbit in 1969, observed that from space the Earth appeared "so small and so fragile and such a precious little spot in the universe" (cited in White 1998: 38). These words captured the sentiments of many who saw, or saw a picture of, the Earth looking like a lone, blue balloon floating in a vast dark sky. The new conceptualization of the natural world as vulnerable and requiring human protection, therefore, was partly grounded in an actual view of the world.

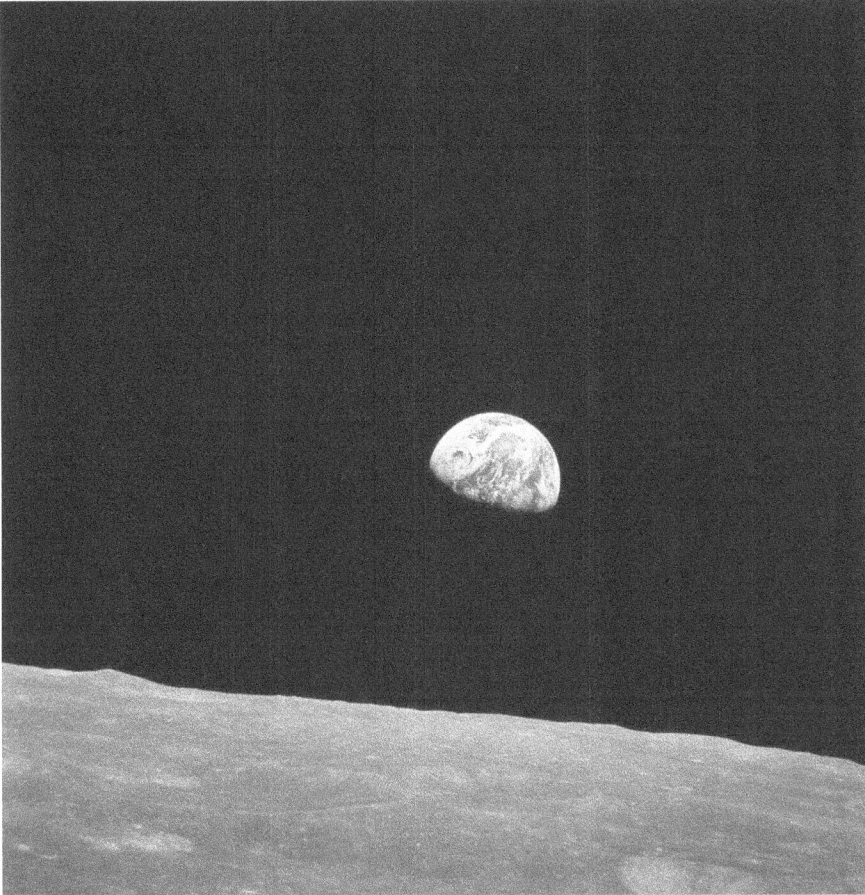

FIGURE I.5: A small planet: a view of the Earth from orbit around the Moon. National Aeronautics and Space Administration.

THE COUNTER CULTURE AND ROCK MUSIC

The environmental movement which flourished in the second half of the twentieth century was part of a larger complex of social and political developments which challenged conventional modes of thinking about and interacting with the world. These included decolonization, feminism, civil rights movements, and anti-war protests. For the older generation, born in the early decades of the century, it often seemed as though society was being turned on its head, with those who were previously "invisible," "silent," and subordinate now insisting on being seen and heard and treated as equals.

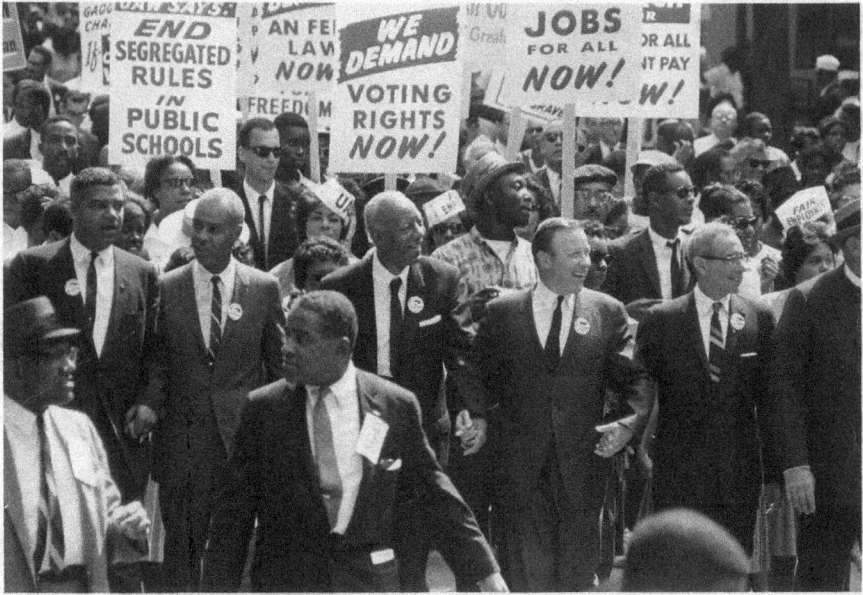

FIGURE I.6: Walking hand in hand: the civil rights march on Washington. National Archives and Records Administration.

One notable instance of this change was the massive 1963 March on Washington for Jobs and Freedom, highlighted by Martin Luther King Jr.'s "I Have a Dream" speech, which focused public attention on the disadvantaged position of African Americans within society. Describing the effect the march had on the senses of both participants and observers, one young woman said: "I saw people laughing and listening and standing very close to one another, almost in an embrace . . . White people [were] staring in wonder. Their eyes were open, they were *listening*" (Euchner 2010: Part 2).

The fact that the event, and others like it, was widely broadcast on television increased its social and sensory impact.

Social reformers often aimed to encourage empathy for oppressed peoples by enabling others to see the world through their eyes. A classic example of this approach is the non-fiction book *Black Like Me*, published in 1961, which conveyed the experiences of a white man passing as black in the Southern United States (Griffin 2004). The author, John Howard Griffin, described how, though nothing of his identity had changed but his skin color, he began to receive what he called the "hate stare" from whites and found his applications for work rejected.

The book helped bring not only a skin color that was supposed to be socially invisible to the fore of mainstream consciousness, but also a voice meant to be socially unheard—for "I" could never be "black" according to the rules of the dominant culture. And, of course, the catch in the title was that the writer was not, in fact, black. As a white man he *did* have the "right" to speak, but the fact that he was using his voice to tell of his experiences as a "black" man confounded social distinctions based on race and positioned skin color as a superficial sensory trait with enormous and unjust cultural ramifications. The "Black is Beautiful" and "Black Power" movements of the 1960s and 1970s attempted to reverse traditional stereotypes and exclusionary practices concerning African Americans by associating positive qualities with a dark skin color (Ogbar 2004; Thomas 2012).

"Counterculture" was the term often used to refer to the broad, youth-centered movement in the 1960s and 1970s which supported new social values, while at the same time rejecting the conventional, middle-class way of life, summarized by one activist as "a fresh-frozen life in some prepackaged suburb, Howard Johnson's on Sundays, Disneyland vacations, the cut-rate American dream of happiness out of an aerosol can" (Robert Alter, cited in Belasco 2007: 62). In opposition to this "synthetic substitute for reality," people were urged to "reach out to each other with noises/gestures/visions to create a new and common reality," as a flier distributed by one countercultural group put it (cited by Kramer 2013: lix).

The sensory manifestations of this quest for an alternative way of life were numerous. One of the most visible everyday signs of countercultural trends concerned changes in hairstyles and dress. Long, loose hair, T-shirts, jeans, mini-skirts, and bright "psychedelic" colors, all signaled a rebellion against the more controlled and formal modes of self-presentation of previous decades and, more broadly, a rejection of conventional social roles and values. Bare feet, in turn, expressed a desire for a greater closeness with nature.

"Unisex" clothing and hairstyles were often taken by the mainstream to represent an unsettling loss of gender distinctions: women apparently wanted to look and act "like men," and men apparently wanted to look and act "like women." This last was also said to manifest itself in the pacifist tendencies of the counterculture, which led to long-haired young men defying brush-cut, gun-wielding soldiers with flowers, opposing "war" with "love" and hardness with softness.

This brings us to the issue of tactile values. The counterculture asserted that the social role of the police and the military was not only to protect and defend, but also to coerce and suppress. "Police brutality" became a widely discussed public issue. The pacifist approach adopted by many social reformers and widely associated with the counterculture, by contrast, implied an unwillingness to employ aggressive forms of touch to dominate others. One popular form of social protest of the time, the sit-in, involved the physical occupation of a site. This tactic would result in the protest's opponents taking on the role of aggressors when they resorted to tactile force to clear the site. The sit-in also had the attraction of simplicity—to protest all one needed to do was to sit.

Non-violent actions such as sit-ins and marches were not the only form in which the desire for social change found expression, however. In the United States, the 1960s were marked by race riots in major cities. Mass riots by protesting students and workers, notably the 1968 riots in France, shook many other countries. A number of countercultural groups began with non-violent protests but, inspired by Marxist ideology and fired by youthful energy and idealism, ended up espousing armed revolution as the only means of overthrowing the political, business, and military alliances which maintained the status quo. The social turmoil of the time—and its extensive media reporting, hence brought the politics of touch to the fore of public consciousness.

The counterculture's questioning of the social institutions of marriage and the nuclear family, and its experimentation with communal living and "free love" (facilitated by the invention of the birth-control pill), brought touch to the fore of public consciousness in another way. At the time, such practices were often seen as evidence of the moral and corporeal laxity of contemporary youth. Blame was frequently placed on the mid-century shift in childrearing practices which had replaced the strict, no-cuddling, techniques advocated in the early decades of the century with an approach mandating tender, hands-on care. The childrearing "bible" by Benjamin Spock, *Baby and Child Care*, had helped revolutionize childrearing by urging parents to hug their children, feed them when they were hungry, and refrain from corporal punishment (see Synnott 2005). The result, some said, was a generation of soft, self-indulgent "flower children" who could not be counted on to discipline their bodies, uphold social values, or defend their country. The debate over tough or tender touch in childrearing continued to the end of the century. However, generally the tender approach won out, with the age-old tradition of corporal punishment in schools, for example, being banned in many countries in the last decades of the century. And while communal living did not catch on, the "sexual revolution" supported by the counterculture ultimately led to widespread changes in public attitudes towards sexuality.

Turning to the sense of taste, this was primarily affected by the counterculture's desire for a more "spiritual," "natural," "environmentally-sound," and "ethical" diet. Synthetic, industrially-produced foods were rejected (at least in theory) in favor of natural or organic foods, which were touted as both healthier and more flavorful. Perhaps the defining taste of the movement was that of granola, a mixture of oats, nuts and dried fruit, which made for a nutritious and "natural" snack.

During this period, vegetarianism, which challenged the values of the "establishment" at the basic level of food production and consumption, emerged as a popular countercultural diet. Francis Moore Lappé's *Diet for a Small Planet* (1971) argued convincingly that meat-eating supported a wasteful use of natural resources. Others saw clear parallels between the exploitation of women and workers and the exploitation of animals for food. Feminist vegetarian groups were founded. Struck by the miserable conditions of farm animals, the prominent advocate for farmworkers' rights, Cesar Chavez, became a vegetarian. In a few decades vegetarianism went from being regarded as a bizarre fad or cult practice with dangerous health consequences to being tenuously accepted as a healthy and morally-defensible alternative to a meat-based diet. Tellingly, when the 1998 edition of *Baby and Child Care* advocated a vegan diet for children, it raised some eyebrows but did not cause much of a stir (Spock and Parker 1998).

The sensory heart of the counterculture was music. The song "We Shall Overcome" was sung by civil rights marchers, anti-war protesters, and striking farm workers, with the line "We'll walk hand-in-hand" expressing the sense of solidarity experienced by agitators for reform. While protest songs and folk music played an important role in giving a musical voice to the counterculture, it was rock music which had the most impact. This was not only, or even primarily, because many rock musicians addressed social issues or made countercultural statements in their songs. It was, rather, the music itself which in multifold ways appeared to subvert conventional social mores. Its strong beat gave momentum to desires for social change or, at least, for excitement. Its loudness provided an immersive environment and also expressed the demand of dissatisfied youth to be heard. The simple structure of most pieces, their frequent authorship by members of the band performing them, as well as the fact that many performers were not trained musicians or singers, gave rock music the aura of authenticity that the counterculture demanded. Rock musicians were no slick, "synthetic," crooners performing cover songs. And although rock musicians were overwhelmingly white, by fusing elements from African American and European musical traditions, their music served as a model for a racially-integrated society. The free-form dance styles which accompanied rock music, in turn, physically conveyed the contemporary craving to be freed from conventional social strictures.

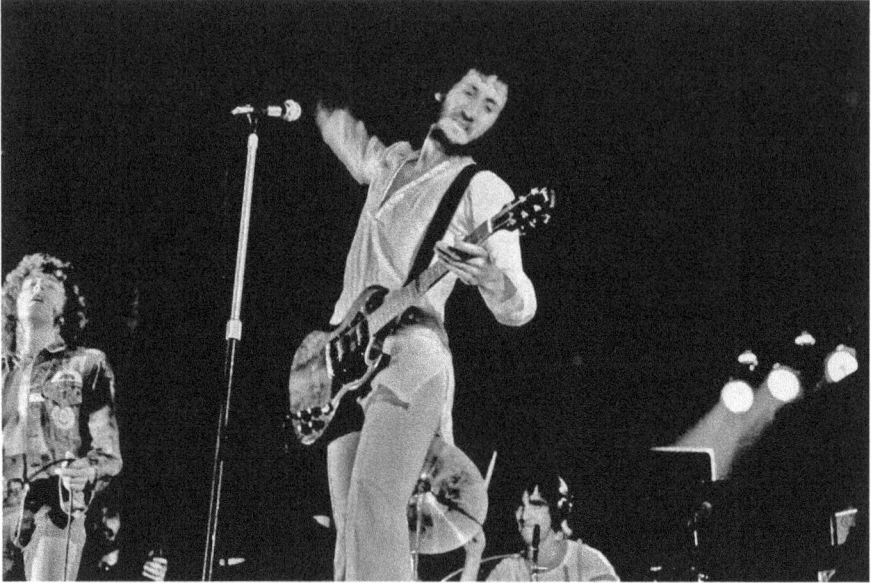

FIGURE I.7: Feeling the muse: the rock band The Who in concert. Public domain.

Rock musicians themselves played an essential role in promulgating the styles and values of the counterculture through their own appearance and lifestyles. The radio became the essential medium for transmitting this musical tidal wave. However, the crowds that gathered for live rock concerts, memorably the 400,000 at the Woodstock Music Festival in 1969, could feel in their numbers the power of a movement whose time had come.

Critics denounced rock music for its seeming power to subvert, mobilize, and disorder. Its so-called African rhythms were said to incite deviations from "civilized" behavior as well as encourage white youth to mix with "coloreds." The "sensuous gyrations" performed by certain singers (notably Elvis Presley) and their dancing fans were said to arouse sexual passions, and again called up comparisons with "savage" sensorialities—one reviewer compared them to "an aboriginal mating dance" (Martin and Seagrave 1988: 62). The fact that rock concerts sometimes ended in brawls seemed to confirm the music's destabilizing effects. While these criticisms convinced some to forswear rock music, others saw them as evidence of its liberating potential.

One aspect of the counterculture frequently associated with rock music was the use of drugs. Along with patchouli oil, the odor of burning marijuana was the defining scent of the movement. Drug use was a form of social bonding, a means of experiencing alternate realities and, in the era of popular psychology, a fast route to the development of "human potentiality." Its promise of non-linguistic revelations had a strong appeal due to the countercultural emphasis on corporeal and spiritual fulfillment (as evidenced, for example, by Aldous Huxley's call for "non-verbal humanities" in *The Doors of Perception*, 1954).

Hallucinogenic drugs such as LSD transformed the user's sensory perceptions, inducing sensations of vibrating colors and shifting shapes, and deepening the experience of music. Such visionary sensations helped inspire the psychedelic artwork popular at the time and contributed to the synaesthetic tendencies of the counterculture, which, in its search for holism, saw rock music as part of a sensory and social totality. Perhaps this synaesthetic tendency was expressed most strongly by Pete Townshend, a member of the rock band The Who, when he spoke of wishing to "translate a person into music" by "feed[ing] information—height, weight, astrological details, beliefs and behavior—about that person into the synthesizer" (cited in Wilkerson 2006: 176). It seemed as though the multisensory fantasies of the nineteenth-century Symbolists were being brought to life (see Classen 1998: Ch. 5).

Drugs (like rock music itself), however, were also associated with escapism and anarchism, and regarded as purveyors of mindless pleasures and instigators of gratuitous violence, with the synaesthetic revelations they promised dissolving into sensory excess. The addictive nature and often harmful physical effects of a number of popular drugs, in turn, alarmed many people both inside and outside the movement.

Another way in which the counterculture sought to access alternative realities was by turning to the East, and particularly, India. India seemed an almost magical land of both spiritual and sensory plenitude. As such it provided a rich range of styles and practices to be reinterpreted in Western settings. The bright colors and swirling patterns of Indian aesthetics made a good match with psychedelic designs. Indian melodies and instruments added "exotic" notes to rock music. "Yoga" and "meditation" provided engaging spiritual and corporeal practices. Fashionable young men sported "Nehru" jackets and Western followers of Krishna dressed in orange robes and chanted Hindu prayers. More substantially, the non-violent protests popularized by Gandhi in India's struggle for independence helped inspire the marches and sit-ins of Western protest movements. Indian traditions of vegetarianism and showing compassion for animals, in turn, were enlisted to support the vegetarian movement in the West. These Western forays into Eastern cultures exoticized the East at the same time as they glorified it; however, they also indicated a

growing openness towards other cultures which helped pave the way for the
late-twentieth-century rise of multiculturalism in the West.

Eventually, in the 1980s, the counterculture lost momentum. On the one
hand, mainstream society eventually incorporated many of the changes advocated
by the movement (particularly as the youth of the 1960s and 1970s grew older
and acquired positions of authority). On the other hand, most supporters of the
counterculture turned out to be not all that radical in their aspirations. Some of
the sensory signs and practices of the counterculture, such as psychedelic art,
walking barefoot, and the scent of patchouli, became dated. Others, such as
meditation and alternative medicines—crystal therapy, therapeutic touch,
aromatherapy—became part of the "New Age" movement. Yet others, such as
yoga and vegetarianism, acquired increasing mainstream recognition.

Rock music continued to be popular to the end of the century, however the
ways in which it was experienced changed. Music television transformed it
into a media spectacle, with a new emphasis on accompanying visuals. At the
same time, radio declined in popularity. (Significantly, the first music video to
be aired on the US music video channel MTV was "Video Killed the Radio

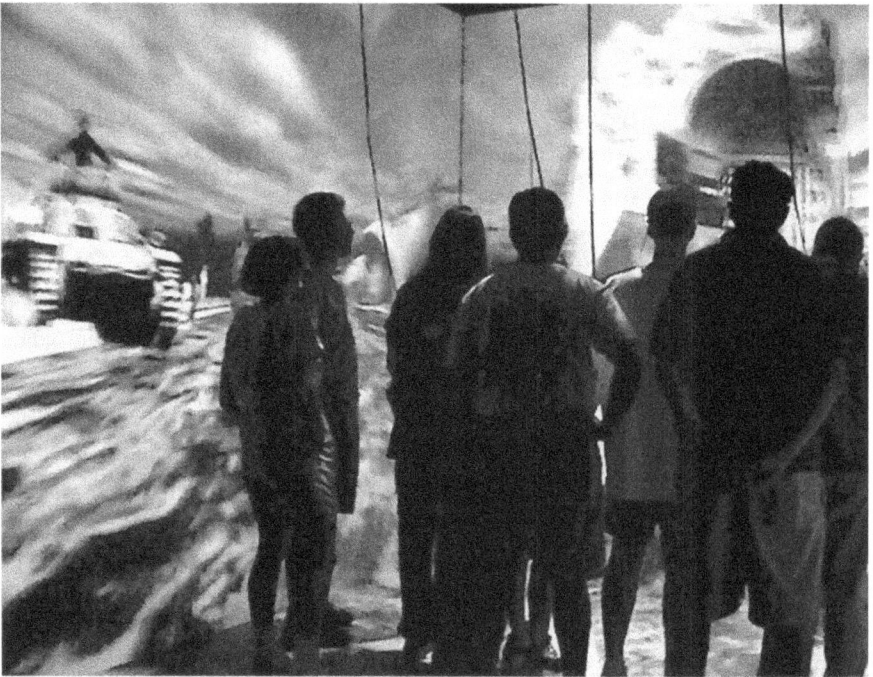

FIGURE I.8: Virtual sensations: "World Skin" virtual reality installation by Maurice
Benayoun. Photograph by the artist. Public domain.

Star" by The Buggles.) The Walkman, a portable audio cassette player with headphones, privatized the experience of music, with users listening to their personal favorites rather than tuning in to the mass broadcasts of a radio station (see Bull 2000).

Unlike the popular music of the 1960s and 1970s, furthermore, which was closely associated with dance, the new music, heard through a portable Walkman, accompanied ordinary, everyday movement—walking, shopping, riding a bus. Dance itself declined as a recreational activity and mode of self-expression in the 1990s. In the early 1970s Susan Sontag wrote that photography had become almost as popular a pastime as dancing (1973: 8). With the spread of digital cameras and the salience of internet imagery, by the end of the twentieth century it had become far more popular. Collective culture itself was in the process of becoming digital, as computer networks made new, long-distance and disembodied modes of connectedness possible. As for the senses, their ultimate destination, a destination for which they had been prepared by the century's succession of technological "wonders," seemed to be the glowing virtual reality of cyberspace.

THE HISTORY OF THE HISTORY OF THE SENSES

The period from 1920 to 2000 was not only one of dramatic and rapid changes in the material and cultural life of the senses, it was also, and as a result, one of important developments in ways of thinking about the senses. These developments occurred within the physical sciences and psychology, and also, although following a different trajectory, within the social sciences and the humanities. Focusing here on the field of history, we see how the roots of this development were grounded in experiences of a changing sensory world, as well as in particular intellectual concerns.

The realization and ensuing theorization of the "social formation" of perception was inspired by two major experiences. One was observing the effects of new technologies and urban and industrial developments on the human senses and sensibilities. The other was encountering sensory difference brought on by exposure to other cultures. Responding to the effects of industrialization on art and influenced by the Modernist movement, Walter Benjamin considered the rise of new paradigms of perception in his 1936 essay, "The Work of Art in the Age of Mechanical Reproduction." "The way in which human perception is organized—the medium in which it occurs—is conditioned not only by nature but by history," he wrote (Benjamin [1936] 1973: 216). (Benjamin echoed here Marx's statement that "the *forming of the*

five senses is a labor of the entire history of the world down to the present";
[1844] 1987: 109.) Two years earlier, in 1934, Marcel Mauss had reflected on
his experience of cross-cultural difference during the First World War (when
soldiers from many different nations were thrown together) to elaborate a
theory of the social construction of the body in "Techniques of the Body"
(Mauss [1934] 1979). Both these essays helped to position perceptual
experiences and corporeal practices as social in nature, and not simply
subjective and private (as psychology would have it) or physiological (as in
biology). They would both influence a range of later twentieth-century scholars
who contributed directly or indirectly to the field of the history of the senses,
such as John Berger (1972) in the case of Benjamin, and Pierre Bourdieu
([1979] 1984) in the case of Mauss.

In the middle decades of the twentieth century, the Annales School of
history rose to prominence in France. Its outlook was in large part a consequence
of the experiential break with the past produced by the new conditions and
ideas of the modern age, which brought out the importance of cultural and
environmental factors in the shaping of history. Lucien Febvre, Marc Bloch,
Philippe Ariès, Robert Mandrou, Jacques Le Goff, and others influenced by the
School, contributed to the development of the history of the senses by exploring
relationships among the mental orientations, corporeal practices, social
structures, and physical environments of previous epochs. Reflecting the
School's interest in the study of "mentalities," Febvre provocatively remarked
that: "a series of fascinating studies could be done of the sensory underpinnings
of thought in different periods" ([1942] 1982: 436).

In the 1960s and 1970s, prompted by the countercultural questioning of
conventional values and perspectives, the philosopher Michel Foucault
contributed to the development of the history of the senses by investigating the
ways in which the body was conceptualized and controlled in modernity by
state institutions (e.g. Foucault [1963] 1973, [1975] 1979). The prominent
role Foucault gave to visual surveillance in this process stimulated a vast
amount of work on the subject and helped arouse interest in the social uses of
the senses. His emphasis on "discourse" and issues of "representation" (echoed
by poststructuralists generally), nonetheless tended to distract attention from
actual sensory experience (see Howes 2003: Ch. 2).

In 1982, however, sensation or *"le sensible"* (the perceptible) gained center
stage as a subject of historical inquiry, thanks to the work of the premier
"historien du sensible," Alain Corbin (see Corbin and Heuré 2000). It was in
1982 that Corbin published *Le miasme et la jonquille—The Foul and the
Fragrant* in English translation (Corbin [1982] 1986)—the first in-depth,

sociohistorical account of a field of sense—in this case, smell in nineteenth-century France. Based on in-depth research and replete with penetrating insights, Corbin's book remains a landmark. He followed it with *Les cloches de la terre—Village Bells* (Corbin [1994] 1998), which delved into the social meaning of sound in the nineteenth-century French countryside.

Meanwhile, in North America, the twentieth-century spread of radio and television, along with the countercultural interest in non-verbal modes of communication, prompted scholars to reflect on the ways in which the media as "extensions of the senses" might shape people's ways of knowing, thinking, and acting. The Canadian Marshall McLuhan (1962, 1964) and his student Walter J. Ong (1967, 1982) highlighted the shifting relationships among the senses brought on by changes in the prevailing technologies of communication—speech (which privileged hearing), writing (which privileged sight), print (which further intensified the role of vision), and finally the electronic media (which reconfigured the world as a "global village" and put everyone in instant "touch"). McLuhan and Ong theorized that the historical privileging of sight over hearing had resulted in a rationalist, linearly-organized society, since sound is more immersive and emotionally compelling than vision, which requires detachment from objects to function.

In the 1990s, these different currents of research came together and were integrated with ideas emanating from the anthropology of the senses (i.e. Howes 1991) to produce a flowering of work in the history of the senses. In an essay in the Canadian journal *Anthropologie et Sociétés*, Alain Corbin ([1990] 2005) reflected on how the history of the senses differed from the history of mentalities (as exemplified by the work of Lucien Febvre), and also offered a range of key methodological considerations for the sensory historian. He urged fellow practitioners to "take account of the *habitus* that determines the frontier between the perceived and the unperceived, and, even more, of the norms which decree what is spoken and what left unspoken" ([1990] 2005: 135). In other words, the key to writing the history of the senses lies in "sensing" between the lines of written sources and delving into the cultural and material environments of the time. In 1993, which was a banner year for the developments we are tracing, the anthropologist Michael Taussig (taking his cue from Walter Benjamin) came out with a "particular history of the senses" in *Mimesis and Alterity* (1993); the philosopher Martin Jay rendered an account of the "denigration of vision" in twentieth-century French thought in *Downcast Eyes* (1993); and, in *Medicine and the Five Senses* (1993), the social historians W. F. Bynum and Roy Porter and their contributors traced the role of the senses in the diagnosis and treatment of disease from antiquity to the present. (This book presented the first domain-based approach to the study of the sensorium—later to be emulated by Bentley and Flynn's *Law and the Senses*, and Bacci and Melcher's *Art and the Senses*.)

In the same year, the cultural historian Constance Classen united history and anthropology in her collection of essays entitled *Worlds of Sense: Exploring the Senses in History and Across Cultures*. Classen's comparative approach presented an important corrective to the technological determinism of McLuhan and Ong's vision of the history of perception by disclosing how there is as much diversity to the ways in which the senses are valued and utilized among oral societies as between oral societies and literate societies. *Worlds of Sense* served as a pioneering model for the history of the senses and would be the forerunner of a number of works in the field by Classen (i.e. 1998, 2012; Classen *et al.* 1994), including an important survey essay in the *Encyclopedia of European Social History* (2001; see also Classen 1997). This body of work, covering many different aspects of social history, made it clear that the history of the senses was not simply a particular sub-field within the study of history, but a new way of understanding historical experience and change through the embodied, sensorial values, practices, and relationships of a given period.

In the twenty-first century, the cultural study of the senses has grown both more international (e.g., Danius 2002; Jütte 2005; Smith 2007) and more interdisciplinary, with scholars from a wide range of humanities and social science disciplines turning to the senses as both object of study and means of inquiry (e.g. Kalekin-Fishman and Low 2010; Pink 2009; Skeates 2010; Vannini *et al.* 2012). This convergence in turn laid the foundations for the emergence of the multidisciplinary field now known as "sensory studies" (Bull *et al.* 2006), which itself regroups not only the multiple disciplines, but also the multiple subspecialties that have crystallized in the interim—including visual culture, auditory culture (or sound studies), smell culture, taste culture, and the culture of touch, as well as the "sixth sense"—a highly-variegated construct (Howes 2009).

The editors of and contributors to the present *Cultural History of the Senses* series, together with other contemporary scholars (notably Mark M. Smith), are all participating in the development of this dynamic, sense-based approach to the study of culture. The present book, and the series of which it forms a part, are, therefore, both a product of the twentieth-century development of the history of the senses, and a foray into the expanding field of sensory studies in the twenty-first century.

The Social Life of the Senses: Ordering and Disordering the Modern Sensorium

TIM EDENSOR

In "The Metropolis and Mental Life," published at the dawn of the twentieth century, the German sociologist Georg Simmel provided an influential account of the ways in which modern cities were settings for powerful new sensory experiences. He drew attention to how urban dwellers were exposed to a radically different sensory world from that of the villages in which they dwelt before they migrated to the city. The urban denizen was subjected to an "intensification of nervous stimulation" in the context of an "accelerated city life" typified by the "rapid telescoping of changing images, pronounced differences within what is grasped at a single glance, and the unexpectedness of violent stimuli" (Simmel 1995: 31). According to Simmel, the urban habitué was induced to adopt a blasé attitude in the face of this hyperstimulation—a rational, distancing measure that formed a shield against overwhelming and rapid sensory impressions, but also inculcated the incapacity to respond to them. This defense accompanied the social reserve and instrumental attitude towards work and interaction with other people that was required by operating within a money economy.

Simmel's value-laden assertions about sensation in the city chime with the sociological contentions of Ferdinand Tonnies, who construed the dualistic terms *Gemeinschaft* and *Geselleschaft* to underscore what he regarded as the contrasting sorts of social relations that obtained in urban and rural spheres respectively. Tonnies conceived of the rural as embodying "the lasting and genuine form of living together" (1955: 37). In a similarly dichotomous fashion, for Simmel, the rural was typified by a "slower, more habitual, more smoothly flowing rhythm" (1995: 31). It was an environment in which sensations could be absorbed and in which social contact was warm and friendly, in contradistinction to the cold, reserved disposition of the urbanite. Such dualistic understanding of contrasting sensations in urban and rural spheres persisted throughout the twentieth century, though subtly changing as I discuss later.

There is no question that advancing urbanization, which could be considered *the* defining feature of the modern age, has produced an almost complete transformation in sense experience. I thus acknowledge that, as Simmel suggests, the conditions of modern life may well have called for distancing strategies to insulate personhood by blocking out powerful noises and smells, and onrushing sights. I shortly discuss how the dynamism of modernity simultaneously continued to provoke an uneven but often overpowering range of sensations as all that is (or was) solid seemed to melt into air (Berman 1982). This "baroque" modernity (Lash 1999) echoed Simmel's depiction of the turn of the century urban environment, which was variously sensed as fleeting, multiple, dazzling, and confusing. However, this very dynamism, and the perceived sensory disorder it produced, also incited a range of increasingly intensive attempts to regulate the environment and facilitate a more disciplined, orderly social and sensory experience of the city. Accordingly, I shall consider how a plethora of technological developments and a range of values and imperatives came to inform the sensescapes of the twentieth century. I further discuss how these regulatory strategies became so powerful and pervasive that they had the unanticipated effect of instigating the active pursuit of *unfamiliar* kinetic, aromatic, sonic, and visual sensations by those who grew dissatisfied with the sterile "blandscapes" that had eventuated across the urban West.

These contradictory modern processes—regulation and the desire for sensory order versus volatility (destructive dynamism) and the quest for sensory alterity—might usefully be thought of in terms of the "Apollonian" characteristics of modernity which affirm "structure, order and self-discipline," and the contrasting "Dionysian" qualities of modernity, productive of "sensuality, abandon and intoxication" (Rojek 1995: 80). These tensions have been highlighted by the proclivities of modern subjects to demand and impose epistemological, social, and spatial order on the one hand, and to long for disorder and transgression on the other. Whilst the dominant urge has been to seek refuge in reconstituted regimes of order in the face of continual change, the desire to transcend regulated minds, bodies, and environments has constantly bubbled just below the disciplined surface of twentieth-century everyday life and found various outlets (Cohen and Taylor 1992), often in spaces and events saturated with unfamiliar sensations.

To explore the tensions between these modern desires for sensory order and sensory alterity, the contrasting values and identities with which they were associated, and the complex ways in which they intertwined and clashed, I investigate four modern spatial processes. Firstly, I look at various strategies to order spaces and bodies, and the overarching regulatory measures that have come to pervade most aspects of social and sensory life in the modern age. While doing so, I also treat some examples that bring out the compulsion to seek out sensory alterity that this sensory ordering provoked. Secondly, I instantiate these processes by examining the project to illuminate space as an ongoing ordering process, but also look at how illumination simultaneously produced an uncanny sensory realm, and how extensive illumination provoked a search for darker spaces as well. Thirdly, I investigate how twentieth-century tourism was a practice through which comfort and familiarity were pursued, but also inculcated the desire to seek out sensual difference and surprise, and thus transcend the normative apprehension of space. Finally, I circle back to consider how these processes played out in the sensory experience of the rural.

SENSORY REGULATION AND THE QUEST FOR SENSORY ALTERITY

The bourgeois moral imperatives and scientific rationality that were first applied to the regulation of the sensorium of the city in the nineteenth century gained more and more momentum over the course of the twentieth century. These included the containment of smell through the construction of sewers and efficient waste disposal, measures to limit smoke, and the creation of urban and national parks to provide compensatory greenery and clean air. This desire for rigorous sensory control was particularly evident in the emergence of the "International" or "Modernist" style in architecture from the 1930s and concomitant drive to sweep away all traces of the past: buildings which predated the twentieth century were conceived as vestiges, outmoded relics of limited use that could justifiably be erased from the landscape. Doyen of the movement, Le Corbusier, contended that the provision of plentiful light, clean air, and space would encourage the rational development of the healthy individual, whose eyes, nose, and ears would be uncluttered by sensory rubbish. The slogans that underlined the rise of the Modernist style in architecture and urban planning resonated with these regulatory desires. Ornament was "a crime" (Loos 2006), living quarters were to be devised to accommodate bodies "efficiently," and the house was to become "a machine for living in." One of the foremost imperatives, as articulated by Le Corbusier (1933), was to "kill the street," thereby ridding urban space of unnecessary distractions and producing linear spaces of transportation that would optimize the movement of people and goods. The street was to become "a machine for traffic," purified of pedestrians and cafés that "eat up the pavement." In short, the ideal modern street was the freeway, conceived as a uniform space of, and for, mobility without obstruction, in virulent contrast to the multifunctionality of the "traditional" or "old modern" street—i.e. the nineteenth-century avenue with its "volatile mixture of people and traffic, businesses and homes" (Berman 1982: 168).

Le Corbusier's machinic episteme was further concerned with the functional and spatial division of the city into discrete parts where people might reside, work, shop, and carry out leisure pursuits, thus preventing "friction" between practices that might otherwise compete in the same space. In Le Corbusier's view, the truly modern city would be "a fully integrated world of high-rise towers surrounded by vast expanses of grass and open space—'the tower in the park'—linked by aerial superhighways, serviced by subterranean garages and shopping arcades" (Berman 1982: 167)

While Le Corbusier's designs were only realized in a few cases, the influence they had on the modern discipline of urban planning was enormous, as Berman (1982) points out. For example, in many Western cities, the delimitation of single-purpose spaces or "zones" produced exactly the segmented city that modernists like Le Corbusier so desired, drastically reducing social and sensual diversity. Such zones have been described by David Sibley (1988) as "purified" spaces, strongly circumscribed and framed to banish ambiguity of function and character. In a similar vein, Richard Sennett (1994: 15) argues that in the latter half of the twentieth century, urban space was reduced to "a mere function of motion," engendering a "tactile sterility" where the city environment "pacifies the body," with car drivers, for instance, using only "micro-movements" to negotiate space. The body was coerced into passive acquiescence and subordinated to the sterile spaces through which it passed as the desire for smooth transit "triumphed over the sensory claims of the space through which the body moves" (1994: 15). Similarly, Trevor Boddy (1992) draws attention to a "new urban prosthetics" that coerced pedestrian bodies into a passive engagement with their surroundings via a system of smooth and sealed walkways, escalators, bridges, people-conveyors, and tunnels. Constituting a comprehensive movement system to link work, recreational, and commercial spaces, these cocoon-like passages produced an aesthetic and material form typified by "incessant whirring," "mechanical breezes," "vaguely reassuring icons," "trickling fountains," and anesthetic qualities like low murmurings and insensate movements. While not entirely devoid of sensual features, these movement systems, with their mild stimulations, were not designed to excite the body either, but rather to simulate urbanity, and also filter out that which might disturb the pedestrian, the glaring sights, disruptive textures, and "troubling smells and winds" (1992: 123–4) associated with the "chaotic" city of the past.

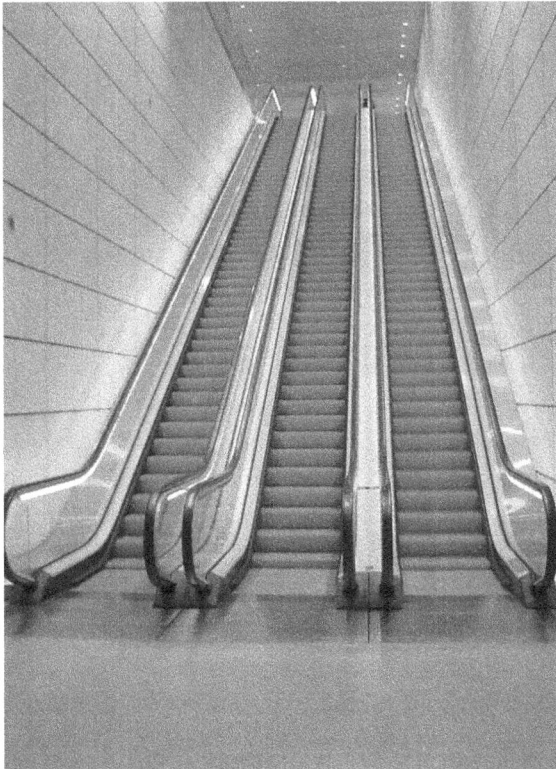

FIGURE 1.1: Smooth passage: escalator at Canary Wharf, London. Public domain.

These spatial functions were intensively managed to secure illusions of orderly permanence and minimize that which might render them the least ambiguous. Smells, noises, textures, and tactility were closely monitored by often invisible maintenance procedures that ensured that waste would be swiftly removed and that the sensory impact of those people who failed to adhere to the prevailing spatial norms would be sharply curtailed. For instance, in the last two decades of the twentieth century, there was an intensification of injunctions against sleeping or resting on benches and floors, which imposed severe restrictions on the movements of the homeless. In the highly ordered single-purpose spaces that became increasingly normative, "loitering" and "hanging out" were strictly proscribed. Graffiti-writing and bill-posting were also intensively monitored to ensure that anything considered to be an "eyesore" or that interfered with the visual order imposed by sanctioned advertisements and signage was speedily removed. Similarly, noise abatement policies attempted to ensure that loud music and "out of place" activities were minimized in residential and commercial zones.

This aesthetic and sensory control over space would appear to have reached its apogee in the increased production of themed spaces from the 1980s. Gottdiener (1997: 73) coined the term "scenography" to refer to the sort of "themed milieu" exemplified by the theme park, shopping mall, festival marketplace, regenerated waterfront, and so-called cultural quarter. Scenographies create the illusion of vibrant living but are actually highly restrictive in what practices they allow, with activities largely confined to browsing, shopping, and dining. It is not that there are no sensations to be had in such spaces, but that the sensations on offer are all carefully managed to produce particular "atmospheres." Carefully selected smells, such as the aroma of coffee or fresh-baked bread, would be released to stimulate "linger time" amongst consumers. Likewise, particular soundscapes of popular music or muzak were deployed to produce an ambience of mild relaxation. Sensory management also extended to the smoothing of floor and wall surfaces to engender a tactile seamlessness so that progress through such spaces was never jarring, always smooth.

Other areas of social life were also subjected to increasingly intensive regulation from the 1920s on. For instance, in 1930s Sweden, the sensory control of space was complemented by attempts to manage the feelings and performance of the body through an educational regime that promoted only "good habits." As Frykman (1994: 68) observes, "Sweden pioneered the teaching of sex education and sexual hygiene in schools . . . an example of the desire to rationalize the body and its drives—to make sensible use of them."

The state did not have to lecture the citizenry about the importance of physical fitness, though, for "Modern" Swedish men and women enthusiastically embraced gymnastics (in particular), and found its regimens liberating. Many voluntary gymnastics associations sprang up in the interwar years. There was talk in the popular press of "the body's revolution" and its role alongside political organizing in the coming to be of a truly "Modern" society. Frykmam quotes an excerpt from a 1934 issue of the journal *Morgonbris* (1994: 72):

> the world must be remade, people's lives must assume other forms . . . in order to endure one must have physical strength, a trained, well-formed body, flexible, well oiled—a machine to live with. This applies to the men. But it also applies to the women, who are violently wrenched out of an indolent existence in a fat corset and tight shoes. Make the body strong and shape it to be living, glad, and harmonious, and the soul will willingly follow in its tracks.

The connection between somatic regulation and modern reflexive projects of self-fashioning can also be seen in the proliferation of sites for the management of the body, including not only gyms and swimming pools, but also massage parlors, nail parlors, and hairdressers. All of these sites were dedicated to the development of selective bodily capacities.

This sensory management extended into private space as well—that is, into the home. From the 1960s, a minimalist aesthetic became fashionable which emphasized purifying domestic space of clutter. This was accompanied by an intensification of habitual procedures and techniques for maintenance, temperature control, and spatial management which were supposed to foster cleanliness, comfort, and convenience (Shove 2004). And finally there was the car which, from the 1980s became perhaps the most sensually controlled environment of all, as "standard" features or amenities came to include first power steering, then power windows, power seats, and so on, with "auditory cocooning" topping the list (Bijsterveld 2010). Valorizing only certain forms of sensual experience, while obviating others, these processes of regulation co-produced a body that could open itself out to certain sensory experiences but would automatically withdraw from others.

However, despite all the ordering processes that transformed many spaces into homogeneous, diluted sensory "blandscapes," the social and cultural dynamism of modernity continued to produce a baroque kaleidoscope of stimulation and diversity. While many of the more powerful stimuli which characterized early twentieth-century life would gradually be managed out of existence, strong sensory experiences could not be entirely eradicated, and continued to co-exist with regulated spaces in an uneven distribution across space and time. As Appadurai (1996) insists, the evolution of modernity is discontinuous and far from homogeneous. Thus, despite the forces of globalization, very different forms of social and sensual ordering often persist outside the West, in Indian market areas or bazaars, for example, which have enduringly provided an exemplary modern space, just not one that has ever been successfully subordinated to Western regulatory schemes.

The Bazaar

As explored in greater detail elsewhere (Edensor 2000a), the bazaar typically constitutes an unenclosed realm that provides a meeting point for a variety of people and multiple activities, mixing together small businesses, shops, street vendors, public and private institutions, and domestic housing. The street is also a site for diverse social activities such as loitering, sitting, chatting and observing, and domestic activities such as collecting water, washing clothes, cooking and child-minding.

The space of the bazaar is typically made up of a variety of overlapping spaces—alleys, niches, awnings, and offshoots—that constitute a labyrinthine structure with numerous openings and passages, enabling a flow of different bodies and vehicles to crisscross the street in multi-directional patterns. Unlike the seamless passages envisioned by Le Corbusier (who, as will be recalled, wished to "kill the street"), in the streets of a bazaar, pedestrians must weave a path by negotiating obstacles, and take account of the other people and traffic that cross their route at a variety of speeds. Walking is thus likely to be a sequence of interruptions and encounters that disrupt smooth passage. Jostling amidst the crowd engenders a "haptic geography" which involves continuous physical contact with other bodies. The confrontation with multiple textures alongside the body and underfoot further compounds the experience of diverse tactile sensations. Visually, the maintenance of a cultivated appearance through control or theming is rare; rather, one encounters an unplanned bricolage of structures decked out with ad hoc signs, contingent and personalized embellishments, and unkempt surfaces and facades. This is supplemented by numerous distractions and diversions offered by heterogeneous activities and sights, and an ever-shifting series of juxtapositions and assemblages of diverse static and moving elements which can provide surprising scenes. Moreover, the "smellscapes" and "soundscapes" of the bazaar are rich and varied. The jumbled mix of pungent aromas, both delightful and repulsive, produce intense "olfactory geographies," and the medley of noises generated by numerous human activities, animals, forms of transport, and performed and recorded music, creates a changing symphony of diverse pitches, volumes, and tones. Accordingly, in such an environment, the senses are excited by a variegated and changing array of stimuli.

While the sensory intensity and multiplicity of a non-Western setting such as an Indian bazaar may seem to most closely chime with the chaotic impressions of urban life recorded by early twentieth-century observers such as Simmel, there are also sites within the modern Western city, such as the street market, that offer alternative ranges of sensory pleasures. Of particular note is the plethora of "wildscapes" (Jorgensen and Keenan 2011) and derelict, abandoned, and ruined spaces that have emerged in the wake of the deindustrialization of many Western cities during the 1980s. These pockets offer a profound contrast to the sensory order maintained elsewhere. Here I focus on the ruin as a site that counters sensory sterility (Edensor 2007).

The Ruin

In contrast to the aesthetically controlled realm of the mall, replete with commodities and coded decor, in the ruin there are numerous objects and forms of matter that provide an alternative visual array. This may be due to processes of decay, where, for instance, fallen masonry, plaster and lath commingle, and paint, wallpaper, and plaster peel off walls to reveal multiple layers of color. In industrial ruins there may be offcuts and residues, or components of products that were never assembled. There may also be matter that spilled during the manufacturing processes, or byproducts like metal shards in addition to all the "stuff" that will have accumulated in the building once it was no longer maintained and ordered, such as animal droppings and corpses, plants, and fungus. Large artifacts such as machines in old factories or furniture in abandoned homes suddenly seem sculptural once they no longer possess a function shaped by the ordering of the production process. Everywhere, the things and fixtures that were formerly confined to their place have been released, and, thus, instead of upholding a particular visual order, direct the gaze to an emergent aesthetics, one that cannot be fixed through endless repair and upkeep but is constantly becoming different.

Ruins can also serve as "aromatopias" (Drobnick 2005: 270) by revitalizing attention to smell. Powerful botanical, industrial, and decaying scents have not been banished and testify to the widespread deodorization elsewhere as well as to the blurring of the organic and the synthetic, the rural and the urban. The

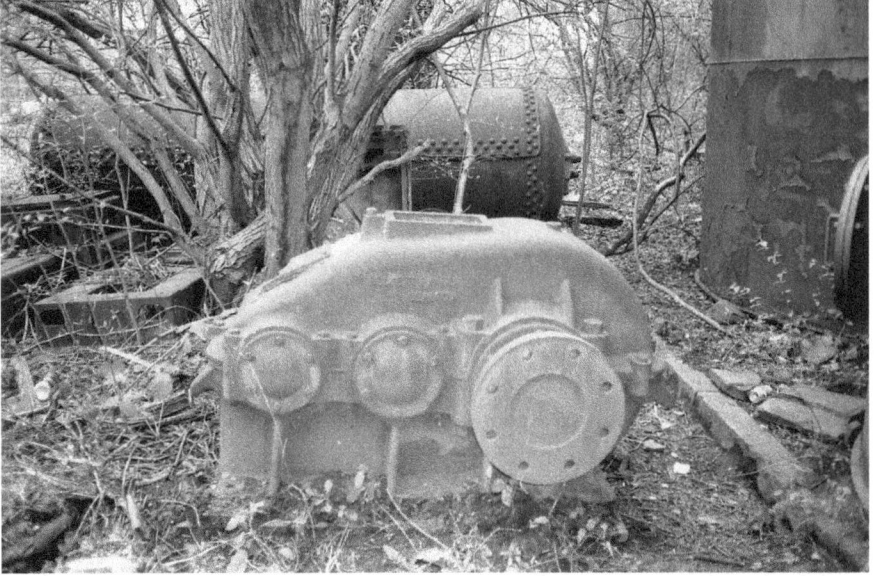

FIGURE 1.2A: Industrial ruin: obsolescent machinery. Photograph by the author.

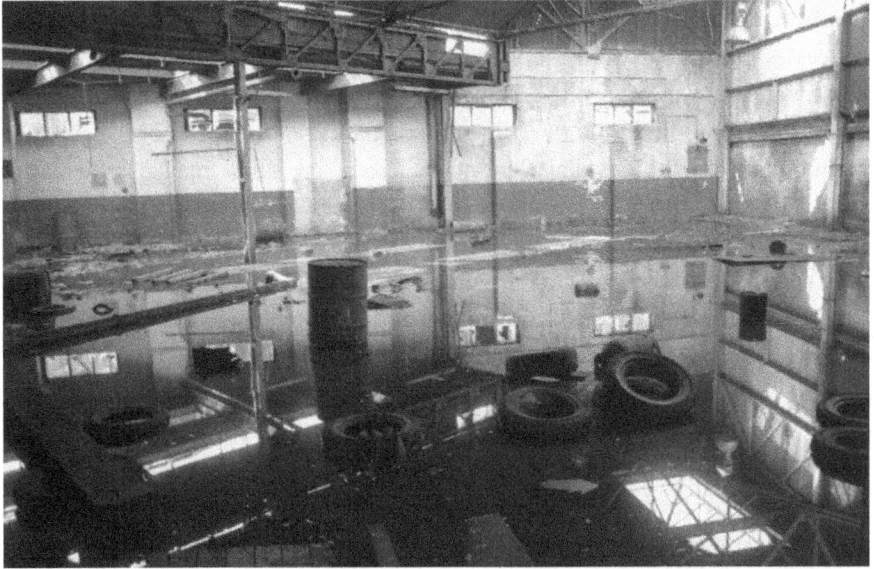

FIGURE 1.2B: Industrial ruin: abandoned factory, alternate sensuality. Photograph by the author.

smell of crumbling masonry, damp plaster, and rotting wood mingles with the pleasant scent of plants such as buddleia but may also combine with the unpleasant stench of petrol and carrion. And though at first ruined sites seem quiet as they block out much of the usually pervasive urban din, they are home to distinctive, often quite delicate, soundscapes, as footsteps echo, wind makes doors creak and slates tumble, birds sing, and flocks of pigeons produce sonic flurries.

Walking amongst a clutter of objects and fragments continually provokes a rich engagement with tactility and texture, and bodies are coerced into adopting unfamiliar somatic maneuvers, crouching and leaning as they forge a path across a chaotic material assemblage. This is not a world of silken sheen or velvety textures, polished surfaces, ceaselessly swept floors, or plush carpeting. Instead, it might contain the splintery surfaces of an old table, shards of glass on concrete flooring, a mulch of decomposing fabric or moldering paper, the cushioning textures of moss, corroding steel and slimy, rotting wooden floorboards. Though this may be experienced as disturbing in its sensual alterity, such spaces also offer opportunities to engage with the material world in a more playful, sensual fashion. Thus, in the derelict space, where there is no surveillance and no prohibition on touching (unlike the museum), things invite touch; they are available to pick up, to stroke, to throw, to smash or pull apart, and thereby release a flood of neglected sense-making capacities. Yet these pleasurable materialities may also be accompanied by more sensually disturbing matter that threatens the body with infection, pain, or falling: viscous puddles of grease, nails sticking out of upturned boards, piles of asbestos.

The body in the ruin by turns recoils or opens itself out to these sensual stimuli, to the abundant textures, to the abject and pleasurable materialities that are absent in more regulated spaces. A number of exhibition curators have explored these tendencies. When Caitlin DeSilvey engaged in the experimental curation of a derelict Montana homestead, she discovered that the diverse residues and artifacts she encountered sparked "simultaneous—and contradictory—sensations of repugnance and attraction" (2006: 320). Justin Armstrong explored a series of abandoned places in rural Saskatchewan, and found that to move about in them was "to follow in the tactile and accumulated wake of History" (2010: 274). In such sites of ruination, the physical traces of the past impress themselves upon the senses in a way that rarely happens at codified, narrated, and anaesthetized heritage sites where the *feel* of the past has been swept away in favor of potted, authoritative narratives (Edensor 2005). A confrontation with rough industrial textures and smells, and the din of the workshop, for instance, is absent from most industrial heritage sites, as clutter is banished and smooth walkways guide bodies along safely organized routes.

Accordingly, in the ruin, the dissolution of sensual familiarity and the advent of sensory surprises may be initially overwhelming, repulsive, or arresting, but it has the potential to provide a stimulating experience by its very distinctness from the familiar, regular, ordered space. Derelict spaces can provoke an often startling awareness of the ways in which we are sensually alienated from the material world because it is impossible not to be immersed in such spaces when visiting them (Garrett 2011). Goatcher and Brunsden (2011) reveal in their account of representation at the vast ruined spaces at Chernobyl, that visual techniques such as photography are inadequate for capturing the deluge of sensory and imaginative experiences that emerge during a visit to that derelict nuclear site.

The Temporary

Besides these ruined sites, there are other sites and occasions where less regulated sensory experiences may be enjoyed, and where different forms of (usually temporary) activity occupy space and disturb its sensory order. Temporary occasions, such as car boot sales, processions and political demonstrations offer an alternative to the usual sensory regulation. Sarah Pink (2007) reveals how the proponents of the slow food movement and *cittàslow*, founded in 1986 and 1999 respectively, call for the senses to be re-educated through a more sustained engagement with the particular affordances of local spaces. An increasing number of music and other festivals across the Western world, starting with the famous 1969 Woodstock Music Festival in upper New York state, have offered temporary suspension of ordinary modes of comfort and cleanliness, and a more intense engagement with sound, other bodies, and movement. There are also forms of subcultural practice that temporarily appropriate or reappropriate spaces, so that apprehension may be altered by the use of drugs, as for instance during the raves of the 1990s in which participants were "hurled into a vortex of heightened sensation, abstract emotions and artificial energies" (Reynolds 1998: xix).

Borden provides a rather Romantic depiction of the practice of skateboarding as "nothing less than a sensual, sensory, physical emotion and desire for one's own body in motion and engagement with the architectural and social other" (1998: 216). Yet he is right to point out how the affordances of regulated space that normally guide the body and senses (e.g. steps, handrails) are inverted by the very different use made of them by skaters, along with exponents of parkour

(Mould 2009). These adventure sports all use space to produce more radical kinetic, sonic, and tactile encounters with urban materiality. Similarly, Monica Degen (2008) has shown how the ordering and recoding techniques utilized in the 1990s regeneration of Castlefield, Manchester, and El Raval in Barcelona, which had the effect of killing or diminishing familiar sensescapes, have been continuously contested by residents and visitors who valorized different sensory markers and a more heterogeneous range of sensations.

While the quest for sensory alterity is ongoing, it is usually marginal in time and space. As Rob Shields has contended, fairs and carnivals with their teeming activities, fleeting and surprising sights, and powerful sensations have persistently been "pruned and replanted at the margins of society" (1991: 86) Moreover, popular desires for the carnivalesque and overwhelming have often been co-opted by advertising and marketing strategists, who produce spaces which appear to promise a cornucopia of sensations and "unconstrained social differences" but only ever deliver a "controlled diversity" (Mitchell 1995: 119). Here, "sites of ordered disorder" (Featherstone 1991: 82) have increasingly satisfied what Chris Rojek calls "the timid freedom of respectable leisure" (1995: 80).

Outside the West, it is also increasingly common to find that "the thrills of the bazaar are traded in for the conveniences of the sterile supermarket" (Chakrabarty 1991: 16) as the relationship between sensory alterity and familiarity is continuously reworked, and such spaces become a site of ongoing struggle between residents and workers on the one hand and technocrats and politicians on the other (Anjaria 2012). Middle-class distaste for the sonic and other sensations that emerge from less regulated realms may result in a moral and sensorial reordering expressed through the construction of walls or fences that hedge in (while screening off) slums (Chandola 2012) but equally, a reterritorializing dis-ordering may subsequently kick in. Fascinatingly, Shompa Lahiri (2011) reveals how Brahmo migrants from Kolkata to London note similarities in the desensualization of space in both cities but also retain memories, rekindled in repeat visits, of highly valued impressions of the taste of street food, the scent of fragrant blossoms, and the sounds of street traders and music that contrast with the more muted sensations of the suburban areas of London in which they reside.

ILLUMINATION—ORDERING THE SENSES AFTER DARK

The process through which space was progressively colonized by illumination over the course of the twentieth century presents a useful case study with respect to understanding the modern project of sensory ordering generally.

"Improved" lighting enabled movement, signified meanings and facilitated forms of oligoptic surveillance, producing value-laden understandings about how people should behave in public space. As a signifying element of the city, revealing certain spaces to vision while concealing others, artificial light figured as "a symbol and a determinant of urban differentiation" (Otter 2008: 335). Electrification was slow to reach rural areas, and within urban areas themselves there was considerable inequality to the distribution of illumination. The gloomy neighborhoods of the poor contrasted with the brightly-lit mansions of the wealthy.

Jakle (2001) has described how lighting norms in the American city perpetrated a spatial hierarchy where the luminosity of streets was largely determined by the heaviness of the traffic on them, and their perceived "importance." Across the United States, the "Main Street" of every town became saturated with the marks of commerce and capital by night, awash with flashing and neon signage identifying retail outlets, fast-food joints, and advertising products. As regards buildings, light was projected onto state buildings, heritage sites, monuments and corporate skyscrapers, inscribing the identities and values of the powerful on space. Accordingly, McQuire submits, a "new 'map' of the city" (2008: 124) was produced in which esteemed buildings were floodlit while others were cast into darkness. Despite the persistence of these inscriptions of power on space, alternative lighting practices persisted, as with the late twentieth century, largely working-class, British festive practice of illuminating houses with an effusion of bright, animated Christmas lights—a pursuit often criticized as excessive and tacky (Edensor and Millington 2009).

Lighting came to define "a new landscape of modernity" (Nasaw 1999: 8). The routines and compulsions formerly dictated by cycles of sunlight and darkness, and the cycle of the seasons, were transcended by electric light, which progressively transformed the city from a sometimes dark and dangerous environment into a continuously illuminated and comparatively well ordered space, in which night-time practices could flourish. But besides signifying power, efficiency and technological progress, illumination also contributed to the uncanny dimensions of modernity through the production of a phantasmagoric realm (Collins and Jervis 2008) that defamiliarized, excited, and eclipsed ordinary ways of sensing. A host of unlit elements could not be perceived, illuminated buildings lost their solidity, light was refracted in puddles and windows, and scale and proportion came to seem illusory—all qualities captured in the chiaroscuro of film noir that emerged in Hollywood in the 1940s and 1950s. Much modern space was thus transformed "into a perceptual laboratory" (McQuire 2008: 114), a dream-like realm of fantasy and experimentation. Light was increasingly used to enchant and excite from the mid twentieth century *son et lumière* show to the 1970s rock concert, where the lighting formed an essential accompaniment to the music. There was also a proliferation of light festivals in urban and rural spaces, such as the world's largest light festival, Fête des Lumières, in Lyon, France, initiated in 1989. Its goal was to produce magical nocturnal landscapes through the judicious use of lighting which, for example, enabled otherwise unnoticed features of the surroundings to be brought to the attention, peculiar illuminated sculptures to suddenly appear out of nowhere, and buildings to be dematerialized by shape-shifting projections (Edensor 2012).

The halflight also attracted its denizens. What William Sharpe calls a "second city—with its own geography and its own set of citizens" (2008: 14) emerged after nightfall to provide a "realm of fascination and fear which inhabits the edges of our existence, crowded by shadows, plagued by uncertainty, and shrouded in intrigue" (2008: 9). Roger Palmer conceives of the night as the "time for daylight's dispossessed—the deviant, the dissident, the different" (2000: 16–17) to engage in oppositional activities; it is the period for pleasure-seekers to escape the strictures of commerce, economic rationality, and spatial regulation that are maintained during daylight hours and seek out "sensualities and sociabilities, aesthetics and the art of resistance" (2000: 453). The sensations and atmospheres of gloom were co-produced by the prostitutes, drug dealers, and musicians who plied their trade and the bohemians who dwelt in shadowy spaces. And, despite the spread of illumination, the twentieth century also contained its own dark realms, the tunnels, cellars, and sewers, and the theaters, cinemas, photographic darkrooms, and ghost trains that were potent because of the absence of light and concomitant solicitation of the non-visual senses.

Finally, the spread of illumination would spark some disaffected elements to band together in praise of darkness. The founding of the International Dark Sky Association in 1988 is a case in point. Its mandate involved identifying and maintaining "dark skies" locations. The latter attracted tourists and astronomers who wished to witness starry heavens without the interference of ambient glow. In these gloomy landscapes, with a paucity of light—except sometimes of the moon and stars—the sensorium was challenged and transformed. For, besides signifying devilry and danger, darkness also symbolizes the ineffable and mysterious. Darkness also stimulates different ways of looking at landscape and the things that stand out in the gloom, such as the silvery shape of a tree, or the glimmer of water, or the thick shadow of a bush. Where the visual sense is muted, hearing becomes accentuated, which results in heightened attention being paid to the murmurs and scuttles of non-human beings and the various sounds of rushing water and wind. Smell too comes to the fore, as the scent of fungi or nocturnal creatures such as skunks and raccoons pervades the air. The body becomes attentive to shifting textures underfoot, a tactile awareness of space that is further enhanced by heightened consciousness of the qualities of the air (humidity, closeness, etc.). Moreover, the absence of light means that a conjectural and imaginative approach to space must be adopted, one that extends beyond the scanning gaze practiced in daylight. With little visual warning of what lies ahead, the feet learn to differentiate between textures, and the body has to anticipate how to walk from moment to moment, not knowing when it will come up against a wall, or a cliff (Edensor 2013).

SEEKING SENSORY FAMILIARITY AND ALTERITY THROUGH TOURISM

I now consider the ways in which tensions between the contradictory modern desires for the regulation of sensation and the transcendence of regulation continue to be reconfigured and redistributed through a practice that underwent significant expansion (under the aegis of globalization) during the last century—namely, tourism (Franklin 2003; MacCannell 1976; Urry 2002).

While analyses of tourism have commonly characterized it as involving a quest for liminality and authenticity—that is, as a movement away from the everyday towards the extraordinary and exotic, most twentieth-century tourist experience was replete with routine, unreflexive habits, common sense, and culturally specific escape attempts from normativity (Edensor 2006). Many of these mundane, iterative practices were accommodated in familiar serial tourist environments, including luxury hotels and resorts, and various themed spaces and enclaves. In these carefully controlled spaces, only preferred activities were encouraged (or allowed). Crucially, such realms were sensually regulated to minimize disruption and provide many (if not all) of the "comforts of home," so that the body was cajoled and cosseted into relaxed ease. Themed designs ensured that there were few surprising sights. Smell was monitored to prevent any traces of sewage, rotting food, or heavy industrial processes from assailing the nostrils while floral scents abounded; the sonic environment was modulated to minimize harsh noises and let in piped music; textures were smooth, and linen sheets, cushioned furniture, and air-conditioning enclosed bodies so they might relax in habituated comfort. Movement was facilitated by clear pathways and shuttle services. Such intensive sensual regulation did not merely epitomize mindless spatial homogenization; it also testified to tourist desires for reliability, comfort, and luxury. In such circumstances, bodies were rarely jarred out of the preferred state of unselfconscious relaxation. Moreover, such spaces were reproduced by the connivance of tourists. Their particular affordances encouraged performative conventions of walking, lounging, and consuming as part of the reproduction of shared cultural norms (Edensor 2001) or a particular form of touristic habitus.

Cultural analyses of tourism initially tended to focus on "the tourist gaze" and how it was supported by the practice of sightseeing and the ubiquity of the camera or video recorder. In "On Safari" (1991), for example, Kenneth Little problematized the tourist perspective by showing how tourists to Kenya were influenced in their selection of what to photograph by images of "wild Africa" they had seen in movies and magazines before coming. Once in Kenya, they would "take pictures to make a record of their trip and to show others back home that 'they were really there'" (1991: 155). As a result, most of their experience of Kenya was "framed" first by the Western images of Africa they carried in their mind's eye, and second by the viewfinder of their camera. It would be legitimate to question whether they "saw" Africa at all. In "On Safari," Little was also concerned to expose the controlling power of the tourist gaze vis-à-vis its object—that is, the African subject. "Taking pictures of other people," such as the "proud Samburu warrior," meant "turning them into objects by subjecting them to the controlling and curious gaze of the photographer" (1991: 155). The Samburu were thereby frozen, objectified, "captured" by means of the camera—and stereotyped, with no chance to speak back, or point out how they were modern too.

Subsequent analyses of tourism have been less concerned with exposing the hegemony of the tourist gaze, and more concerned with bringing out its multiplicity. For example, Urry (2002) has documented how alongside the "romantic" sightseeing solitary gaze, there exists the "collective" and "anthropological" gaze. Urry's insight has been extended by Jordan and Aitchison (2008), who note how the tourist gaze is frequently gendered and sexualized, and by Maoz (2006) who introduced the idea of the "mutual gaze," which involves a more nuanced relationship between tourists and hosts. Furthermore, as Degen *et al.* remark, visuality is often "multimodal: that is, visual experiences are frequently accompanied by aural, tactile, and oral experiences" (2008: 1909). There are in fact a host of tourist practices which accentuate other senses besides sight, and other sensory combinations besides the audiovisual, in the quest for sensory alterity. This highlights how tourism might be more broadly considered as a key twentieth-century practice for sensory enhancement. For instance, Pau Obrador-Pons avers that naturist beach tourism is "a way of accessing the world through the body and a sensual disposition" (2007: 128) that cultivates a focus upon "the feeling of the sun caressing the skin, the sensual movement of the naked body into the seawater and the unpleasant infiltration of sand into body orifices" (2007: 134). Discussing hill-walking and climbing, Katrin Lund (2005) highlights how touch and tactility are imbricated with other bodily sensations, including muscular exertion and tension, mobility, balance, and the effects of temperature and soreness.

As the century progressed, the quest for sensory unfamiliarity appears to have intensified. The search for immersive sensation was evident in the sensory whirls produced by participation in tourist action sports such as bungee jumping and white-water rafting, and the thrills provided by the ever faster and higher white knuckle rides of amusement parks (Sally 2006). The tourist sensorium was further expanded through a host of other somatically enlivening endeavors, including trekking adventures, mountain biking, and wilderness canoe trips, all practices that promote visceral excitation and may cause exhaustion and pain (Cloke and Perkins 1998). Stephanie Merchant (2011) has revealed how scuba divers develop new sensory skills, especially in the domains of touch and hearing, as they discover that the senses that they usually rely on are unreliable or redundant when negotiating underwater space. Though such experiences may be alarming and awkward, these sensations are also thrilling in their difference. Arun Saldanha (2002) has documented how the Goan beach raves which attracted worldwide attention (and interest) in the 1980s, combined the sounds of music, smells of sweat, kerosene, and cannabis, sight of the moon and swaying coconut trees, tactilities of moving bodies, sand underfoot and humidity—all augmented by the stimulating effects of sense-enhancing drugs—to produce an intensely sensual experience at variance to everyday apprehension.

The search for a more sustained immersion in sensual and cultural otherness is also exemplified through forms of backpacking experience that became progressively more popular throughout the twentieth century, and were often motivated by the desire to acquire cultural capital. Movement through the often sensually rich, socially diverse, and cluttered materialities of heterogeneous honeypots—often akin to the Indian bazaar areas discussed above—with their rough textures, undulating pavements and dust and dirt, often stretched the backpackers' habitual ways of sensing. In their travels, backpackers had to confront all sorts of unfamiliar materialities: animal noises, religious sounds, uneven textures, powerful and unidentifiable smells, unfamiliar sights. For example, on the first day of my own visit to an Indian village during a backpacking holiday, the startling vision of yellow frogs, the sight of large flocks of large fruit bats flying overhead, the smell of bidis and buffalo dung, the cries of peacocks and snatches of Bollywood music all combined to produce an initially unsettling but thrilling sensory alterity.

In the search for sensual otherness, the tourist body recoiled or welcomed these alternately abject and pleasurable sensual stimuli. According to a recent study, at the start of their trips through India and Thailand, many female backpackers did not want to be sheltered from harsh sensations, expecting, even desiring, physical pain and repellent smells, dirt and noise, for to be able to cope with such sensations produced self-pride and also garnered cultural capital. Despite this disposition to embrace the sensually repugnant, travel over a longer period promoted a tendency to modulate sensory experience. Thus, while adventure tourists may initially want to plunge into sensory alterity and face up to disgust, they tend to adjust their disposition towards sensation over the period of travel, mixing physical hardship and sensory onslaught with visits to comfortable hotels and air-conditioned restaurants (Edensor and Falconer 2012). And while these same backpackers were often eager to sample challenging local fare at the outset of their travels, later they modulated their eating experiences by mobilizing both *neophobic* tendencies to avoid unfamiliar tastes and *neophilic* inclinations to try different tastes (Cohen and Avieli 2004).

Accordingly, many tourists tried to balance their desire for sensory familiarity with a quest for alterity in a single trip. However, culturally different sensory dispositions could clash at particular destinations. In a more global context, in 1993, British package tourists at the Taj Mahal complained that the numerous Indian tourists at the site were too noisy and paid insufficient visual attention to the mausoleum (Edensor 1998). Throughout the century, international tourism became an exemplary site at which esteemed sensations and the cultural values that informed them could be confounded or challenged. Yet as I have inferred above, under contemporary conditions of globalization, the tastes, smells, sights, and sounds of otherness might be resisted in the making of new sensory markers of gender, class, and ethnicity—or alternatively, become domesticated and made familiar, as with the "ethnic quarters" that pervade Western cities, as I discuss in the final section.

SEEKING SENSATIONS IN THE RURAL

The tensions that circulate around the modern desires for sensory regulation and alterity, and the way in which sensory values were mobilized to foster the perception of distinctions between places, are acutely exemplified in the complex understandings and practices that have continued to focus upon the rural. As discussed at the start of this chapter, Simmel contrasted the overwhelming sensorium of the modern city with the more stable, allegedly authentic sensory setting of the village and the countryside. The desire to escape the sensually chaotic city for the privileged sensory realm of an idyllic rural setting permeated the twentieth century. In everyday thought, the rural was seen as more "natural" than the city, and in a rural setting the body was supposed to respond more "naturally" to its environment, dropping its self-consciousness and performative dispositions, adjusting to slower rhythms,

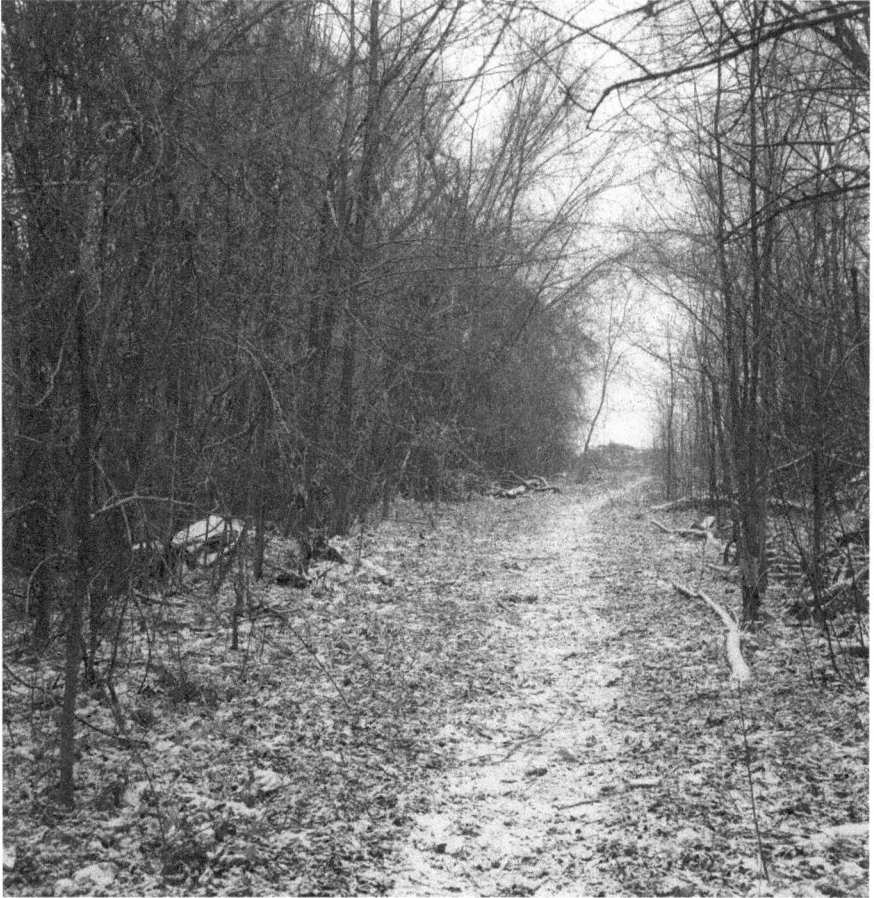

FIGURE 1.3a: Nature walk: November snow on path, from the series *Sur la trace du renard*. Photograph by Louis Perreault.

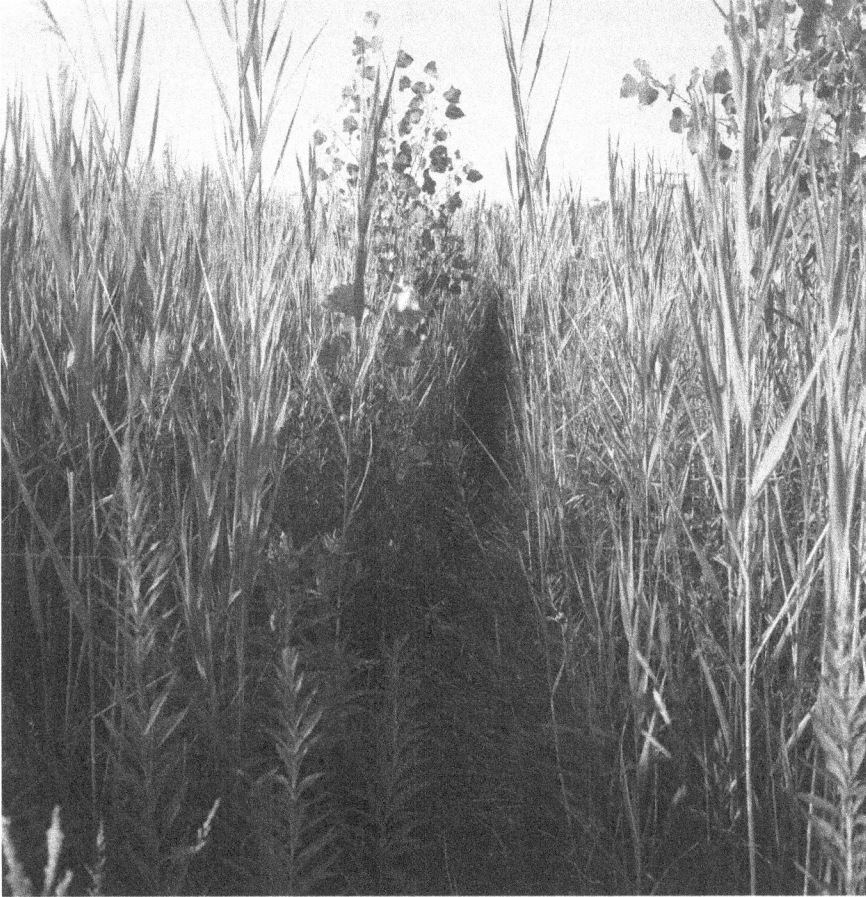

FIGURE 1.3B: Nature walk: through the tall grass, from the series *Sur la trace du renard*. Photograph by Louis Perreault.

opening out to sensation rather than having to be shielded from over-stimulation. The rural has remained a location where freer practices and more "natural" sensations may be sought (Neal and Walters 2007). For instance, those drawn to walk in the countryside continue to be motivated by widespread cultural notions that walking stimulates the dulled urban body into a sensual excitation away from urban noise, polluted air, and unsightliness (Edensor 2000b).

However, the same regulatory processes that characterized twentieth-century urban planning and governance have been steadily extended into rural spaces. This is exemplified by attempts to maintain visual order in particularly esteemed environments such as the Peak District National Park in northern

Derbyshire and surrounding parts, designated in 1951, where new building developments are carefully monitored to ensure that they accord with specified architectural styles and landscapes are preserved to maintain a mooted historical continuity. This fixing of the visual and material qualities of space preserves the myth of an unchanging "natural" landscape and has been underpinned by the post-productionist values of rural gentrifiers who have increasingly populated the countryside since the 1980s (Burton 2012). Similarly, the ramshackle appearance of new-age travelers and their vehicles in the British countryside in the 1980s led to stringent rural policing to restore order by banishing those regarded as out of place and offensive to the senses. These forms of regulation are also entwined with discourses about sensation that are mobilized to justify "essentialist views of inferior or superior places" (Drobnick 2002: 37). In this sense, the countryside was conceived as a privileged setting in which the sensory intrusions of such non-traditional rural dwellers were not welcome (Cloke 2006). The same un-welcome was extended to the non-white migrant groups that had come to populate the cities of Britain from the 1960s whenever they ventured into the countryside. The rural thus served as a venue from which to express judgments about the inferiority of the spaces, practices, and bodies of others according to sensory criteria, where noise, smell, appearances, and textures were key markers of cultural difference.

Yet despite these entrenched cultural discourses, it is also obvious that the specific affordances and configurations of rural space do offer very different sensations to those experienced in most urban realms. Echoing the points made about the ruin above, walking through woodland or hill country enlivens the body as it is coerced to move in non-linear fashion over rough terrain, agricultural smells suffuse the atmosphere, there is no rush of visual impressions, and soundscapes tend to be less cluttered. Moreover, the rural provides environments in which darkness can be enjoyed, away from the over-illuminated city, and where the visceral sensory experiences of adventure sports may be staged.

Indeed, these actual differences and the consistently dichotomous conceptions of the rural and the urban continued to stimulate an increasing diversity of endeavors that pursued sensory alterity in the rural towards the end of the twentieth century. This ensured that the countryside became a highly contested realm, as a host of competing recreational pursuits sought to escape urban regulation and injurious sensations (Macnaghten and Urry 1998). For instance, the adrenaline-fueled rush of speedy descents down hillsides by skiers and mountain bikers, and the airborne surges of hang-gliders contrasted and competed with the more deliberate, subtler sensory attunements to the rural desired by walkers and birdwatchers.

CONCLUSION

In this chapter, I have argued that a key modern impulse has been to forge an orderly and predictable world and that this has entailed the regulation of the senses across space. However, I have also contended that this came at a cost to sensory diversity and excitement, producing sterile, over-regulated spaces and unstimulating blandscapes. I suggest that this regulation exemplifies Jacques Rancière's notion of the "distribution of the sensible" (2006), through which the powerful organize sensory experience. This perpetuates a situation in which certain ways of perceiving and feeling establish the conditions for what it is possible to sense and thus what it is possible to communicate. However, this distribution, as Mark Paterson asserts, is "continually shifting and culturally variable. It varies according to a society's rules or proscriptions as well as technological mediation and physical environment" (2009: 771).

This continuous transformation is characteristic of a capitalist modernity that ensures that most things do not endure for long (Berman 1982). Buildings, industries, fashions, and policies have emerged and crumbled throughout the twentieth century, and huge human and cultural flows have moved through and across space, transforming the sensescapes of everyday life and providing unfamiliar, often disturbing, and frequently exciting sensations. Moreover, because processes of economic growth, politics, and planning have been uneven and spatially diverse, certain spaces continue to exist as less regulated, multisensual realms, such as certain rural environments, ruins, and Indian bazaars. In addition, many people reacted against sensory homogeneity by seeking out marginal sites and events that lack ordinary sense-making infrastructures, and engaged in activities that transcend or confound normative sensory experience.

The persistence of highly regulated urban spaces that constrain sensory diversity testifies to the relentless processes of maintenance and policing at the heart of modern life. But despite the effectiveness of such schemes, unbidden sights, sounds, textures, and smells lurk, waiting to burst out and invade orderly sites, disrupting sensory experience as the "old, earthy environment . . . persistently breaks through the cracks in the pavement" (Howes 2005a: 37).

CHAPTER TWO

Urban Sensations: A Retrospective of Multisensory Drift

ALEX RHYS-TAYLOR

The twentieth-century city underwent a cascade of intertwined social, political, technological, and economic revolutions, all of which combined to radically alter the spectrum of sensoria that filled the everyday life of the century's urbanites. At the same time, the great revolutions of the century are reflected in the sensibilities through which urbanites made sense of this diversifying sensual maelstrom. Zooming in and out of various perspectives on the city, while moving through disparate locations, this chapter develops a retrospective of the changes within the sensoria and sensibilities of the twentieth-century city, taking the city of London as its homebase.

VERTICALITY

In 1895, a 95-meter high ferris wheel was erected at Earl's Court in West London as part of the great Empire of India Exhibition. In many respects the towering feat of engineering formed the opening bracket of a century of tumultuous change in the city. On New Year's Eve, 1999, the centurial bracket was closed with another, brand new, ferris wheel 40 meters taller than the last.

As midnight struck, the wheel became the centerpiece in the millennial city's spectacular riverside display of lasers and fireworks—rippling circles of blue, red, and yellow reflected in the murky Thames beneath it. Three months later, in March 2000, the ferris wheel (the EDF London Eye, formally known as the Millennium Wheel and the British Airways London Eye) was finally open for the public to ride in. Since then, the colossal circle of steel and glass has attracted over 3.5 million people a year. With a ticket to ride in one of the wheel's spacious ellipsoid booths, visitors are able to experience many of the sensations that typified the twentieth century. Tightly sealed within the hermetic security of a reinforced glass capsule, passengers are lifted up in a movement that feels like a slowed down version of the first moments of air flight. At a height of 135 meters into the sky above London, passengers can see up to 40 kilometers in all directions and are afforded an elevated panoptical view of the city that echoes the view favored by modernity's urban master planners and surveillance specialists. The constantly changing perspective during a ride on the Eye typifies a century in which people, culture, politics, and economics were in constant motion, while the slow turning action of the spoked wheel creates the appearance of a giant clock, its hands turning in time with the inexorable metamorphosis of the modern city and the sensoria that fill it.

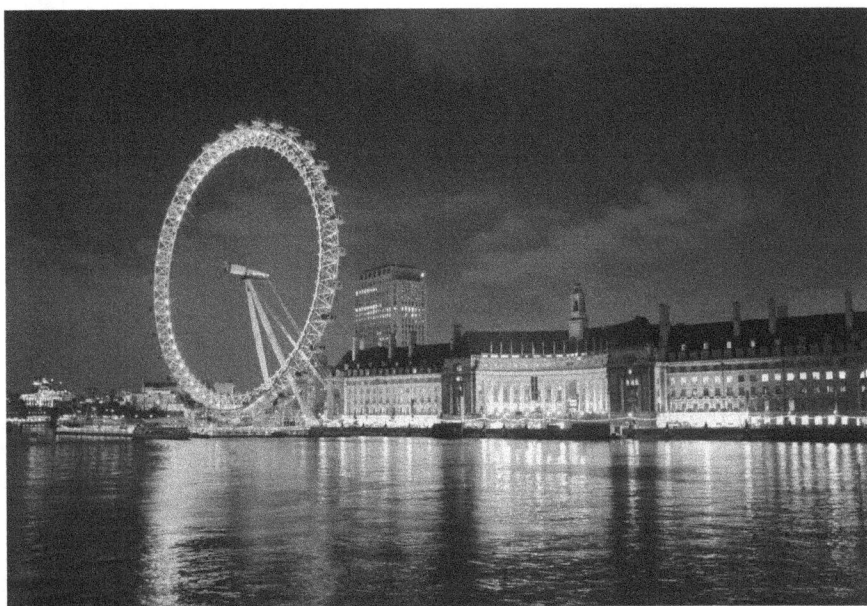

FIGURE 2.1: The London Eye at night. Photograph by Mike Peel. Public domain.

The silhouetted skyline visible through a glass capsule is itself a quintessentially modern way of experiencing and representing the city, requiring both twentieth-century architecture to create the view, and the sensibility of a modern urbanite to understand what the hieroglyph means. As cartographic historian Simon Foxell outlines (2011: 56), up until the late nineteenth century, the favored way of looking at and representing London was as it appeared to the sailor that sidled up into the city along its river, landmarks unfurling like a scroll. New York, similarly, was frequently represented "as it looked when one approached it by sea from the harbour" (Taylor 1988: 225). By the end of the nineteenth century, however, "the approach to the city by rail and road began to encourage a new perspective on the city, silhouetted against the sky" (Taylor 1988: 225). The popularization of cameras with which to immediately capture a totalizing image of the city, as well as the invention of new vertical buildings types, visible from afar, ensured that the skyline would become the dominant way of imaging a city's identity. In the last decades before the millennium, the view from Waterloo Bridge (immortalized in the Kinks song, "Waterloo Sunset") was so important to selling the city that it had effectively become a "protected vista" (Gassner 2010: 142–55), all architectural obstructions to the crown jewels of the towering financial district to the east of the giant wheel, and the gothic spires of parliament to the west, forbidden.

While London's signature skyline transformed constantly over the course of the twentieth century, the most notable difference between the millennial view over London and the view from atop the ferris wheel the century before is that one is even able to *see* the city from a distance. For a steady 300 years previously, the air that enveloped the streets of London had grown steadily more opaque, particularly during the odd fog or "pea-souper." In the wake of the Great Smog of 1952, which was responsible for over 8,000 deaths, and led to the passage of the Clean Air Act (1956), the acrid exhalations of industrial London started to lift, drift away, and henceforth fester over the cities of the global South. As the last of the pincushion of nineteenth-century chimneys collapsed, the only fumes visible from the giant ferris wheel are the recalcitrant yellow haze of vehicular exhaust fumes and the odd puff of smoke billowing out of an incinerator. The same could be said of many cities in Europe and America in which the gradual dissipation of the clouds of particulate matter from mid-century on signaled—visually, olfactorily—the shift from manufacturing and export towards a knowledge-based service economy.

Across the metropolitan centers of Europe and America, for each cluster of chimneys that had collapsed, a bolder histogram of vertical lines had started

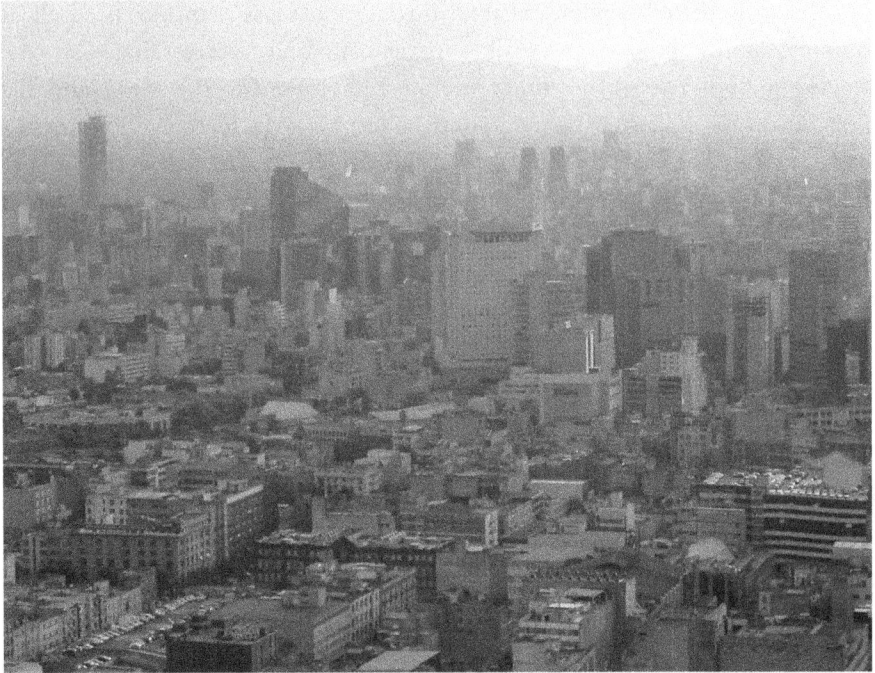

FIGURE 2.2: Mexico City in smog. Photograph by Christian von Wissel. Public domain.

biting at the sky above the city. While the millennial skyline of London was increasingly dominated by commercial buildings, the buildings that gnawed on the horizon for most of the century had been housing. The same could be said for many of the twentieth century's cities: from the peripheral high-rises of France's banlieu (Wacquant 2007: 229–31) and Sweden's förorter (Hammarén 2010: 211–17), to the post-shanty housing of Hong Kong (Castells *et al.* 1990) and the communal behemoths of the Eastern Bloc, the social and economic mulch of the century sprouted clustered forests of beige and slate, growing steadily taller with each decade.

While the internal mechanics of each "machine for living" (Le Corbusier 2008: 151) would differ significantly depending on the local ecologies in which they were embedded, the "brutalist" aesthetics of these towers' exteriors—the bold uniform concrete lines and colossal surfaces—allude to deeper socio-structural affinities between modern cities of the twentieth century; an affinity that told a wider story about modernity. In his remarkable essay on architecture and the senses, *The Eyes of the Skin*, Juhani Pallasmaa (2005: 71) contends that "the timeless task of architecture is to create embodied and lived metaphors that concretise and structure our being in the world," to materialize and eternalize "ideas and images of the ideal life." Religious buildings had historically been designed, for instance, to materialize a sense of a majestic, divine being. On the whole, however, the species of "being" concretized through most premodern architecture was of a scale that an individual could grasp with his own senses: the family, the community, and the city quarter. The various arrays of monolith that chewed at the skyline of the twentieth-century city, however, constituted attempts to hail a very different type of being—one in which the individual was part of a whole far larger than the family, neighborhood, or even city. Dwarfing the city dwellers standing in the shadows beneath them, the being that the new brutalist architecture concretized was that of the modern nation: a writhing colony of "rationalized" activity.

In the first instance, the UK's suburban sink estates and inner-city developments were devised as part of a scheduled effort of social and spatial containment (Gartman 2012: 213), a Keynsian investment aimed at transforming working-class bodies into equal participants in the modernizing economy. Private toilets and bathrooms, multiple bedrooms, larger floor areas, fitted kitchens, and designated green spaces were all part of an attempt to create a fitter, more productive and less unruly workforce. Presented as egalitarian interventions, in many respects the new mass housing represented the apex of architecture's involvement in the problems of population and health (Foucault 1980: 148–9). In some places the bold, modernist, geometric aesthetic of the exterior provided a powerful signifier that tapped into mythologies of progress and development. In the UK, however, the valorization of the utopian aesthetic was thwarted by the contours of local culture and social history. The working-class communities who were first decanted into the angular new dwellings feared the loss of community in their stacked abodes— the inability to bump into neighbors, to see who was coming and who was going, and to hear what was going on outside (Young and Willmott 1992: 151). Bourgeois conservative critics (Scruton 1995), on the other hand, feared that abandoning the vernacular classicism of Victorian and Georgian structures would lead to a diminution of national and regional identity. The greatest obstacle to the valorization of the modernist aesthetic, however, emerged from within the obdurate sensibilities of the middle classes, alongside whom many of the century's boldest and most brutal public housing projects sprung. It might not, however, have been the design of the buildings themselves that was at fault. Any aesthetic developments associated with working-class living, it seems, be they low-rise vernacular terraces or monolithic blocks, were likely to be met with stinging disparagement by the suburban middle class, a wide group

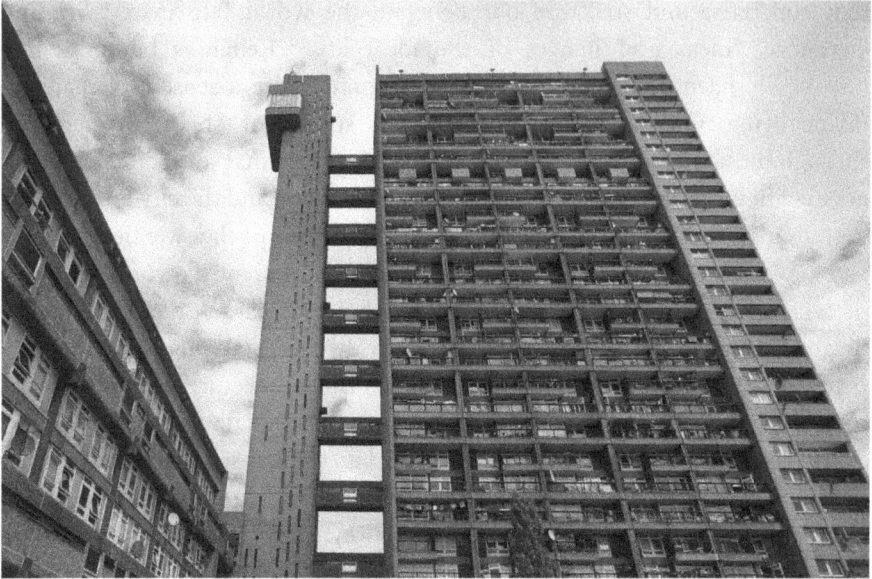

FIGURE 2.3: Brutalist architecture: Trellick Tower designed by Ernö Goldfinger. Getty Images.

united in their drive to distinguish themselves from the urban masses. Bourgeois conservatism, working-class fear and middle-class disgust combined with poor upkeep, spectacular fires and rotting concrete (Levy 2002) to ensure that the towering blocks scattered across the British urban skylines would be stigmatized for much of the century.

Across much of Europe and America, where the ascending dwellings were more commonly found on the urban periphery than in city centers, the stigmatization of mass housing structures was not as immediate. In mainland Europe and Scandinavia in particular, an initial alliance between property developers, the state, and forward-thinking middle-class urbanites that identified with the modernist aesthetics initially made mass housing popular with a cross-section of society (Hammarén 2010: 212; Wacquant 2007). However, it took little time for the pioneering tenants of these "machines for living" to latch on to popular criticism of master-planned modernism (Jacobs 1989). By the end of the century, sensibilities had thoroughly shifted, and the brutalist visual aesthetic, once associated with the bold and brave march of the rationally planned city, instead connoted alienation, delinquency, danger. In the United States, the failure of "the projects" intersected with the epidermalized nature of class ensured that the stigmatization of public housing also bore traces of racism. Furthermore, as with many aspects of twentieth-century American life, the racialized symbolism of public housing was globally exported and tinted perceptions of public housing around the globe, irrespective of the demographic make-up of the context in which it was embedded. French commentators spoke of the ghettoization of suburban France, despite the ethnic heterogeneity of its inhabitants (Wacquant 2007). British tabloid journalists put their notorious story-telling skills to work painting bold caricatures of the arrival of the deviant cultures from Harlem and the Bronx into the estates of inner-city Britain (Hall *et al.* 1978: 19)

SENSATIONAL MACHINES

While over the century a profusion of housing towers would take tenants closer to the stratosphere, the first inhabited structures to truly graze the clouds were spectacular edifices that grew out of the fertile commercial world of mid-century North America. Distinguishable from the colossi of housing by their opulent glass skins and even greater height, the tallest commercial buildings were so high that the average person strolling around downtown New York or Chicago simply couldn't see the top of them. Chicago's 1969 John Hancock Center stood at 100 stories high, while New York's Empire State Building (1931) stood at 102. Beneath them, pedestrians were left wandering roofless corridors with nothing for orientation other than reflections of themselves in glass-curtained lobbies. From inside the skyscraper, however, there was no such vertiginous alienation. From the inside, the new glass places of commerce afforded the powerful with the ability to see the city as they had long imagined angels to have done. Higher than any previous steeple, tower, or monument, the elevated perspective made it possible to see the organizing logic of the city's infrastructural skeleton: pedestrians moving in silent swarms along pulsating arteries, trains slithering between concrete blocks, strings of automobiles oozing along the raised asphalt belts that ran above and below the city.

As they appeared to those afforded with the angel-eye view of the sixtieth floor corner office, the rhythmic movements of masses were a testament to the success of the modern city's new god: the master planner. Most twentieth-century cities were subjected to some degree of infrastructural master planning and were partially subsumed to the "rational" calculations of metropolitan population density, mobility, profitability, and growth (Jacobs 1996: 426). The most infamous of all the century's master-planned projects were those undertaken in the United States by Robert Moses. Moses' vision was central to the redesign of the green spaces, housing, and even the coastlines of the modern

US. His notoriety, however, derives from the colossal new highways such as the Cross-Bronx Express Way which, between 1948 and 1972, ploughed through the old suburbs of New York in an attempt to connect the financial and "cultural" center of Manhattan to the new high-density suburbs.

Whether they were embraced or resisted, such gargantuan projects necessarily came with a maelstrom of new sights, sounds, sensations, and feelings. Which of these sensations the city dweller experienced, however, was necessarily contingent on their social location in the city. Moses' expressways were the physical manifestation of a growing symbiosis between the national economy and the internal combustion engine. As mass-produced consumables, cars were central to the advancement of capitalism. Fleets of cars and trucks and vans also allowed for faster modes of production, allowing greater access to human and material resources and expanding the city into its peri-urban belt. To urbanites, however, the automobile was more than a solution to equations of distance, time, and efficiency. For the first time in history, automobiles endowed humans with the experience of supernatural speed and mobility. As Filippo Marinetti waxed in the opening paragraphs of his "The Founding and Manifesto of Futurism" ([1909] 1972: 39–41), automotive speed offered a set of truly novel sensations that spilled over into a mix of excitement and fear. Rushing landscapes, growling motors, shuddering chassis, the weightiness of acceleration, and the metallic scent of engine oil and steel— all were integral to the "geometric and mechanical splendour" of the century (Marinetti [1919] 2002: 90).

To be sure, these were exciting and addictive sensations. Like their contemporary, the roller-coaster, a large part of their pleasure seemed derived from the sense of mortality they produced within the speeding body, the heart-pumping, skin-tingling effects of adrenaline being the body's response to impending doom. In distinction to the simulated sensations of the theme-park ride, however, the excitement of the speeding automobile derived from a very real proximity to death. By 1955, forty-seven years since the first mass-produced car rolled off production lines, the US Department of Health calculated that automobile deaths were the number one cause of mortality amongst men aged 20 to 29, with 421,460 "man years" lost each year (Norman 1962: 14). Such statistics, however, made little impact on the city dweller's hunger for sensational automotive transport in North America, or elsewhere. From the trundling early Fords and perfunctory Soviet motors, to the snorting "hot rods" of Los Angeles boy-racers, the sensations of speed, comfort, and personal encapsulation soon became second nature to city dwellers the world over.

Of course, those who could afford it might glide over the surface of the city in the hermetic sensory bubble of the automobile. By 1953, when the New York Transit Authority consolidated a number of earlier private lines, the vast majority of the century's New Yorkers—like Muscovites, Parisians, Berliners, Tokyoites, and Londoners before them—surfed daily through the city on public transit. Admittedly these commuters shared the vestibular experience of acceleration with their car-dwelling counterparts. The inner-ear is, however, where the similarities ended. The sights, sounds, and smells of public transport were entirely different. The "public" aspects proved particularly testing to urban sensibilities, with transit systems bringing strangers and their concomitant sensoria into unusual proximity with one another on a daily basis. Subjected to the tactile and olfactory reach of strangers, the social distinctions of the city were actively worked out on the move, with perceived epidermal and olfactory differences regulating the degrees, direction, and types of contact between commuters (Maines 1977). The development of subterranean transit also tested commuters' senses in new ways. Ushered into homogeneously tiled burrows, and spun around until they didn't know which way was up, the paucity of visual cues with which to orientate themselves turned commuters into urban moles, reliant on proprioceptive memories of the body's movement through space to navigate the daily commute. The resulting experience of the city above ground was also altered. The philosopher and architecture critic Brian Massumi (2002: 178–84), for instance, remarks on having mistakenly believed his east-facing office window in Montreal looked north—the result of daily dependence on subterranean transit.

Looking down from the zenith of high-rise structures revealed elements of the city's infrastructural scaffolding. However, it was when eyes turned upwards that they glimpsed the foundational grid out of which the late-modern city would emerge. By the end of the millennium, the ceiling above virtually every city was joined up by webs spun by rumbling engines floating from horizon to horizon. In the early days of aviation, the contrails joined the dots between the cities in neighboring countries, shoring up regional associations. As engine noise grew, the vapor trails lengthened to link up continents, from London and Paris to New York and Tokyo. Viewed from above, the contrails offered an ephemeral blueprint for the late century's networks of global control and power. At the immediate ends of each contrail grew new types of spaces that, on the interior, were increasingly disconnected from the *terroir* of the locales in which they were embedded—transitional spaces between nations and cities colored with a globally homogenized soundscape of announcements, bells, trundling suitcases, the smell of twenty-four hour breakfasts and duty-free

perfume, caricatured by Mark Augé (1995) as "non places." If on the interior
the sensorium of the airport was dislocated from its local setting, on the
exterior the sensoria of airports suffused their locale with the roar of jet
engines, a sound that vaporized the distinction between public and private.
Amongst the loudest of modernity's mechanized noises it was the turbines and
propellers of airplanes that pushed national governments into the development
of anti-noise regulation, to protect what Hillel Schwartz (2003) would refer to
as "the indefensible ear."

Of course, the ambient hum of airports was far from the only set of novel
sensations experienced by a newly airborne humanity. From Icarus to Peter
Pan and Da Vinci's doodles, literary history suggests that human beings have
long been haunted by dreams of flying. However, the sensational actualization
of this dream was entirely new to the century delivered of *homo volans*. Again,
Filippo Marinetti's futurist poetry paints a vivid portrait of these novel
sensations:

> Up high! Open Sky! Here I am resting
> On the air's elastic laws! Ah! Ah!
> I'm hanging straight over the town
> and its intimate chaos
> Of houses set out like obliging chairs! . . .
> I sway gently like a bright chandelier
> over the town square, table set
> with many steaming plates, cars,
> whose sparkling glasses pass
> electrically!
>
> Marinetti [1919] 2002: 43

That it is the Italian polemophile who writes the most vividly of the century's
new sensations, reminds us of the most profound way in which the sensations
of the century were shaped by aviation. It was Marinetti's fellow countryman
and pilot, Lieutenant Cavotti, who in 1911, cheered on by the Futurist poet,
dropped a grenade from his plane as he flew over the oasis of Tagiura outside
Tripoli (Lindqvist 2001: 76–9). As the first aerial bomber, Cavotti incarnated a
new relationship between cities and the skies above them. Cities were no longer
defensible fortresses, and citizens were no longer bystanders in international
warfare. From the excitement of children watching dog-fighting pilots draw
fluffy loops in the summer sky (Francis 2010; Murphy 2005), to the impending
doom signified by the howls of the "doodle bug" bomb or the roaring

tomahawk missile, the senses bore shocking witness to the technological evolution in the delivery of high explosives.

In the immediate aftermath of the Second World War, the streets of London were checkered with dusty piles of bricks and burnt timber. Absent buildings created new lines of sight between hitherto separated streets while remaining buildings bore fresh shrapnel wounds. By the end of the millennium, however, there were only the subtlest traces of such devastation—breaks in the vernacular rhythms of nineteenth-century terraces where new property developers and speculators "repressed the ancestry of violence" with new buildings of red brick and glass (Ferro in Kenzari 2011: 60). The same was true for many of the century's bombed cities: Taguira, Guernica, Dresden, Naples, Pyongyang, and Hanoi. In each location, the only real traces of bombardment were the sensational memories etched in the synapses of their citizens.

STREET SOUND

As the millennial tourists on the London Eye rise up above a glittering Thames to view the city, what they see before them is a remarkable landscape chiseled by the political, technological, and social tectonics of modernity. And, as is the habit of visitors to such attractions, they wait until they are at optimum height, lift a small camera to their eye, and take a picture of the view. It is no coincidence that the view was so photogenic. The twentieth century's favored mediums of photography and film both seemed to have an affinity with the city. As urbane city dwellers learnt to present their best side to the camera and to pout and pose, the cities of the twentieth century learnt to make very particular aspects of urban activity "visible" to the eye of the lens. Yet in fact, only a tiny percentage of modernity's legacy is discernible from within the sealed and controlled environment of the ferris wheel's glass carriages, and even less so within the mono-sensory frame of a photograph. The majority of changes that the twentieth century brought to the city, and to the sensibilities of city dwellers, are only discernible when passengers step out of the capsule and venture into the aromatic and sonorous clamor of the street.

If from on high the rhythmic circulation of vehicles around the modern city might have the appearance of a symphonic totality, the sensorium that the pedestrian walking beside a congested city street in the latter half of the twentieth century had to suffer bordered on cacophonous anarchy—an intense competition between mechanical and electrically-generated noises. These sounds only grew louder when the weighty infrastructure of the modernizing city underwent construction or refurbishment. As a young man growing up amidst the mid-century dust, floodlights, and jackhammers of Robert Moses' mid-century Cross Bronx Expressway, Marshall Berman (1982: 290–2) likens the master planner to the figure of "Moloch" in Allen Ginsberg's "Howl": "a sphinx of cement and aluminum [that] hacked open . . . skulls and ate up their brains and imagination, . . . whose buildings are judgement, . . . whose eyes are a thousand blind windows" (Ginsberg 1959: 9). For city dwellers in neighborhoods beneath the new expressways, the new infrastructure severely disrupted the relatively settled sensory rhythms of the street.

The century did not, however, start so noisily. As the nineteenth century closed, John Dunlop's invention of pneumatic rubber tires and the pioneering of new asphalt road surfaces offered city dwellers a potential reprieve from the growing clamor of clopping horse shoes and wheezing steam engines. At least they did when the inventor first attached the tire to his son's bicycle (Best 2004). Attached to the wheels of an automobile, however, any noise reduction gained through improved traction between asphalt and rubber was lost due to the drone of combustion engines and the infrastructural maintenance upon which they relied. As the century rolled along, automobiles also became platforms for a whole new set of amplified sounds, each effecting temporary changes in the urban ecologies through which they passed. Mobile subwoofers were the favored medium with which young men in cities everywhere—from the low riding crews of Mexico City and Los Angeles, to the window rattling Bangla-Boys of East London—territorialized their streets with a proud masculinity. In the case of East London, such sounds often shared sunny days with the saccharine chimes of nomadic ice-cream vans which shattered the masculine ideal and brought mothers and their daughters scuttling outside while turning even the toughest man-sons into ice-cream slurping boys. The soft chimes of ice-cream vans produced a sense of "safe" urban space by coloring the air with sugary childhood memories, while the subwoofers scented the streets with territorial pissing. There were other sounds, however, that colored the urban landscape with fear. Les Back observes that by the mid-1960s the burble of London's roads was increasingly disrupted by the terrifying wails of police sirens (Back 2007: 116–22). However, as Back notes: "[t]here is nothing inherent in the tones of the sirens themselves that produces this [fearful] effect." Toddlers, he reports, sometimes dance as rhythmic sirens hurtle past. Rather, the association with fear is an artifact of modern processes of socialization and "has a history which aligns the sound to a state of emergency and domestic threat" (Back 2007: 119). From warnings against Zeppelin bombers and the blitzes of the Second World War, to the sporadic red alerts and rehearsals of the Cold War, the mechanized cry came to signify threats to the individuals and communities in London as elsewhere. Attached to emergency vehicles, by the end of the century sirens would propagate a constant state of emergency to the city's streets; integral to what Back refers to as the development of the twenty-first century "phobocity."

Sirens, like the sound of the engines that shuttle them through the city, are what most twentieth-century city dwellers might have referred to as "unwanted sound," or rather, *noise*: the auditory equivalent of Mary Douglas' "dirt"— matter out of place (Douglas 2002). Like an unruly teenager who gradually turns the volume up on his stereo despite his neighbors' requests to turn it down, the unwanted noise of the modern city crept up year on year. Songbirds were compelled to sing at higher and higher pitches so as to pierce the cacophony (Slabbekoorn and Ripmeester 2008). No doubt the volume of human conversation rose also. Other sounds were totally vaporized by the mechanized sounds of the street. It was, for instance, still vaguely plausible that a child born in nineteenth-century East London might be able to hear the famous bells of St-Mary-Le-Bow's church a mile or two away, an "auditory marker" (Corbin 1998) that defined him as an official "cockney" (Ackroyd 2001: 61). By the end of the century, however, only those within 20 or 30 meters of the church, that by then was sandwiched between large office buildings, could hear it above the mechanical hum of passing motors and the shriek of sirens. For birds and humans alike, aural orientation and communication in cities would come to need new strategies.

SHIFTING WINDS

As the volume level of unwanted noise crept up around aurally adaptable urbanites, there were other changes taking place right under their noses. On days of better air quality, an inventory of a neighborhood's late century aroma-scape—a spatial and temporal thumbprint—offered an index of local lifestyles and demography. On a road such as North East London's Kingsland Road, for instance, the nose would encounter the doughy, smoky spices of the jerk chicken bagel joint, the charred meat of the ocakbasi grill, the compound of bleach, beer, nicotine, whisky, and urine that lingered in the doors of pubs, the caffeinated clouds that billowed out of coffee shops, the nutty tang of fresh chips sprinkled with vinegar, the seductive meaty sweetness of a popular burger outlet, the wisps of star anise and garlic that crept out of a dim sum restaurant, and the sweet turpentine smell of mangoes and melons offered at a fruit stall. Thought about objectively, the smells offer tangible evidence of the increasingly cosmopolitan life of an inner-city location. In such a picture, the street appears as a laboratory for the mutation of cultural sediments and the production of new flavors born of the increasingly transnational reach of the modern city and its inhabitants. Yet as much as the nose seems well suited to objectively index the cosmopolitan material culture of the modern street, for the twentieth-century city dweller, the experience of smells was never objective. Rather, the nose offered a direct passage to reservoirs of subjective and culturally derived meaning.

This enduring nuance of the human sense of smell—that is, the tendency to load particular smells with culturally, biographically, and politically contingent meanings—played out in many different ways in the twentieth-century city. As the work of Nadia Serematakis (1994) and David Sutton (2001) demonstrates, smell and taste were both incredibly important for modernity's many migrants, many of whom tried to rekindle a sense of home through seeking out smells or flavors from past and distant moments. Even the most diluted hints of a biscuit, a fruit, a herb, an aftershave, a spice—the faintest embers of a past existence—enabled the dislocated body to rekindle home in the midst of what was often an inhospitable environment. The ability of smells to attract cultural meaning, however, also left aroma amenable to the highly negative cultural connotations that emerged through the power struggles between the various factions brought together by the modern metropolis. Thus, while the aromas of difference might not be offensive themselves, as Constance Classen (1992: 134) writes, "the odour of the other ... often serves as a scapegoat for certain antipathies toward the other for whom ... an animosity [is felt] for unrelated reasons."

In British urban centers, for instance, smells were enmeshed in the simmering antipathy between the upper, middle, and working classes. As George Orwell (1958: 128) outlines in *The Road to Wigan Pier*, reflecting on the prejudices ingrained in him by his upper middle-class background: "You thought of those nests and layers of greasy rags below, and, under all, the unwashed body, brown all over (that was how I used to imagine it), with its strong, bacon-like reek ... The smell of their sweat, the very texture of their skins, were mysteriously different from yours." The landscape of smoky pubs and oil-coated kitchens clearly marked the bodies of the laboring classes and provided a tableau of sensoria against which the hegemonic sensibility of the upper and middle classes was able to define itself. This was nothing new to the British culture. For centuries prior to the modern city, the spatialized division of labor was marked by smell. London, like many other British and Northern European cities, was designed around the principle that the poorest should be located in the east—that is, downwind from the financial district and residential quarters of the wealthy. With the east side of the city already historically the favorite for tanneries, cemeteries, plague burial pits, pig farms, the docks, and their workers, the spatialized division of labor in the city simply became more pronounced amidst the furnaces of industrializing England.

With such a distinctive olfactory signature, myths and anxieties about the laboring classes were readily attached to the material space in which they lived, leaving wealthier city dwellers living in perpetual fear of the day that the winds would shift. Even as industry drifted elsewhere and the sewers were paved over and submerged, the residual patterns of segregated habitation ensured that there were still plenty of odors that were taken as signifiers of poverty. However, instead of being the literally dirty stench of toxins and sewage, the signifiers shifted to become the food smells and odors of working-class domestic life itself. Of course, such sensoria were in no respect as dangerous to life as the erstwhile smog. Yet the persistence of the class structure ensured that they were treated with equal disgust. Moreover, as much as the middle classes upheld a regime of distaste with which to identify and stigmatize working-class people and space, they also continued to develop their own regime of taste; a concoction of odors and flavors with which they colonized urban space. It is telling, for instance, that Sharon Zukin referred to the 1980s regeneration of Bryant Park in Manhattan as "gentrification by cappuccino" (Zukin 2010: 247).

Appealing to the noses of the upper middle classes has in fact been integral to the "success" of many gentrifying regeneration projects. Nowhere was this more obvious than in the area surrounding Spitalfields Market in East London. A busy wholesale fruit and vegetable market since the seventeenth century, the area's evening aromascape was, for much of the twentieth century, characterized by the ethylene smell of ripe bananas, the earthy mud of potatoes, and the spiky scent of coriander, smells that drew in hungry vagrants who gathered around burning oil drums outside the market in the evenings. In 1989, the wholesale market, which sat very close to the expanding financial district, was closed down and relocated to the outskirts (see Jacobs 1996). By the end of the millennium the market was well on its way to being re-odorized in tune with the British bourgeoisie's attachments to the aromatic boulangeries and fromageries of their French counterparts. Successfully re-scented, the old scavengers' playground would, in coming years, host some of the most expensive real estate in Europe. As Monica Degen has demonstrated, deliberately intervening in, and "refining," the sensorium of urban space was integral to the transformation of erstwhile industrial urban landscapes, from Baltimore, through New York to Berlin, Barcelona and Manchester (Degen 2008). In each instance, the initiatives were part of a combined effort by planners, politicians, and businessmen to make the urban landscape more

economically profitable amidst the shift towards post-industrial economies. In
each instance the sensory redesign was intended to create an ambience that
would draw in new types of people. At the same time, however, such activity
also fueled new forms of social and spatial exclusion from those spaces (Degen
2008: 133–61). Today, in the aforementioned Spitalfields Market, a beggar
that approaches the young couples breakfasting alfresco under the tarpaulin of
the new patisserie is not able to offer a "good morning" before being forcefully
moved on by the area's new private security force.

Without a doubt, the class antagonisms of the twentieth-century city were
partly anchored in the nostrils and tastebuds of city dwellers, and this in turn
had an impact on the sensory ambiences of urban space and the meanings
given to it. In Europe and North America, however, the recent history of urban
smell, taste, and tactility is also one of racist and xenophobic tension. That
these aspects of urban experience should be so routinely embroiled in
xenophobia might not be obvious at first. As Les Back points out, race, and
racism especially, have tended to "operate within ocular grammars of
difference" (2007: 119). However, the optical tonality of skin has long
interacted with the ways in which the other senses detected difference and the
meanings ascribed to it (see Smith 2006). "I just didn't fancy going in there if
you know what I mean. I just thought it stank" says a 93-year-old Londoner,
winking conspiratorially as he recalls his youthful anxiety around the smell of
garlic emanating from one of London's early Italian bistros. Such sentiments
are echoed in complaints surrounding the aromatic "cultural quarters" such
the world's many China Towns (Adamson *et al.* 2009: 32, 39), or white
working-class anxieties about the growth of East London's Bangla Town. They
are also analogous to earlier Londoners' anxiety about the Sephardic practice
of deep-frying fish in batter, or the wide assortment of minorities accused of
stinking of onions over the centuries. It was partly through the meaning
ascribed to such fragrances by twentieth-century xenophobes, that entire
neighborhoods became coded as utterly Other, no-go areas—faint spices and
novel odors on the breeze threatening the body of the "indigenous" urbanite
and the culture that lived through her. Not least of the consequences of the
olfactory stigma attached to ethnicized urban space was the emergence of an
intense ambivalence amongst a myriad of new arrivals to the twentieth-century
city about the odor of their habitus (see Manalansan 2006: 41–52); a painful
irony given diasporas' dependence on the aromatic kernels around which they
attempted to rekindle a sense of home.

While the recent history of the city is one punctuated with racist violence, it
remains remarkable how many times over the course of the century the smells

and flavors that were initially identified by the nose as different and laden with pernicious myth and exotic fetish, eventually osmosed into the everyday sensory rhythms of the majority of the city's residents. The millions of curries, lasagnas, chicken kievs, chow-meins, and salt beef sandwiches consumed in London alone towards the end of the century were evidence of evolution in a very local form of multiculture. Even more significant than the way modern city dwellers grew accustomed to new flavors that osmosed from their neighbors' kitchen was the extent to which different essences mixed and merged into new local dishes. The jerk chicken bagel, which first appeared in parts of London at some point near the end of the 1980s, is particularly indicative of the occasional culinary creolization that took place between the various migrant communities upon whose cheap labor the modern city was built. Like the Franco Sephardic fusion food the British came to call fish 'n' chips, or the legendary local innovation of the chicken tikka masala, jerk chicken bagels would, by the turn of the millennium, be readily incorporated into the city's vernacular culture. Such morsels demonstrate that the aroma-scape of the modern inner-city street, especially in London's poorer areas, was one of continual "multicultural drift," which Hall and Back (2009) define as a gradual change that takes place within the sensibilities of urban citizens as a consequence of the various migratory waves that lapped at the shores of the city. While this combination of sensoria is that of a multiculture peculiar to a given location and moment in London, analogous developments could be heard, tasted, and smelt across the century's interconnected cities. Consider early twentieth-century Tokyo where the new dishes, pork and chicken tonkatsu *karē*, combined the powdered curry spice mixes favored by the British merchant navy with the old Portuguese traders' practice of frying in breadcrumbs. The result was a new dish for Tokyoites visiting new Western themed restaurants (Robertson 2005: 421), and which, ironically, by the late twentieth century, became a popular dish through Europeans and North Americans seeking a taste of Japan. Or consider, for that matter, millennial Glasgow where local dishes such as the haggis pakora combine the local taste for offal and deep-fried food with Asian batter mixes and spice to produce a set of flavors and textures that reflect the increasingly transcultural history of the previous century.

MECHANIZED ENCHANTMENT

The delectable flavors and scents of the internationalizing urban street were far from the only novel odors that appeared on the increasingly limpid air of the century's avenues. Other revolutions were also taking place within the nostrils of urbanites. By the end of the nineteenth century, perfumers had amassed large repertoires of aromatic compounds and were well versed in creating elegant and artistic infusions of rose, violet, ylang ylang, and jasmine, as well as dab hands in the application of an assortment of musks, extracted from the dried internal organs of rats, large cats, and rare deer. Most of their creations were, however, incredibly exclusive owing to the expense of procuring highly concentrated amounts of rare ingredients. Exclusiveness, however, started to dissipate when, in 1881 a chemist called Paul Parquet procured a large amount of "a freshly minted synthetic ingredient called coumarin" (Turin 2006: 26–8). While the compound was previously available in natural form, "to have it pure and cheap, allowed him to use a big dose and to get a different effect altogether" (27).

Coumarin was only one chemical compound to be synthesized and made available to mass production. In the wake of the advances made by the likes of Rutherford, Bohr, and Curie in the field of chemistry, a cascade of compounds oozed out of the vats and cauldrons of the century's industrial chemists. These chemicals had a variety of uses and many had a profound impact on modern life. They provided the vivid bases of new paint pigments, enhanced crop yields, and allowed for the production of chemical weapons. Many more of these compounds comprised the faceless muscones, aldehydes, and turpines binding the jasmine rose and sandalwood notes of 1921's Chanel No. 5—or the proto-metrosexual cedar-wood, vanilla, cinnamon, and citrus notes of 1937's Old Spice.

Throughout the twentieth century, a shifting kaleidoscope of synthesized fragrances served as the key signs and signals within the period's increasingly

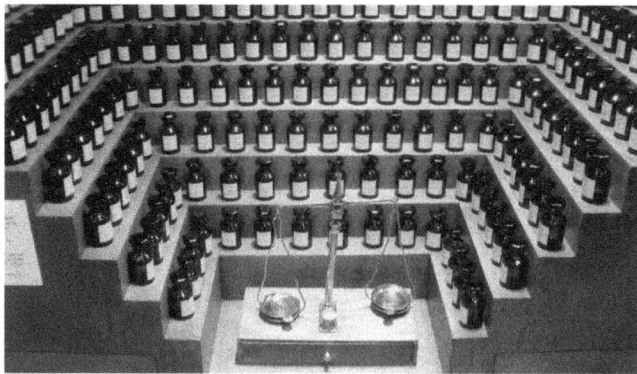

FIGURE 2.4: "Perfume organ," Fragonard Perfume Museum, Paris. Photograph by Nico Paix. Public domain.

commodified rituals of courtship. To hijack Walter Benjamin's famous thesis, on the work of art in the age of mechanical reproduction, the evolution of chemical science allowed for the synthesis and mass reproduction of complex compounds, allowing them to be consistently reproduced and delivered to the masses, robbing the original works of olfactory art of their magical "aura" (Benjamin 1969: 211–45). However, Michael Taussig argues, it would be a misreading to take Benjamin's account of mass produced art's loss of aura as an account of the triumph of capitalism's cold rationality over the "magic" of the pre-modern sensibility (1993: 24–30). As much as it might seem that the landscape of the modern city alienated the individual from her senses and mystical pre-modern sensibility, Benjamin also felt the mechanization and commodification of sensation was part of a radical reawakening of sensuousness. Modernity was the era in which, Benjamin writes, blasé urbanites "whom nothing moves or touches any longer, are taught to cry again in film" (Benjamin 1986: 86) and where "science and art coalesce to create a defetishizing/re-enchanting modernist magical technology of embodied knowing" (Taussig 1993: 24).

NOCTURNAL SENSATIONS

Nowhere was this retooling of urban sensibilities more pronounced than in the night-time of the modern city. It was when the sun had set that the most revolutionary profusion of new sensations emerged. As Craig Kolofsky (2011) records, by the end of the nineteenth century the colonization of the night-time was already well underway, with lighting technology progressing swiftly from the gloom of gas lamps through the white light of arc lamps to the warm candescence of light bulbs. By the start of the twentieth century, electrical infrastructure around the world's metropoles was quickly developing, fully illuminating the sides of the cities that faced away from the sun. Many cities would only again know darkness in the blackouts of war. Everywhere else, the night constituted a newly colonized land open for both labor and leisure (Kolofsky 2011: 5).

Electrical illumination itself quickly developed into a spectacular art form; nowhere more spectacularly than in the various applications of another by-product of industrial alchemy—Andre Claude's (1935) neon bulb. From the Las Vegas strip and Times Square, through London's Piccadilly Circus and Hamburg's Reeper Bahn, to Shibuya Crossing in Tokyo, the cool blue backdrop of the night-time was lit up with a crackling kaleidoscope of invitations to consume burgers, ribs, pizzas, popcorn, pop icons, musical sensations, dance troupes, films and, of course, sex. Such illuminations, Benjamin contended, were powerful not for "what the moving red neon sign says—but [for] the fiery pool reflecting it in the asphalt" (Benjamin 1969: 86). The city dwellers' seduction by the warm light on sweaty tarmac was just one example of what Benjamin saw as a typically modern reawakening, and transmogrification, of the senses through a sensuous relationship with the mechanized nature of modernity. This re-enchantment of the senses at once accounted for the new urban citizenry's underlying infatuation with speed and destruction, but also its literal worship of film stars and the ascription of magical powers to the newly commodified sensations of popular music and fashion.

The shift in city dwellers' obsessions and fantasies marked profound religious transformations taking place across the urban night, where the vestigial trusses of piety were shaken off with an assortment of Charlestons, hoochie-koochies, jitter bugs, stomps, shimmy-shams, shakes, electric slides, and twists. The perceived profanity of these new forms of liberated body movement was particularly pronounced across Europe and America due to the fact that, from jazz through rock and roll, to punk and hip-hop, popular dances and concomitant youth cultures emerged from an (occasionally physical) exchange between the hitherto segregated descendants of "black" slaves, and "white" Europeans. The "syncopated synergy" (Ware and Back 2002: 169–96) of twentieth-century urban culture was often in stark contrast to the strict epidermalized tactile protocols of the eighteenth and nineteenth centuries (Jordan in Malnig 2009: 28; Smith 2006). As such there was constant effort on the part of conservative social reformers to prohibit the nightly resurrection of Satan in the dance hall (Girodano 2008). Such efforts, however, were often to little avail. As each decade passed on, the increasingly leisurely lives of modern urban youth were filled with the exchanges of muscle memories and movement systems. Such exchanges would not, however, have happened were it not for the fact that the twentieth century saw the city increasingly filled with a sonorous polyphony of voices and melodies, amplified by the new technologies of sound reproduction. From 1920s electric gramophones and the transistor radios of the 1950s to the cassette decks popularized in the 1970s and CD players from the 1990s, technology allowed for the hi-fidelity sound tracking of public and private spaces throughout the city. The popularity and profitability of the "light" music played on such devices led a scornful Theodor Adorno to cite Aldous Huxley asking, "who, in a place of amusement, is really being amused?" (2002: 288). The reproduction of the public's favorite sounds certainly enabled profit to be channeled back to the archetypal capitalists who sat atop increasingly centralized and powerful record companies. But the electronic machinery of sound recording and reproduction, along with the sounds that they relayed, must also be credited with getting people's feet tapping in ways that freed them from the predictable rhythms of the Old World. Not only did mass-produced music help shake off the vestiges of the past, it also made erstwhile urban culture less local, as bass lines, lyrics, licks, and riffs circulated between and within cities, plugging urbanites into the pulses of elsewhere and broadening the horizons that urban life threatened to eat up.

CONCLUSION

To be sure, there were few better ways of capturing the spectacular economic growth and ambition of the twentieth-century city than taking a ride in the London Eye and photographing the skyline. However, a great many more legacies of modernity were also discernible within city dwellers' everyday lives. As urban economies grew across the twentieth century, cities took their citizens both closer to the clouds and deeper underground than they'd ever been. Urbanites hurtled through space, some even through the sky, at the fastest speeds humanity had ever experienced. Illuminated nights were full of a rainbow of new sounds, scents, and shuffles. At a glance the city of the twentieth century was filled with many of the most exciting and pleasurable experiences that humanity had ever known. But the sensations of the city also endowed citizens with a growing sense of alienation and dislocation, filled them with the terror of war, the fear of the other and often left them sleepless and irritable. An oscillation between horror and ecstasy, the history of the twentieth-century city is one of material, political, and social edifices constantly changing through their circuitous relationships with city dwellers' sensory experiences. Some of these new sensations, such as those that accompanied modern warfare, were shocking and horrific. Others, such as the bombastic spectacle of music, lasers, and fireworks that illuminated the London Eye on the eve of the millennium, induced delight. A great many more of the new century's sensations were less obvious and emerged somewhere within an urban matrix of olfactory, culinary, kinesthetic, and tactile crossroads: the local high street, the market, the school, the pub, the club, the inside of a car, the bedroom. All of these locations were wellsprings of multisensory drift, sites where the sensibilities of city dwellers and the sensoria that fill their lives changed gradually, under the aegis of repetition and habit. Such drift, however, does not merely passively reflect the colossal technological, political, social, and economic history of the twentieth-century city. The ways in which urbanites "made sense" of their environment fed back into the city and impacted on its physical, social, and economic topography. As the giant ferris wheel turned with the millennium, none of this was due to change. The senses of city dwellers would in the future be taken to new heights, experience new horrors, and be bombarded with an increasingly dense battery of sights and sounds. But for the most part, all of the changes that would unfold in the early twenty-first century were elaborations of those that appeared amidst the breathtaking sensuousity of the urban century before.

CHAPTER THREE

The Senses in the Marketplace: Commercial Aesthetics for a Suburban Age

ADAM MACK

The Walt Disney Company keeps a light burning in the window of the apartment that its founder maintained on Main Street, USA, the gateway to his world-famous theme park on the outskirts of Los Angeles, California. The "antique-style lamp" reflects well Disney's desire that his guests begin their adventure with what the company advertises as a stroll through the "quintessential small town of middle America in the early 1900s" (Walt Disney Company 2012). In 2011, visitors spent around $79–85 for one-day passes to Disneyland, passing through the restaurants and shops of Main Street before they made their way to the park's action-packed rides (Walt Disney Company 2011). Before they enjoyed the wind in their hair on "Dumbo the Flying Elephant," or listened to dozens of animatronic children intone "It's a Small World," they encountered sensory information designed to lift the burdens of modern life, even as they enjoyed the hospitality of the world's largest media conglomerate, as measured by revenue.

As guests wander Main Street, Disney advertising explains, "sounds from the past fill the air" including "train whistles and barbershop quartet tunes [as well as] the *clop-clop* of hooves as horses draw colorful street cars down the road." The sight of the horse cars complements the gas street lamps to further the "nostalgic ambiance" of the vintage architecture. Lest guests skip breakfast to beat the crowds, the "scent of freshly baked goods and other tempting aromas waft from the windows" of eateries like the Plaza Inn, where hungry park-goers can dine with Minnie Mouse and friends in the once-daily "character breakfast." For adults who want to get the kids to the rides straightaway, "rich coffees" help them through the morning, while "sugary ice cream cones" provide a boost in the afternoon. When day's end arrives, as they make their way to the expansive parking lot, Main Street, USA, again hits their senses. Stomachs full from ice cream and other treats, Disney tempts park-goers at the "old-time Victorian general store," one of the many shops offering bright, plush, and soniferous merchandise so that they can "take home a piece of the magic" (Walt Disney Company 2012).

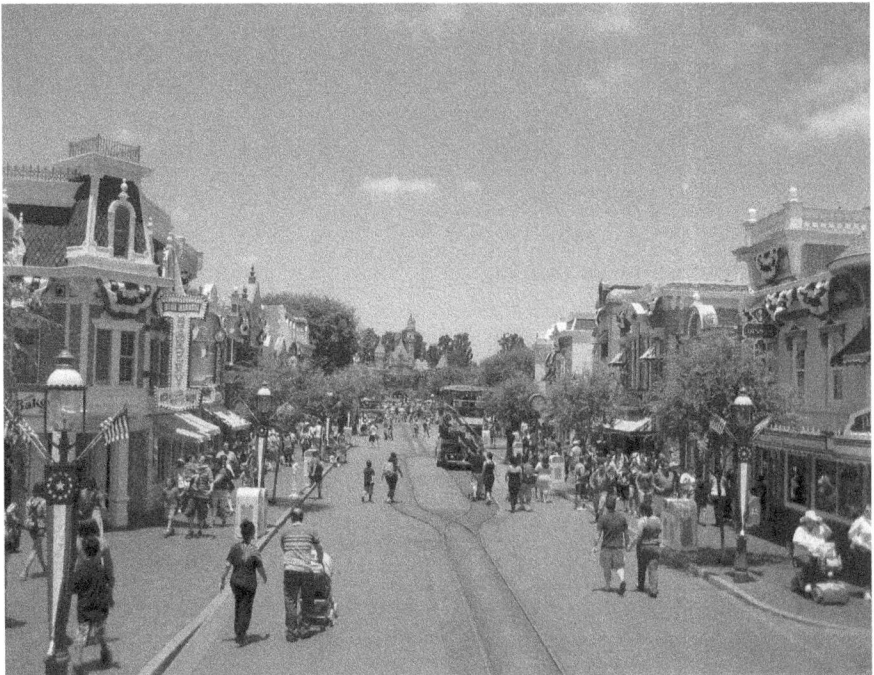

FIGURE 3.1: Main Street, USA at Disneyland, California. Photograph by Alfred A. Si. Public domain.

One irony of the Disney Company's effort to bathe Main Street, USA in sensory information synonymous with an idyllic past of small towns is that sophisticated computer technology orchestrates the entire show. A correspondent from *Wired* magazine, a technology monthly, discovered as much when he toured the backstage areas of Florida's Disneyworld, twin to the Los Angeles park, located outside Orlando (Kirsner 1998). Here Main Street represented merely one corner of the "most sophisticated virtual world ever created," far more convincing than even the most advanced video games. "Disney has the kind of control over visitors' experiences—what they see, smell, hear, and feel— that videogame builders can only dream of," wrote the amazed reporter. Even the simple flowerbeds that treat guests' eyes and noses rely on a computerized irrigation network hooked into the park's weather monitoring system— ominously named "One Control Center"—that records temperature, wind, and rain conditions to measure watering levels. One Control Center also relays minute-by-minute weather conditions so that park managers know when to close outdoor rides, and when they need to quicken the pace of Main Street's twice-daily parades to avoid rain. Should the foot traffic on Main Street drown out the sounds of the piped-in muzak, acoustical engineers are there to "subtly increase the sound" as the park fills with people over the course of the day (Kirsner 1998). Main Street's sensory environment seduces visitors precisely because it offers a predictable, secure, and sanitized setting for family play. Every year millions of people from around the world stroll Disney's Main Street in parks in the USA, Europe, and Asia. Only in Japan has Disney altered the formula (Yoshimi 2001). In Tokyo Disneyland (the company's first overseas park, opened in 1983) visitors enter through a "World Bazaar" corridor that, ironically enough, illustrates the global reach of US consumer culture by featuring the same nostalgic model of the American small town found in the parks in California and Florida. The whole operation delivers a hefty profit, too. In 2000, Disney's theme park division boasted earnings greater than its movie studio, generating more than 40 percent ($1.5 billion) of the company's operating profit (Hirsch 2000).

Historians have long documented the central role that Walt Disney and his theme parks played in the rise of modern American consumer culture. Steven Watts, in an illuminating analysis of Walt Disney's films, argued that the creator of Mickey Mouse might be "the most influential American of the twentieth century" (Watts 1995: 84). Similarly, the urban historian Eric Avila gives Disneyland title as "the most significant landmark in American cultural history" (Avila 2004: xv). Business theorists have added to the praise, crediting Walt Disney as the chief forerunner to the twenty-first-century marketing wizards who "stage" memorable experiences for consumers. They see Disneyland as the original institution in what they call the modern "experience economy" because the theme park goes beyond simple amusements to place customers in "a living, immersive cartoon world" (Pine and Gilmore 2011: 3–4). My introductory discussion of Main Street, USA, expands on those judgments by highlighting how Disneyland embodies another crucial development in the history of the modern marketplace: the increasingly sophisticated and centralized effort to engage all five of the senses to sell goods and services in a suburban context.

The anthropologist David Howes has suggested that the effort to appeal to the five senses grew ever more intense over the course of the twentieth century. The "sensual logic of late capitalism," he writes, has pushed merchants to "engage as many senses as possible in its drive for product differentiation and the distraction/seduction of the consumer" (Howes 2005b: 288). This chapter takes up Howes' insight by exploring the effort to seduce shoppers' eyes, ears, noses, tongues, and skin in the context of the post-1920s USA, the nation that, in the words of the historian Victoria de Grazia, set the "global norms for a market-driven consumer modernity" in the second half of the twentieth century (2005: 5). The thematic emphasis is the displacement of the industrial city by the suburbs as the center of commercial gravity, with particular focus on the mass retailing and popular amusements industries as spearheads in the development of a commercial aesthetic that recast the sensory hallmarks of urban consumption for the suburban age. Regional shopping centers and malls, supermarkets, and theme parks changed marketplace aesthetics by delivering the sensual thrills of urban consumption in a sensory context that simultaneously evoked the social homogeneity, predictability, and security unique to the suburban ideal. Their operators continued the longstanding focus on women as key customers, but in ways that valorized the middle-class, suburban family as the nation's key economic unit. As merchants created a new sensory landscape that focused on the suburban family, the marketplace itself increasingly revolved around what Avila aptly terms the "privatized, public experiences" endemic to late twentieth-century consumption in the USA and beyond. Merchants delivered pleasure, family fun, and security by domesticating the marketplace; that is, by extending the suburban home into semi-public, commercial spaces to undergird a series of conservative cultural values (Avila 2004: 213).

DECENTRALIZATION AND DEPRESSION

Although business observers in the 1920s saw evidence that the marketplace of the future would be outside industrial cities like Chicago and New York, the men and women who chased the sensory thrills synonymous with the decade's consumer culture found them chiefly in urban areas. New York's Coney Island is a case in point. Its enclosed amusement parks continued to dominate the leisure industry decades after their construction around the turn of the twentieth century. Thousands of New Yorkers flocked to the seaside resort to escape the confines of the city proper and to enjoy the pleasures of food and drink, racy shows, and mechanical rides in the decade before the Great Depression. Coney Island's attractions encouraged consumers to thrill in the sensory dissonance that served as a funhouse mirror of the city streets. "Coney Island and its generation of cultural institutions," Avila reminds us, "invited audiences to revel in the dissonance, vulgarity, and exuberance of urban industrial culture" (Avila 2004: 112–13). Unlike later theme parks of the Disney variety, Coney Island served as a meeting ground for pleasure seekers of a wide range of economic, ethnic, and national backgrounds. Inside, park-goers abandoned restraint for an experience that transformed the jarring physical hallmarks of modern urban life, including socially heterogeneous public spaces, into pleasurable thrills (Sally 2006).

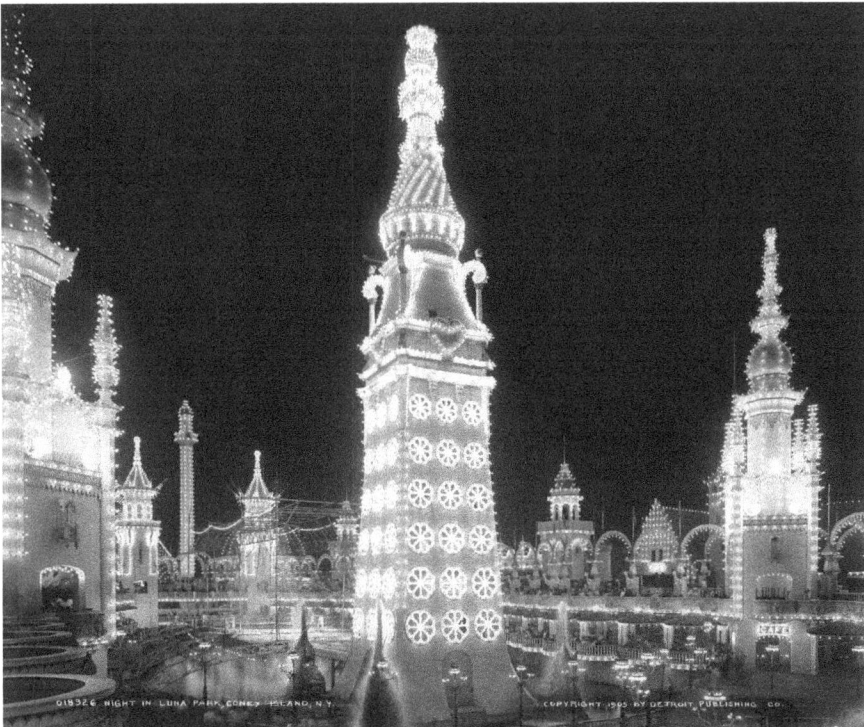

FIGURE 3.2: Luna Park, Coney Island, at night. Public domain.

Visiting Coney Island meant negotiating an overwhelming amount of sensory information designed to generate spending. Spectacular visual displays, composed of the same dazzling electric lights that gave Broadway its title as the "Great White Way," flattered visitors' sense of sight even before they smelled the beer and peanuts. Luna Park, based on the "Trip to the Moon" exhibit at the 1901 Pan-American Exposition, offered some of the most impressive vistas. Thousands of electrical bulbs covered its rides and towers to create a fantasyland of illumination, especially striking after dark (see Figure 3.2). Designers reconfigured the display every season to parallel the dynamic landscape of the Moon and to evoke the themes of novelty, abundance, and technological progress that animated urban consumer culture. The park's ever-changing electric lighting, the performance theorist Lynn Sally argues, presented visitors with a visual landscape that mirrored the city itself, inviting them to imagine urban transformations as exciting and pleasurable (Sally 2006: 299).

At the same time, Coney Island went beyond visual spectacle to transform the nature of spectacle itself into an experience that electrified all the senses. Sally argues that the seaside resort summoned visitors to cast off Victorian invocations of sensorial restraint, "to recognize, to revel in, and to celebrate themselves as sensuous beings" (Sally 2006: 305). The mechanical rides delivered not-so-subtle sexual thrills as they forced screams of delight and threw together men and women (often strangers) in ways that transgressed the norms of modesty in public spaces. Even more, the mechanical rides gave factory workers, who spent their days executing highly repetitive and monotonous tasks, a chance to reconnect with their senses. Sites of consumption like Coney Island thus provided the intense forms of kinetic experience that promised to ease what critics like Karl Marx saw as one of the cruelest tolls of industrial labor: the sensory alienation that reduced workers to actors with the most basic sensory desires (Howes 2005b). Mechanical rides, Sally argues, "brilliantly invoked the very markers of industrial capitalism—mechanization, standardization, the giving of the body to the machine—while inverting the power structure inherent in such a system to reconfigure pleasure seekers' experience of both industrialization and leisure" (Sally 2006: 302). In this way, the rides delivered a rush to the senses that turned the deadening toll of the industrial machine back on itself.

Sally proposes that the appeal of the cacophonous crowds and rides helps explain the failure of one of Coney Island's parks, Dreamland, built as it was to provide the type of respectable and restrained amusements more like the ones marketed later in the century by Disney. "While thrill seekers may have wanted a respite from the chaos of the metropolis," she suggests, "they may

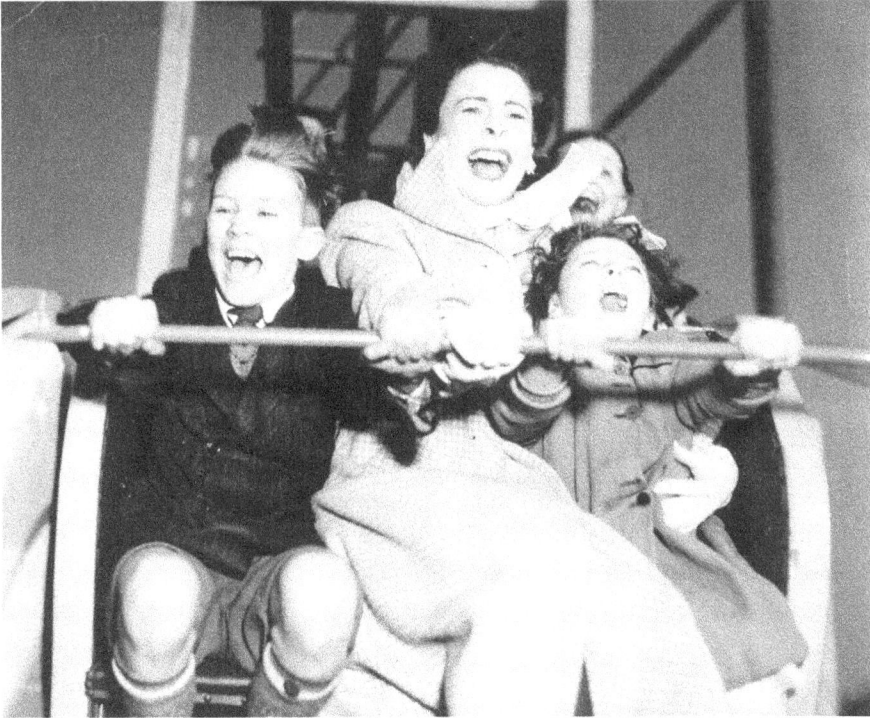

FIGURE 3.3: A family enjoying the thrill of a switchback ride. Photograph by Keystone. Hulton Archive/Getty Images.

not quite have been looking for the clean, orderly, suburban getaway that Dreamland promised" (Sally 2006: 300). A devastating fire in the second decade of the twentieth century sealed Dreamland's fate, but not before its rivals, Steeplechase Park and Luna Park, proved the appeal of amusement parks that recast the cacophonous sounds of the city street and the mechanical keynotes of the factory into a sensory landscape that a wide range of consumers engaged with as a form of entertainment and fun (Sally 2006).

Within the industrial city itself, a series of new marketplace institutions emerged that appealed to the senses to celebrate technology's quiet efficiency as well. The third decade of the twentieth century witnessed an explosion of chain stores in the USA, as urban and suburban neighborhoods became dotted with shops operated by firms like The Great Atlantic and Pacific Tea Company (A&P). Chain stores first emerged in the late nineteenth century, but it was not until the 1920s that they became a truly national phenomenon, numbering as many as 37,000 individual units by the end of the decade. A&P, the leading grocery chain, operated more than 15,000 of the small outlets (Lichtenstein 2009: 18). Unlike the individually owned and operated neighborhood groceries, A&P practiced the new "scientific retailing" in which distant, corporate management mandated uniformly designed stores and cash-and-carry sales. Self-service, the most significant innovation in mass retailing in the nineteenth century, expanded in the twentieth century into the chain groceries. First introduced in the US South by Piggy Wiggly stores in the 1910s, self-service quickly spread to other chains to further transform the shops into what the inventor Thomas Edison termed the "machines for distribution" that generated profits by moving mass volumes of merchandise at a low markup (Strasser 1989: 203; Tedlow 1990).

Self-service fundamentally changed the sensory landscape of mass retailing because it silenced the aural salesmanship that had long shaped the relationships between grocers and their customers (Bowlby 2001). Romantic memorials to the old-fashioned grocery store celebrate the intimate relationships between buyers and sellers, but they ignore the economic and social realities that often made those relationships sources of tension and anxiety. When grocers queried customers about outstanding credit balances, pushed alternative goods or brands, or haggled over pricing, they nettled shoppers' ears and strained personal relationships. By contrast, self-service shops offered no credit, allowed customers to select their own brands from open shelves, and used fixed prices—the same for every customer. Those policies worked because they gave shoppers, chiefly women, a refreshingly impersonal relationship with grocers. Self-service no doubt attracted customers with the economic benefits of low prices, but the new format also strengthened shoppers' sense of agency by allowing for the direct, hands-on inspection of merchandise (Classen 2012; Deutsch 2002). In self-service stores, the silent lure of the package hushed the clerk's hard sell.

Food manufacturers responded by designing packaging that caught consumers' eyes. Self-service thus changed the visual landscape of the grocery market, as shelves featured stacks of cans, jars, and boxes emblazoned with a national brand name as well as appetizing pictures of the contents. Food manufacturers filled the pages of grocery trade journals with advertisements promising that their eye-catching packaging could make the silent sell by symbolically reaching out and grabbing consumers' attention. Chains like Piggy Wiggly ensured that customers gave each and every shelf a glance by designing their shop floors in a linear, "assembly line" fashion, complete with turnstiles at the points of entrance and egress (Tolbert 2009). The transformation of the store itself into a sales vehicle encouraged shoppers to survey the shop floor more closely than ever before, but the other, non-visual senses were also taken into account. The main trade journal for independent grocers used its pages, for example, to demand that stores smelled of the retailing efficiency popularized by the chain companies. "It would seem that in a food store," *Progressive Grocer* suggested, the "governing sense of smell would be of greatest importance." It urged readers to eliminate "S.O." (store odor) because it suggested a lack of sanitation as well as crude, backward business practices. "Clean, fresh smelling stores attract better, more profitable trade" of the type that frequented the chains like A&P, it counseled (Mack 2010: 827–8). Here the trade journal described how the pleasing smell of the store itself—even the sterile nose of cleanliness—took on greater significance, just as new packaging sealed off growing numbers of products from shoppers' senses of smell and touch.

If self-service wrought major changes in grocery stores by making shopping more efficient and impersonal, the grand department stores accelerated their strategy of treating the eye with urban "palaces of consumption" in the decade before the Great Depression. New York's Macy's added multiple stories to its downtown store in 1922, doubling its square footage to 1.5 million. By the early 1930s, as Macy's gained control of an entire city block, it boasted the largest department store in the world (Leach 1993: 280–1). At the same time, however, a minority of department stores followed the lead of the chains by opening multiple, smaller ("branch") stores outside the central city. Chicago's Marshall Field's set up new outlets in the suburban communities of Evanston, Lake View, and Oak Park to attract the growing population of automobile owners who preferred shopping close to home over the commute to the downtown retailing district. The success of the experimental branch stores—combined with the plummeting downtown real estate values and sales receipts wrought by the Great Depression—convinced other dry goods merchants to look to the suburbs as the ideal location for future branches that they believed would thrive with the return to prosperity (Dyer 2002: 608–10; Longstreth 2010: 110–16).

As the economic stress of the Great Depression pushed dry goods merchants to expand outside the downtown business district, it also encouraged independent food retailers to challenge the dominance of the chain groceries by opening the first supermarkets. The original supermarkets beckoned to Depression-weary consumers from the outskirts of urban areas with no-frills stores and bargain-basement prices. Big Bear stores, opened in 1932 in Elizabeth, New Jersey, exemplified the new retailing format. The "wild animal" moniker alluded to the store's effort to "slash" prices, often relayed in advertising that pitted the average shopper against profit-hungry big business. Big Bear borrowed

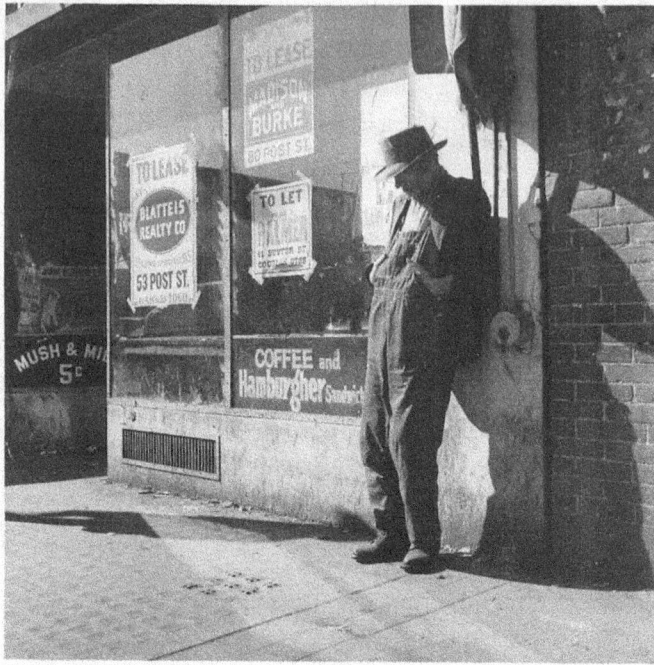

FIGURE 3.4: Store closings during the Great Depression. Photograph by Dorothea Lange. Franklin D. Roosevelt Presidential Library and Museum.

the self-service format that permitted the chain groceries to reduce labor costs, but it further reduced overheads and prices by housing its stores in huge, often abandoned, buildings with none of the amenities that shoppers would come to expect in later supermarkets. Big Bear's low prices attracted thousands of bargain-hungry shoppers, so much so that local police had to direct traffic at the store in its opening weeks. By the mid-1930s, as the Depression took a heavy toll on jobs and wages, independent retailers had opened 1,200 of the early "warehouse" stores, mostly on the East Coast (Mack 2010: 818–20).

The sensory logic of the warehouse supermarkets revolved around the festive atmosphere of large crowds and bargain-hunting. Big Bear's owners encouraged the loud, chaotic atmosphere of shoppers rifling through merchandise piled high on the rough, pine tables. They furthered the carnivalesque atmosphere with publicity that included cash giveaways and promotions like "penny sales" in which they offered dozens of items for a mere cent. Though industry observers disagreed about the long-term viability of the warehouse format, many argued that the type of bargain-hunting revelry found in Big Bear stores appealed with special force to women. Female shoppers looking for bargains "love crowds," one industry analyst wrote. He explained that women were "thrilled by the carnival atmosphere" at stores like Big Bear, concluding that they would gladly shop at future supermarkets wherever they opened (Mack 2010: 819).

The author's choice of metaphor—carnivals—is telling because it highlights how Big Bear rejected the lush aesthetic of the department store and the assembly-line efficiency of the chain grocery for the sensorial dissonance of bargain-hunting. Big Bear's sensory profile called to mind the crowded din and the physical jostling found in the bargain basements of department stores, where an occasional scuffle over a sale item was not unheard of. Yet the location outside of the central business district also gave the stores the sensorial signatures of the county fair or even the circus. The controlled chaos at the warehouse supermarkets washed over consumers' senses to evoke carnival barkers, games of chance, and even Coney Island's invitation to thrill in the crowd, albeit in a far less spectacular fashion. Above all, Big Bear and the warehouse supermarkets overloaded consumers' senses in ways that invited them to abandon restraint and thrill in stealing a bargain in the midst of the national economic crisis, an appeal that worked with special force on working-class shoppers unable to afford the luxuries of the department stores downtown.

Yet the larger grocery retailing industry, much like its dry goods counterpart, came to no consensus about the size, shape, and sensory profile of the ideal store, despite the success of Big Bear *et al.* Warehouse supermarkets proved that self-service worked on a large scale, but industry leaders habitually shied away from competing on the basis of price alone. Mass retailers believed that low prices failed to cultivate loyal customers over the long term because rivals could always offer better deals. Even more, however, they found the warehouse aesthetic wanting, arguing that a return to prosperity would render stores like Big Bear mere gimmicks. Considering themselves experts on the needs and desires of female shoppers, grocery retailers argued that a combination of the large-scale self-service of the warehouse stores with the palatial aesthetic of the department store promised to lower food prices and provide the type of sensory pleasures that post-Depression consumers craved. Mass retailers of all types would look to the suburbs, where members of the new middle class, on the mend from more than a decade of economic exigency and world war, craved security.

THE POSTWAR SUBURBAN MARKETPLACE

After 1945, American consumers enjoyed a booming economy and the end of the spending restrictions created by the economic depression and the Second

World War. Yet the demographic shifts of the war years gave rise to a marketplace geography that grew ever more bifurcated, as cities took on growing numbers of racial minorities and "white flight" fueled a booming suburban population. White flight reflected the social tensions that pushed members of the expanding middle class to isolate themselves against the perceived dangers of urban life by moving to the suburbs (Avila 2004). The burgeoning Cold War further inflamed postwar anxieties by raising the terrifying prospect of atomic holocaust and internal subversion. Middle-class Americans, as the historian Elaine Tyler May argued, responded by seeking shelter and security in the nuclear family. Nestled in suburban homes, they surrounded themselves with the deluge of consumer goods produced by American manufacturers to enhance familial bonds and shield themselves from threatening forces (May 2008). The marketplaces that sprouted around them featured sensory environments that reflected the emphasis on security by synthesizing the aesthetic lures of the downtown department store with the social homogeneity and predictability synonymous with the suburban setting.

Postwar commercial geography saw the rise of the suburban shopping center, an edited version of the urban retailing district. As automobiles became more prevalent and enabled suburban consumers to shop closer to home, avoiding the parking problems of the downtown retailing district, developers built places like the Bergen Mall and Garden State Plaza in Paramus, New Jersey, just outside Manhattan. The new, ersatz "downtowns" (i.e. shopping centers) provided commercial goods and services as well as spaces for local gatherings, promoting themselves as a "new kind of consumption-oriented community center" (Cohen 1996: 1055). Downtown department stores in New York City and Newark, NJ, met the competition by fully embracing the branch store concept introduced in the 1920s. As a result, the decentralization of retailing capital that started in the depression decades continued in the 1950s, as suburban shopping centers rose or fell on the strength of their one or two department store "anchors." By the mid-1970s, branch outlets generated more than 75 percent of all department store business in the USA (Cohen 1996: 1067).

As developers folded the central institution of the urban retailing district into the shopping center, they created a sensory landscape that reflected the emphasis on the privatized, public experience of suburban consumption. Whereas nineteenth-century consumers encountered department stores on chaotic downtown streets, the postwar branch outlets beckoned to them from privately owned and centrally controlled plazas. Developers in Paramus mimicked the layout of the urban retailing districts by placing shops on either side of a central walkway, but they added abundant parking, private security guards, and standardized architecture to create the visual predictability and homogeneity absent downtown. The shopping centers further echoed the suburban ideal by sparing consumers the discordant soundscape of the city streets. They hushed the rumble of delivery trucks with special tunnels and dedicated areas for unloading, while centrally programmed muzak quelled the other street noise that developers thought incongruent with suburban leisure time (Cohen 1996: 1056). Shopping center administrators saw the presence of certain people—vagrants, racial minorities—as grating to middle-class sensibilities so they used less direct means to exclude them from places like the Garden State Plaza and Bergen Mall. The simple lack of adequate public transportation discouraged visits by shoppers without access to private automobiles, often poor urbanites. Even more, however, the indirect exclusion inherent in the presence of high-end retailers, their elaborate sensorial merchandising, and their pricey merchandise set the shopping center and its stores firmly within the aesthetic values of their suburban context (Cohen 1996: 1059–60).

Suburban supermarkets illustrated how merchants used elaborate multisensory merchandising within individual stores. The earlier debate about grocery store formats dissolved after the Second World War as business opinion converged around the idea that large, upscale supermarkets furnished the perfect vehicle for chain companies like A&P to court the middle-class market (Deutsch 2010). Postwar supermarkets represented a basic continuity in retailing practices because they combined the efficiency of the 1920s chain groceries with the visual allure of the urban department stores. Yet they also broke sharply with the past by using the sensorial pleasures of food to whet shoppers' appetites to stimulate spending.

Cast in gendered terms, grocers dedicated themselves to flooding their stores with the pleasant smells, tastes, and textures of food because they viewed female shoppers as especially prone to the emotional pull of the nose, tongue, and skin. The appeal to women's proximate senses rested on longstanding stereotypes that cast the female sensory apparatus as fundamentally irrational (Classen 2005). In addition, it banked on the age-old associations between women, food, and desire (Korsmeyer 1999). The popular understanding of suburban life in the 1950s, invariably pictured to resemble the family television shows of the era such as *Leave it to Beaver*, seldom accounts for the value postwar actors placed on a healthy sexual relationship between man and wife. Yet historical studies clearly demonstrate that suburbanites prized sexual intimacy, as long as it remained confined to the home (May 2008). When supermarket operators used the sexual sell, they extended the private sphere of the home into the marketplace on intimate terms. The underlying message suggested that women might fill the erotic or sexual voids of their lives when they shopped for their family's groceries. In providing female shoppers an intimate "private" experience in a public space, supermarkets echoed the larger cultural emphasis on security by acting as a safety valve for marital discontent, and by extension, the suburban domestic ideal (Mack 2010).

With few salespeople on the shop floor, supermarkets depended on the sensory landscape of the store to express the cultural values that retailers wanted customers to associate with their businesses. Noise control measures typified how supermarket operators synthesized social order and consumptive excitement in aural terms. The use of in-store muzak—a strategy that became synonymous with mass retailing, as the opening discussion of Main Street, USA indicated—muffled the noise of shopping carts, cash registers, and restocking. While earlier grocers often played radios to drown out unwanted noise, supermarket companies hired music service providers to create a centrally programmed soundtrack. The homogenous aural landscape evoked retailers' emphasis on order and predictability, even as they played up musical metaphors of seduction to provide an exciting romantic tease. Trade press

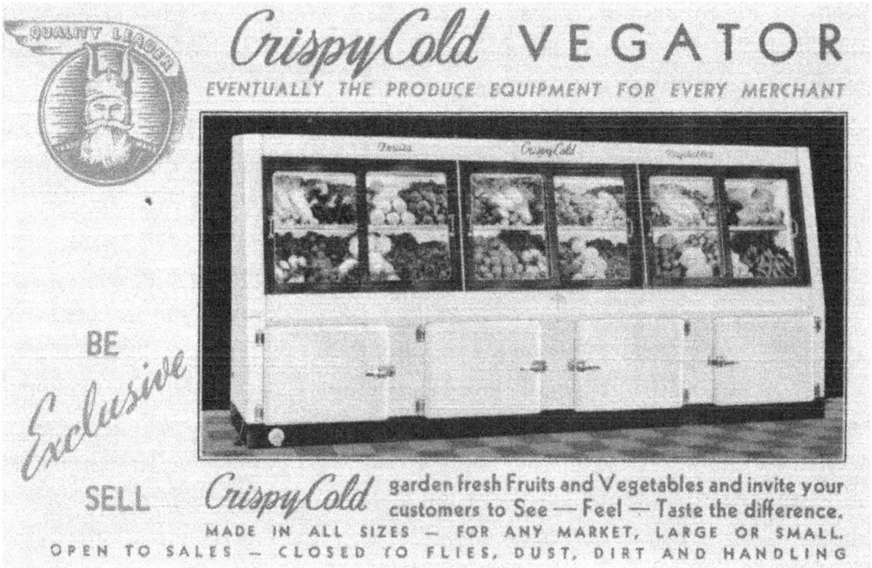

FIGURE 3.5: "See—Feel—Taste the Difference": advertisement for the Crispy Cold Vegator, *c.* 1940. Getty Images.

authors urged supermarket operators to avoid engulfing their stores with the loud, raucous sounds of rock and roll. Supermarket seduction involved none of the youthful hip thrusting of Elvis Presley, a form of musical expression that raised the specter of uncontrolled female sexuality and interracial sex. Retail surveys indicated a preference for the softer tunes—"I'm in the Mood for Love" was a popular, and telling, example—that eased the mind of the harried housewife to help her imagine food shopping as a romantic adventure in which male grocers showered her with attention. The overall metaphor, often relayed literally in newspaper advertising, portrayed supermarket managers as grocery store Casanovas who worked their romantic magic with pleasant lighting, soothing music, and of course, the mouth-watering foods that distracted women from the monotony of their daily routine (Mack 2010).

The produce section provided the most explicit material to expand the metaphor of erotic excitement in the supermarket. Here supermarkets elevated the importance of tactile and olfactory merchandising to bank on the natural beauty of fruits and vegetables. Unlike earlier grocers who allowed customers to handle merchandise to counter suspicions of poor quality, produce managers encouraged consumers to handle, squeeze, and smell their wares for the positive "appetite appeal" that they believed moved the items from the bin to the shopping cart. Since produce typically sold without a brand name, supermarket operators believed that customers held them directly responsible for quality, so much so that individual stores could succeed or fail on the basis of their fresh fruits and vegetables alone. New forms of cooling technology (air conditioning, advanced cooling bins) ensured that customers' hands felt crisp, fresh produce and that their noses never smelled hints of spoilage (see Figure 3.6). Much like the metaphors of seduction that trumpeted store amenities like soothing muzak, the language that advertised individual fruits and vegetables carried a strong sexual charge. Here words like "plump," "juicy," "ripe," and even "ready to use" carried double meanings that cast the supermarket as a place that female shoppers could privately—in public—find the type of erotic sensory stimulation that might have been missing from the home (Mack 2010).

If supermarkets sold themselves as places where the routine work of food shopping became a private pleasure, postwar theme parks cast a day of family play as a tamer, but equally reassuring, treat for the senses. Disneyland, the successor to Coney Island in the amusement industry, opened in 1955 in Anaheim, a little over ten miles from downtown Los Angeles. More than 160,000 people visited in the first week, paying between $1 and 50 cents for general admission as well as additional fees for parking and rides. In less than two years, the park averaged more than 10,000 guests every day of the year,

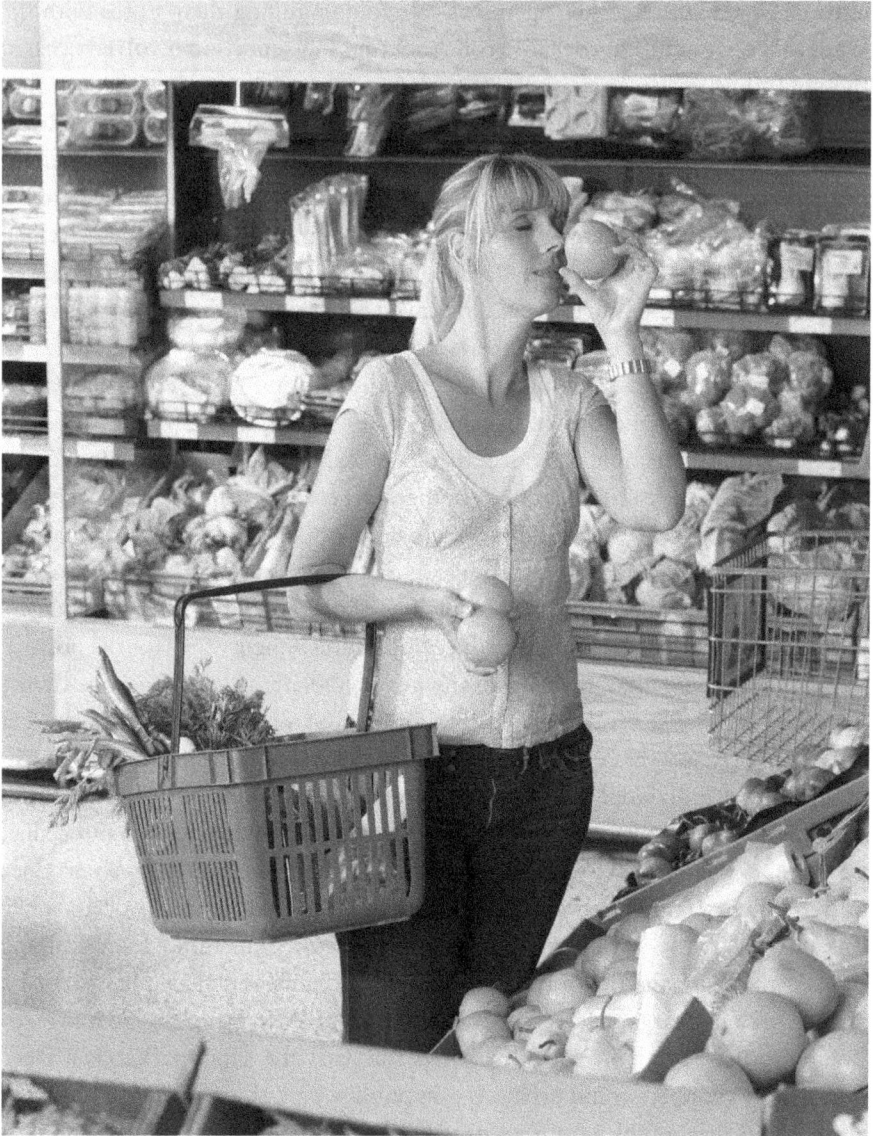

FIGURE 3.6: Seductions of the senses in the supermarket. Photograph by Ulrik Tofte. Hulton Archive/Getty Images.

making it one of the nation's leading tourist attractions (Hill 1955: 17, 1958: 1). The national media heaped praise on Walt Disney as a master of marketing illusions who gave the nation's families a world apart from the strains of modern urban life. "The visitor walking through its conventional turnstiles, like Alice passing through the Looking Glass," the *New York Times* raved, "leaves the world of reality behind, and enters a never-never land" (Hill 1959: 11).

Disney believed that his never-never-land sheltered visitors from the reality outside its gates, but he also built the park to promote the cultural values embodied in other institutions of the suburban marketplace. Earlier amusement parks like Coney Island served not as model, but as foil. In place of the sensorial chaos of crowds and carnival barkers, Disneyland greeted visitors with the placidity of Main Street, USA. The same reporter who applauded Disney for creating a never-never land described Main Street, USA in terms similar to those still used in the company's advertising. When he entered Disneyland, the reassuring sights and sounds of an idyllic small town hit his senses, including the "grassy, flower-bordered town square, a band playing and a train chuffing and clanging at an old-time depot" (Hill 1959: 11). In contrast to the disorder and grime of the urban street, the manicured town square stayed perfectly clean, modeling the sanitation and the uniformity long synonymous with the suburban social order. Disneyland provided baby-changing stations and dog kennels to keep the most odiferous waste from offending the noses of park-goers. Employees earned praise for quickly spotting and removing even the smallest pieces of litter. When Main Street, USA's band took breaks, music wafted from speakers to dampen the noise of the crowds, furthering the emphasis on orderly, clean, and safe family fun (Hill 1959).

Perfecting the sensory logic of Disneyland required more than simply eliminating the sights, sounds, and smells reminiscent of disorderly city streets. The park's overall layout, much like suburban shopping centers, rested on an organization of space and vision to underline its attention to social order (Avila 2004). All visitors to Disneyland arrived and departed through one walkway (Main Street, USA) that guided them to a central hub where they took paths to the park's other themed "lands" (Frontierland; Adventureland; Fantasyland; Tomorrowland). The visual order continued within the "lands," as Disney placed all utilities underground to prevent the street wires from interfering with the visual markers of the particular theme. Park designers carefully determined the heights and shapes of the main structures so that none of the lands could be easily seen from anywhere else within the park. To reduce the chaotic sights of the crowds and the unwieldy lines that often formed around popular amusements, Disney mandated uniformity and visual structure by channeling customers through fences of carefully drawn, winding queues. Attendees found none of the visual hodgepodge that mirrored the city streets at places like Coney Island; instead, their trip to Disneyland unfolded around a set of clear themes, each reinforced in visually discrete sections of the park, where they never had to elbow their way through a crowd to reach the attraction of their choice (Avila 2004: 106, 122–4).

Walt Disney distanced his park from its urban predecessors by stressing visual order, but he also echoed the sensory landscape of the suburban marketplace by providing excitement and thrills. Disney shied away from the type of mechanical rides that twirled and jarred visitors for the sake of pleasure alone, electing to dilute the sensual thrills with didactics (Avila 2004). In "Autopia" (Tomorrowland) children took the wheel of a miniature car to zip around a model freeway system where a "twelve-mile-an-hour whirl beside a neophyte young driver engenders, without much imagination, all the excitement of a real-life highway adventure" (Hill 1958: 1). Here the adventure's real-life qualities included the sensation of speed as well as a primer on the highway systems that undergirded the expansion of the suburbs across the nation. At another one of Tomorrowland's most popular attractions, "The Rocket to the Moon," riders felt Disney's version of space travel as they sat in the "vibrating hull of a simulated rocket" during a launch (Hill 1958: 1). As the sounds of rocket engines roared through speakers and movie screens projected unfolding images of the takeoff, the ride worked on the senses of touch, sight, and hearing to simulate flight. At the same time, it celebrated technological progress in the context of a growing space race with the Soviet Union, rallying American visitors around the patriotism endemic to the early Cold War. The patriotic implications of Disney rides became clear to the media when, in moments played out at various outlets of consumer culture in the 1950s and 1960s, visitors from communist countries enjoyed American pleasure spots. Such was the case at Disneyland in 1958 when a group of Russian visitors "abruptly dropped their studied taciturnity to ride gleefully" on the park's circus train, an act that laid bare the contrast between the consumer-oriented freedom of democratic capitalism and the regimentation of Soviet communism (Hill 1958: 1).

Avila's study of Disneyland's racial politics demonstrates that the park's attractions reflected its creator's notion of progress as the expansion of consumption, technological advancement, and the re-subordination of minority groups who had become more visible in public life during the Second World War, especially African Americans (Avila 2004). Disney's emphasis on racial hierarchies could be seen at Main Street, USA, where an absence of any black "people contact" employees throughout most of the 1960s labeled the "quintessential small town of middle America" as white. It also emerged in non-visual sensory terms in venues like Frontierland's "Aunt Jemima's Kitchen" where park-goers met an actress who played the famous black cook and regaled them with songs of the Old South that celebrated a romantic notion of antebellum race relations. At nearby Adventureland, the racial stereotypes again hit the ear, as speakers played a recorded soundtrack of "the sounds of native chants and toms-toms" that marked the section of the park as one where they might encounter the "wild animals" and "native savages" of the African jungle (Avila 2004: 134–5). Both the Aunt Jemima figure and the drumbeats echoed earlier exhibits at World's Fairs (Aunt Jemima made her debut at the 1893 World's Columbian Exposition in Chicago) that cast non-white people as exotic and primitive. In the context of southern California, home to rising conservative political stars like Ronald Reagan, sensory stereotypes that cast African Americans as primitive foreshadowed the racialized politics of the New Right (Avila 2004: 137). Stereotypical representations of the African-American sensorium at Disneyland, in other words, reassured conservative activists that a return to the prewar racial order made sense. In the decades after the 1960s, Disney's promotion of the conservative political values of the New Right with marketplace aesthetics received further emphasis, this time by Wal-Mart, a company whose size and sales exceeded even those promoted by Mickey Mouse.

THE MARKETPLACE IN THE TWILIGHT OF THE TWENTIETH CENTURY

In the closing decades of the twentieth century, Arkansas-based retailer Wal-Mart opened thousands of giant outlets—"SuperCenters"—that housed a discount department store and a supermarket as well as medical, automotive, and other services all under one roof. The original Wal-Mart, opened in 1962 in Rogers, Arkansas, followed in the footsteps of the chain stores of the 1920s and the warehouse supermarkets of the Depression era by offering consumers bare-bones shop floors and markedly low prices on household merchandise. By the end of the 1970s, the company's low prices, superior supply chain management, and emphasis on the small town markets neglected by other retailers, helped it emerge from its base in the Ozarks region to become a national chain with sales over $1 billion (Lichtenstein 2009; Moreton 2009). The Arkansas chain then claimed a series of retailing laurels unmatched in the history of modern retailing. By the second decade of the twenty-first century, Wal-Mart stood as the world's largest company. It operated more than 3,000 SuperCenters in the USA to become the nation's largest grocery retailer (Warner 2006). Consumer product vendors flocked to its headquarters in Bentonville, a rural outpost with an increasingly global catalog of corporate tenants including Coca-Cola, Pepsi, and Disney (which headquartered its retailing operation there) as well as high-end restaurants and a world-class art museum (Stodola 2011).

Even as Bentonville attracted cosmopolitan cultural institutions, its main benefactor thrived by appealing to rural customers with a conservative political and social ethos. Wal-Mart dominated global retailing by exploiting the most recent advances in communications and supply-chain technology, but it simultaneously maintained an emphasis on "Main Street" values of an evangelical Christian variety, including a distrust of sensualism. Inverting the marketing practices of the nineteenth-century urban department store and the postwar supermarket, Wal-Mart offered none of the titillating sensory cues intended to stimulate spending. SuperCenter customers gathered their groceries and socks in stores that were, the historian Bethany Moreton explains, "ostentatiously stripped-down, no frills places lacking in sensual ambience" in which the corporation intended to recast consumption as selfless, Christian service to the family. The "gridlike aisles and glaring fluorescent bulbs mapped order, abundance, and, ideally, cleanliness, but not [the] mystery and exotic allure" that invited individual gratification or sensual pleasure (Moreton 2009: 88–9). Wal-Mart provided its chiefly rural and working-class customers with a private, non-sensual shopping experience through which mass consumption became safe and even venerated as an expression of the conservative, Christian family values that New Right leaders like Reagan, Newt Gingrich, and George W. Bush extolled on the political stage (Lichtenstein 2009; Moreton 2009).

Wal-Mart's identity as an evangelical Christian company with aesthetically sterile stores helps to explain the unfashionable aura it maintained among urban and middle-class shoppers (Lichtenstein 2009). The Arkansas chain's chief rival, Minneapolis-based Target, also established in 1962, chased the upscale bargain hunter with the sensorial merchandising techniques of its mass retailing predecessors. Target boasted far fewer units than Wal-Mart, but its reputation for attractive, airy stores and stylish merchandise earned it a wide following among younger, college-educated shoppers. In 1995, the company opened its first SuperTargets, a combination discount store/supermarket that treated the senses with bright produce, high-quality bakeries, fresh sushi, and Starbucks coffee outlets, on-site (Rowley 2003). Almost two decades later, the company introduced CityTargets to court affluent urbanites. Reversing the decentralization of retailing capital that started in the 1920s, the chain kicked off the expansion by opening a CityTarget in Chicago's bustling State Street shopping corridor. Housed at 1 South State Street, a historic building designed by architect Louis Sullivan, Target earned plaudits from design critics for working with preservation officials and maintaining the "aesthetic integrity of one of the nation's great works of architecture and projecting the visual brand of one of the nation's biggest retailers," all in the name of good design ("Retailer Right on Target" 2012). The unit featured long, open windows along the busy street, affording views into the store that revived the long moribund tradition of window shopping in the city center. It is far too early to measure the success of the new format, but the effort to maintain the integrity of the turn of the century architecture and window shopping suggest CityTarget may help mass retailing's commercial geography come full circle.

At the same time, however, the rise of the suburban super mall indicates how the effort to attract consumers with a privatized, centrally managed sensory landscape intensified at the dawn of the new century. By the end of the 1970s, commercial developers faced a design crisis as the proliferation of enclosed shopping malls rendered appeals based on particular stores or convenient locations insufficient by themselves to attract new consumers. Developers responded with ever-bigger malls that combined the pleasures of shopping and theme parks (Deutsch 1992). The emphasis on blending retailing with family amusements is best illustrated by the largest shopping mall in the USA, the Mall of America (MOA), located in Bloomington, Minnesota, just outside Minneapolis. Opened in 1992, MOA advertises itself as no mere shopping mall; instead, it is a "destination attraction," well known as a vacation spot for tourists from around the nation and the globe (Mall of America 2012: 6). Forty million visitors patronize MOA every year, wandering its 4.2 million square feet to shop at 520 stores. Yet MOA distinguishes itself not on the basis of size alone, but on the proliferation of entertainment options. On top of a full complement of bars, restaurants, and movie theatres, MOA operates the nation's largest indoor "family theme park," Nickelodeon Universe, which sits on seven acres of central atrium space and offers twenty-seven different rides and attractions (see Figure 3.7). There is also a 1.2 million gallon walkthrough aquarium (Sea Life Minnesota); an eighteen-hole miniature golf course; and a wedding chapel, which has hosted more than 5,000 marriage ceremonies (Mall of America 2012).

The sensory landscape is an expanded version of the ersatz downtowns of the postwar shopping center. MOA advertises itself as a "city within a city," including as it does an entertainment quarter (bars, restaurants, theaters), a park (the central atrium), and of course a retailing district, which is organized around four, three-level "avenues," each of which distinguishes itself through visual and other cues (Karasov and Martin 1993: 23). Like the shopping centers of the 1950s, MOA provides a secure sensory environment that revolves around a synthesis of thrill and social order—a "facsimile of urbanity,"

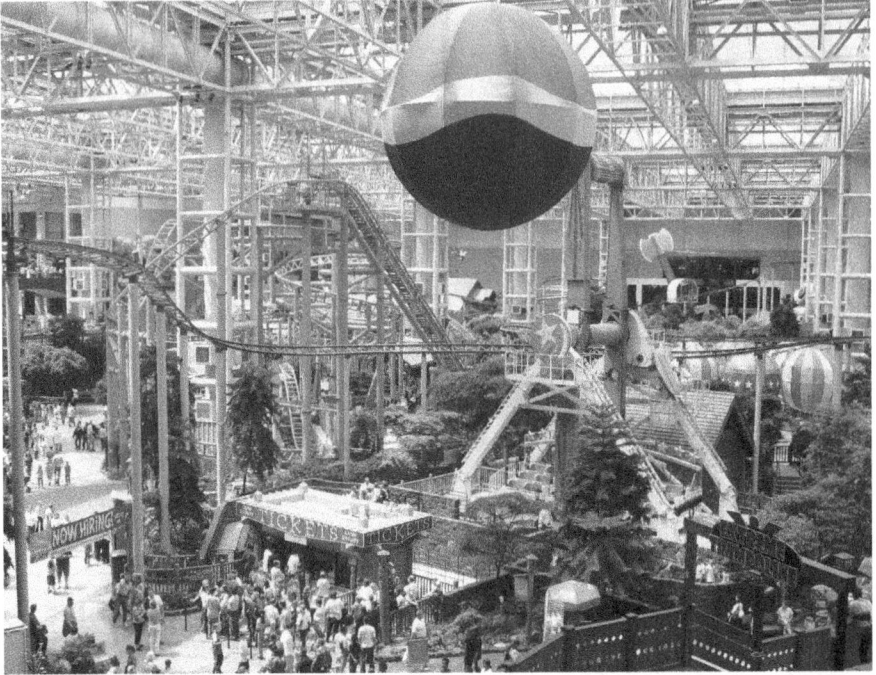

FIGURE 3.7: The amusement park at the center of the Mall of America. Photograph by
Jeremy Noble. Public domain.

according to the communications scholar Jonathan Sterne (Sterne 1997: 27).
Among the most remarkable features of the predictable landscape is how MOA
shuts out the bitter cold of the Minnesota winter without a central heating
system. MOA advertises that its "weather" is "always a perfect 70 degrees," a
comfort level maintained with 1.2 miles of skylights and the residual heat from
lighting fixtures as well as visitors' bodies (Mall of America 2012: 11). The
control of MOA's soundscape is also centrally modulated to evoke predictability
and order. Sterne's study of the retailing background music at MOA indicates
how its flow is managed as an "environmental factor" that is weaved into the
mall's infrastructure, much like its power supply or grounds-keeping (Sterne
1997: 22). The MOA soundtrack includes soft muzak for the retailing avenues,
a "steady singing of digital crickets" that wafts from speakers under the
amusement park, as well as the "foreground" music that plays in the individual
stores, all of which is intended to extend shopping time by raising the acoustic
tempo at points of the day in which shoppers tend to lag, and to slow it down
when they are the most excited. "It is an aesthetics of the moderate: not too

exciting, not too sedate," and thus pitch perfect as a synthesis of excitement and control (Sterne 1997: 22, 30).

The mall's soundscape is also closely policed to quiet the noises of groups that administrators deem threatening to middle-class sensibilities. MOA's security system far exceeds individual guards to include bike patrols, a K-9 unit, and an undercover Risk Assessment Mitigation unit. The mall also houses a sub-station of the Bloomington Police Department, whose officers work closely with the private guards in training and crime prevention (Mall of America 2012: 15). Despite MOA's emphasis as a destination attraction for middle-class families and tourists, some of the most enthusiastic patrons in its first decade were teenagers of diverse racial and ethnic backgrounds. The mall's management looked askance at the young patrons, many of whom congregated along the retailing avenues and in the central atrium. The subsequent attempts to manage their sonic conduct manifested in signs that banned "loud, boisterous behavior" posted where consumers might think such noise entirely appropriate: outside the indoor amusement park. Sterne points out that the juxtaposition of the signs banning "boisterous behavior" surrounding the spots where teens gathered—and not in the entertainment quarter where drinkers congregate in and around bars—revealed how the noise control policies constituted "pretexts for enforcement of social boundaries rather than clearly delineated rules" (Sterne 1997: 43). The policing of behavior that rankles the ears of middle-class adults is also reflected in MOA's controversial parental escort policy, which forbids persons of sixteen and younger from frequenting the mall on weekends after 4 p.m. without an escort over age twenty-one, and that further requires the escort to produce a state-issued ID card when confronted by mall security, or face ejection (Mall of America 2012: 14).

Finally, it is worth noting that certain features of the mall's soundscape have become consumer products in themselves, as the case of Victoria's Secret lingerie store indicates. Sterne notes that the classical foreground music in Victoria's Secret works alongside a plush visual aesthetic and decorations that reference London to portray the store as "European" in origins and spirit (Sterne 1997: 36–7). The "European" sensibility is intended to reflect the cultural refinement that can be purchased by middle-class consumers in the form of the underwear, lotions, and perfume on sale. In recent years, Victoria's Secret has sold recordings of its in-store music program to millions of patrons in CDs complete with liner notes that provide a primer on the featured European composers and other trivia (Sterne 1997: 37). The lingerie retailer, in other words, marketed the products through which middle-class consumers displayed refined tastes, and packaged the store's sonic aesthetic as an instructional device on culturally refined music. The result is a reversal of the pattern by which merchants have extended sensory values of the suburban home in the marketplace; in this case, Victoria's Secret permits shoppers to extend the store's aesthetic values back into their homes.

CONCLUSION

Between 1920 and the opening decades of the twenty-first century, mass merchants created a synthetic marketplace in tune with suburban sensory values. Institutions like shopping malls and discount supercenters combined the functions of the urban department store, the food shop, and the amusement park under one roof. At the same time, the sensory context of the marketplace changed from one in which individual stores competed with the sights, sounds, and smells of public streets to one in which the merchants invited consumers to privately-owned and centrally-controlled plazas to shop free from the dangers and uncertainties of urban spaces. The sensory landscape promoted consumption by bathing all five of the senses with both excitement and reassurance. The cumulative effect was to suggest to middle-class shoppers that they never really had to leave the safety of their homes to participate in the marketplace.

CHAPTER FOUR

The Senses in Religion: Pluralism, Technology, and Change

ISAAC A. WEINER

In a 1933 report, New York City's Noise Abatement Commission proposed a remarkable myth of origins for modern noise. "One hundred and fifty years ago," its story began, "the world was like a quiet valley whose inhabitants, over many centuries, had built up a civilization to their liking. Here the arts flourished and the crafts. Most men lived on the soil and there were no machines. Church bells could be heard for miles on a Sunday morning and the singing of birds was everywhere." But that idyllic world had long since vanished, the report continued, replaced by the "ominous rumbling," "steam whistle war whoops," and "horrible clanking" of "a horde of barbarian machines." Man had entered the industrial age, and "resistance was vain" (Flexner 1933, II: 2–3).

While there is much that was notable about the Commission's account, most striking was its assumption that church bells belonged to the pre-industrial past, rather than the modern mechanical age. Its history of noise doubled as a secularization narrative, taking for granted that religion would be drowned out by the forces of modernity. The Commissioners were not alone in thinking this way, of course. Academics used to assume that religion would wane in influence over the course of the twentieth century. Secularization paradigms dominated scholarly thinking about religion and modernity. Moreover, as Sally Promey and Shira Brisman (2010: 182), among others, have argued, "The weight of secularization theory settled disproportionately on the material practice of religion." That is, if religion did not fade away altogether, scholars expected that it would at least become more individualized and intellectualized, more invisible and inaudible. They posited a developmental model of civilization that assumed steady religious "progress" from the primitive practices of ancient pagans to the mature interiorized faith of Protestant Christianity. Religion might endure, they allowed, but only if it "overcame" its need for material and sensorial expression. Modern religion would not make any clamor.

Religion did not disappear, of course, nor did it retreat to a private, spiritualized realm. Instead, the twentieth century witnessed religion's remarkable persistence and even resurgence. This unexpected trend extended to its material and sensorial dimensions. Religion has never been merely a matter of belief, after all, but of how those beliefs have been acted out, how they have been mediated by and expressed through particular "sensational forms" (Meyer 2009). Religions have shaped how individuals think and feel, but also how they see, hear, taste, touch, and smell. Religious differences have been as much about different styles of practice and different ways of sensing the world as about rival dogmatic theologies.

This chapter analyzes important shifts in the religious sensorium over the course of the twentieth century, that is, changes in how the human senses were used and regulated in religious contexts, focusing especially on how this history unfolded in the United States. Far from offering an exhaustive account, it touches on key figures, groups, and movements that affected the ways religion was practiced, sensed, and experienced, both in the public realm and in private. It moves from the Fundamentalist-Modernist debates of the early twentieth century to mid-century notions of moral consensus and middle-class respectability, to the fragmentation and pluralization of the 1960s and beyond. Along the way, it calls particular attention to the impact of new media technologies, shifting political alliances, and expanded transnational exchanges. Each of these important themes gave rise to and was shaped by shifts in what we might describe as the dominant sensory order. As we will see, and contrary to widespread assumptions, the religious senses were never diminished in the modern world so much as they were continually refigured and re-formed.

RELIGION MODERN AND UNMODERN

Between 1910 and 1915, the California oil magnates Lyman and Milton Stewart financed the publication of twelve paperback volumes, known collectively as *The Fundamentals: A Testimony to the Truth*, which they promised to distribute "to every pastor, missionary, theological professor, theological student, YMCA and YWCA secretary, college professor, Sunday school superintendent and religious editor in the English-speaking world" (Marsden 2006: 119). Written by a group of prominent evangelical theologians from the United States, Canada, and Great Britain, *The Fundamentals* laid out and defended key conservative doctrines, such as the inerrancy of the Bible, the virgin birth of Christ, and the authenticity of miracles. More generally, the booklets aimed to counter the influence of liberal or "modernist" tendencies within Protestant Christian thought, which sought to reconcile Christian faith and teachings with the modern world. The publication of *The Fundamentals* would come to be regarded as a pivotal moment in the early twentieth-century contests between Christian modernists and "fundamentalists," who responded to the social, political, and intellectual upheavals of the modern age in very different ways. Although neither movement was ever unified in its claims, they came to represent opposing poles in broader debates about social evolution, human nature, and the authority of modern science.

Fundamentalists did not only contest their opponents on matters of theology, nor did they appeal only to their audience's intellects. Many conservative evangelical preachers, though certainly not all, also cultivated distinct performative *styles*, which sought to liberate Christianity from what they perceived as the overly effeminate mores of late-Victorian liberal culture (Lofton 2006). Adopting explicitly gendered language, they advocated for a more masculine, "muscular" Christianity, and they worked to embody this ideal through their own carefully crafted public personas. Most notable in this regard was the American Presbyterian preacher Billy Sunday, who promised that he would "fight till Hell freezes over" and gained international renown for his highly theatrical oratorical style. As he preached, Sunday would flail his arms, stomp his feet, hurl invectives, and throw chairs at his audiences, heaping his scorn on unrepentant sinners and theological liberals alike. Although his means were primarily visual and auditory, his histrionic performances were meant to appeal to all of the senses. "There is no 'in a degree,' 'to some extent' or 'as it were' business about the hell that Bill Sunday preaches," his biographer Elijah Brown noted. "He pulls off the lid so that you can almost feel the fire and smell the smoke and hear the gnashing of teeth" (Brown 1914: 145). Sunday's revivals were multisensory events, visual, aural, and olfactory spectacles, which seethed with primal potency and masculine virility. These tactics could not be neatly separated from the theological message that he preached. A "true minister of the gospel," argued Sunday's

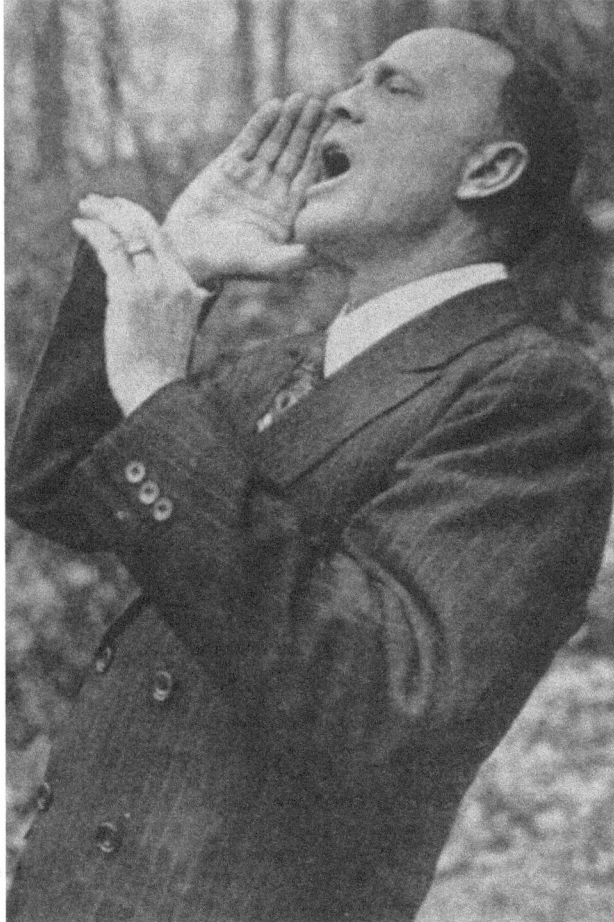

FIGURE 4.1: Billy Sunday preaching. Public domain.

contemporary, Baxter "Cyclone Mac" McLendon, had "a knowable, feelable, tellable, seeable, tasteable case of old time, backwoods calico religion" (Barr 1928: 245). To know the gospel, McLendon suggested, was to feel it in one's bones, to see it and to taste it. Conversely, then, to imbibe God's word was also to comprehend it. Evangelical preachers of the early twentieth century drew little distinction among these different registers of cognitive, affective, and sensorial understanding. Knowing the truth, feeling the truth, and sensing the truth all went hand in hand, eye to eye, and heart to heart.

Sunday, McLendon, and their peers insisted that theirs was an "old time" religion, a restoration and reinvigoration of God's eternal truth. Their sermons were infused with backwards-looking nostalgia, which served to associate the sensuality of their performances with a return to the past. Appealing to their followers' senses was itself a vehicle for reclaiming old habits and values. In this way, they ironically aligned themselves with cultural modernists who similarly interpreted the embodied and multisensorial dimensions of religion as remnants of the past, though they evaluated their worth in very different ways. Many early twentieth-century artists and anthropologists, for example, celebrated the traditional practices and ceremonial dances of Native Americans and other indigenous peoples as spiritually authentic, primitive, and pristine, untouched and uncontaminated by the onslaught of "modern civilization." Enamored by them on this account, they often worked hard to protect and preserve indigenous rituals, but their patronizing assumptions also located them squarely in humanity's past (Wenger 2009: 59–94). This was an attitude shared, in part, by those cultural theorists who posited an evolutionary trajectory culminating either in religion's displacement by modern science or, at the very least, in its de-materialization. For each of these varied actors, religion's sensorial, material, and kinesthetic components functioned as clear markers of its "old-timey" primitivism.

Yet if conservative preachers promoted themselves as throwbacks to the past, they also remained very much of their moment, fully entrenched within the modern world. This was particularly evident in their sophisticated use of new communication technologies, which had important implications for the modern religious sensorium. Acoustic devices such as radios, loudspeakers, and phonograph players offered highly effective means for religious evangelizing, extending the preacher's acoustic reach and dramatically expanding the size of his or her potential congregation, even while creating an artificial distance between them. Fundamentalist preachers such as Charles E. Fuller and "Sister" Aimee Semple McPherson exploited the popularity of commercial radio during the 1920s and 1930s to broadcast their "old-fashioned" religion across the United States. By the 1940s, Fuller's *Old Fashioned Revival Hour* was the most popular radio program in the country. Radio also figured prominently in giving voice to inter-religious conflict and could target audiences that might not otherwise choose to listen to a given message. "Judge" Joseph Rutherford, for example, president of the Watch Tower Bible and Tract Society, the organizational arm of the Jehovah's Witnesses, broadcast combative and inflammatory speeches throughout the 1920s and 1930s in which he derisively berated Roman Catholicism. Not to be outdone, the fiery Catholic priest Charles E. Coughlin grew famous during the 1930s for his potent mix of religious and political messaging until he was finally forced off the air on account of his anti-Semitic and pro-Nazi rhetoric (Hangen 2002: 30–6).

Radio broadcasts relied on auditory means to stimulate their audience's religious imaginations, in line with Protestant Christianity's historic emphasis on hearing the word of God. By reaching potential converts wherever they were, radio religion diminished the physical or tactile experience of being among others as they encountered the gospel. Yet the most successful preachers made adept use of multiple forms of media that would appeal to all of the senses. From her base at the Angelus Temple in Los Angeles, for example, McPherson produced daily radio broadcasts, illustrated sermons, and elaborate stage performances with colorful sets, costumed actors, and outlandish props. She drove around the nation in a "gospel car," an automobile adorned with banners, biblical passages, and other mottoes. And she enthusiastically embraced the media of film, explaining to one reporter that "the talking picture is the greatest agency for the spread of the Gospel since the invention of the printing press" (Babcock 1930: 84).

Other conservative Christians were initially more ambivalent or even apprehensive about film's evangelical promise. The experience of seeing the word, rather than merely hearing it, heightened Protestant anxieties about idolatry, concerns which extended to the theatrical stage, as well. As visual culture scholar David Morgan has argued, "Film encouraged a different way of seeing. Like secular theater, it redeployed audiences as private consumers whose reason for viewing was personal entertainment in the form of visual absorption, not edification." For its Christian critics, film risked reducing the biblical message to a matter merely of "private amusement or aesthetic enjoyment" (Morgan 2007: 173). Yet over time, Fundamentalists and other conservative Christians largely came to embrace the medium, in part for its utility in overseas mission work. Several churches even began to use film devotionally, incorporating clips from popular and religiously-themed movies into their services and liturgies (Plate 2008: 82). Never solely a visual medium, film elicited a wide range of embodied responses from its audiences, including shudders, jumps, and jerks, laughter, tears, and cries. With the advent of 3-D (and eventually "4-D") technology, viewers sought ever more tactile forms of interactions with the images before them. As in religious rituals more generally, "the perceiving body in the screening space" was always "an active body, perpetually in motion" (Plate 2008: 60).

By mid-century, television rose to even greater prominence as the medium of choice for enterprising ministers, deployed most effectively perhaps by Billy Graham, whose mass revivals and prayer meetings sparked an evangelical resurgence. Television offered the illusion of immediacy and intimacy, permitting the viewer to participate, in real time, in the spectacle of a preacher's performance. It could reach its intended audience in the comfort of their own homes, reasserting a link between public faith and domestic values. While primarily a visual medium, it, too, could appeal to other senses as well. The televangelist Oral Roberts, Jr., for example, asked viewers "to place their hands on their television sets to touch his own palm raised before the camera," a technique he learned from his father, who had previously invited listeners to place their hands on their radio sets as they listened in their living rooms (Morgan 2007: 223). In so doing, these charismatic speakers sought to overcome the limitations of their respective media by re-establishing a physical, tactile connection with their audiences.

Roberts came out of a Pentecostal tradition that was widely known both for its sensory forms of knowledge and for its strict regulation of those same senses. Emerging over the first few decades of the twentieth century, Pentecostals were distinguished most clearly by their practice of glossolalia, or speaking in tongues. Interpreted as a sign of their sanctification or Holy Ghost baptism,

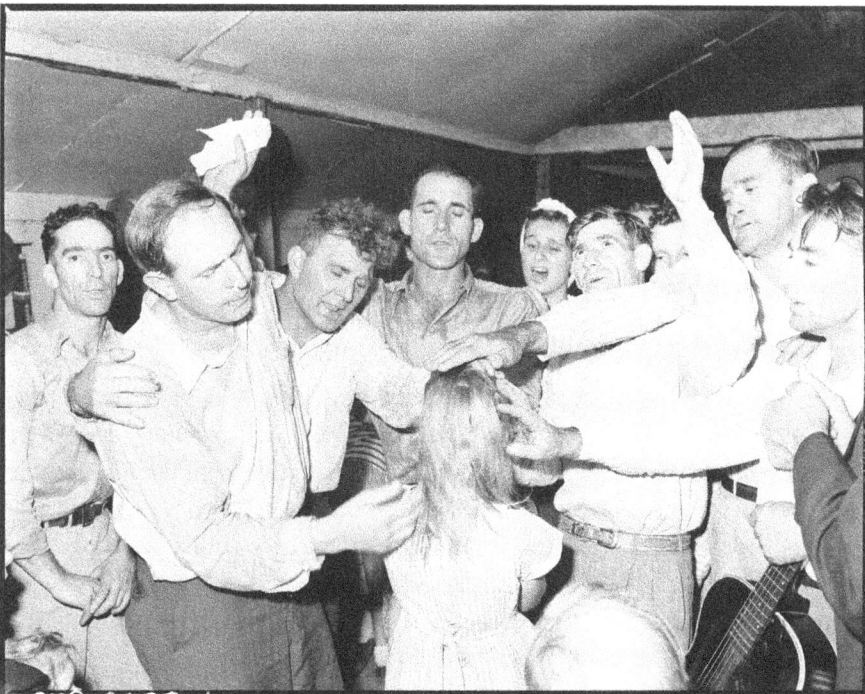

FIGURE 4.2: Laying on of hands, Pentecostal church, Harlan County, Kentucky. National Archives and Records Administration.

Pentecostals experienced the gift of tongues as accompanied by intense physical sensations, most commonly described in first-person accounts as feelings of searing heat, uncontrollable shaking, or jolts of electricity. Pentecostals also practiced distinct forms of divine healing, which often involved the laying of hands directly on those who were sick or infirmed. In so doing, healers tangibly anointed their patients as if with the material substance of the Holy Spirit. While word-centered Protestants often expressed suspicion or even distrust of the human senses, Pentecostals valued these sensory experiences and practices as revealing the real presence of the divine and as offering genuinely authentic forms of religious knowledge.

Regulating the senses also served an important social function for early Pentecostals, marking them as distinct and set off from middle-class American society. Pentecostals observed a remarkable number of social proscriptions and moral taboos, which religious historian Grant Wacker has argued can best be organized "into categories pertaining to the mouth, eyes, ears, body, and genitals." They avoided particular foods and drink and refrained from engaging in idle or frivolous talk. They censured the reading of "novels, newspapers, and comic books," and they refused to listen to "worldly music." They worried about "superfluous items of adornment, including watches, rings, hat pins, neckties, and brass buttons," and they condemned lust, licentiousness, and other forms of sexual impropriety, despite popular and derogatory stereotypes that associated their "fanatically" exuberant worship services with suspicions of sexual deviance (Wacker 2001: 121–30). These prohibitions enacted rigid social boundaries between Pentecostalism and other Protestant sects, distinguishing Pentecostals even from other conservative evangelical Christians. Their moral regulations often elicited scorn and contempt from those who did not share them, but they also played an important part in helping Pentecostals negotiate their ambivalent position in the modern world. The early "saints," those who had experienced sanctification and Holy Ghost baptism, lived always both in the world and out of it at the same time. They longed for direct contact with the divine while always remaining solidly grounded in the times in which they lived. As with the other groups that we have considered thus far, as well as for immigrant communities such as the Irish or Italian Catholics and East European Jews, whose North American numbers swelled during the late nineteenth and early twentieth centuries, carefully regulating the senses played a key role in negotiating their fraught encounter with and transition to modernity. Religion was not to fade away, as many of its critics eagerly expected, but its sensory dimensions were to grow increasingly contested, both within and across a range of disparate traditions.

MID-CENTURY CONSENSUS AND ITS LIMITS

In 1923, the United States Supreme Court decided that Bhagat Singh Thind, a Sikh from the Punjab region of India, was not eligible for US citizenship. According to US law, naturalization could be extended only to "free white persons" or those of "African descent," and the Court had previously determined that such designations did not apply to Chinese or Japanese immigrants, who were understood to belong to the "yellow" race. Asian Indians, however, occupied a more ambiguous position, for racial theory of the time classified them as "Caucasian" and thus potentially as "white." But in his majority opinion in *United States* v. *Thind*, Supreme Court Justice George Sutherland made clear that he could not accept this contention. "In the endeavor to ascertain the meaning of the statute," he wrote, "we must not fail to keep in mind that it does not employ the word 'Caucasian' but the words 'white persons,' and these are words of common speech and not of scientific origin." Thind's racial status was not a matter of biology, Sutherland elaborated, but of common sense, and he took it as self-evident that no one would ever mistake Thind or his progeny for being white. This was because Asian Indians were fundamentally dissimilar to the millions of other immigrants that American society had absorbed over the preceding decades. "The children of English, French, German, Italian, Scandinavian, and other European parentage," Sutherland explained, "quickly merge into the mass of our population and lose the distinctive hallmarks of their European origin. On the other hand, it cannot be doubted that the children born in this country of Hindu parents would retain indefinitely the clear evidence of their ancestry." By virtue of his appearance, his culture, and his religious heritage, Sutherland concluded, Thind could never become American, for visual and behavioral markers would always cast him as irreconcilably other. His essential and incontrovertible difference was a matter of common sensory perception, not scientific genealogy.

The *Thind* decision authorized an assimilationist notion of American identity that conflated racial, religious, and nationalistic categories (Snow 2004: 268–73). One year later, the US Congress moved toward codifying this conception in law by establishing a strict quota system, which effectively curtailed the inflow of immigrants for the next four decades. By mid-century, mainstream notions of American religious identity gradually expanded to include those outside of the Protestant fold, yet they continued to be shaped by a distinctly assimilationist model. Following the trauma of the Second World War and the Holocaust, many liberal religious leaders began speaking of a

"Judeo-Christian tradition," which sought to emphasize that which Protestants, Catholics, and Jews shared in common. Each tradition came to be perceived as offering an equally legitimate way of being both religious and American. Each, so the theory went, had become "accepted as a normal part of the American Way of Life" (Herberg [1955] 1983: 257). As the sociologist Will Herberg famously wrote in 1955, "The three great religious communions— Protestantism, Catholicism, and Judaism—constitute the three great American religions, the 'religions of democracy'" ([1955] 1983: 246).

The construction of a "Judeo-Christian" religious mainstream was shaped, in part, by Cold War era politics and as a response to secularizing trends in Western Europe. Americans stood united in their opposition to "godless Communists" and celebrated the shared faith that undergirded their self-perceived national superiority. Political leaders such as President Dwight D. Eisenhower trumpeted a vaguely defined, highly personal, interiorized notion of faith, which sublimated the more particularistic beliefs and practices that might divide Americans from each other. This imagined moral consensus was predicated on a sharp distinction between that which was publicly tolerable and privately permissible. Religion could form the basis of national solidarity, in other words, only to the extent that its embodied, sensorial, and material dimensions could be reduced merely to matters of cultural preference, rather than understood as obligatory, binding, or more deeply constitutive of personal and communal identity.

The religious upswing in postwar America took place predominantly in the suburbs, and the mass suburbanization of American society also contributed to a new sensory order. In many ways, the suburbs seemed more sterile than the cities that second-, third-, and fourth-generation immigrant families had left behind, with their highly standardized, cookie-cutter subdivisions and greater distance among homes. Automobiles transported parishioners directly from home to house of worship, linking together the two primary sites of mainstream religious life and necessitating large church parking lots, which further separated these institutions from their surrounding environs. As the congestion and cramped conditions of urban living faded into memory, the sights, sounds, and smells of religious devotion proved less likely to spill over into the common spaces of public life. Its sensory cultures grew more tightly contained and compartmentalized.

During the postwar decades, thousands of new churches and synagogues were built in American suburbs, and their designs were shaped by and gave material form to the values of their congregations. They, too, made possible certain kinds of sensory experiences while foreclosing the opportunity for others. Architectural styles tended to be relatively conservative. While several congregations did experiment with modernist designs, they continued to maintain that a church should "look" like a church, their sacred purpose made manifest through their familiar visual appearance. "The House of God must be distinctive," one how-to manual explained in 1949. "It must be at once recognizable as a church. The exterior design must indicate, even to the casual observer, that this is not an auditorium, a theater, a post office or a library, but a church" (Anderson 1949: 39). Inside the building, many congregations introduced innovative seating arrangements, which tended to be more democratic in their spatial organization, reflecting the spirit of the times. They downplayed the hierarchical separation of clergy from laity, even within many Catholic parishes, and experimented with circular, hexagonal, and elliptical designs (Allitt 2003: 34–6). Some Orthodox Jewish synagogues, meanwhile, were divided over the question of whether men and women should sit separately or together during services, and a few notable disputes even ended up in civil court. Mixed seating evolved into a strict denominational boundary, emerging as a primary point of differentiation between Orthodoxy and American Judaism's other branches (Sarna 2003: 257–62). Debates about who could be seen, heard, and touched during religious worship raised important questions about a community's openness to change and exposed internal fissures that otherwise might have remained imperceptible.

Eventually, the suburban automobile culture of postwar American life also gave rise to the creation of megachurches, which transformed popular assumptions about how religious institutions were supposed to look and feel. With their sprawling campuses, open concourses, and cavernous auditoriums, megachurches lacked many of the traditional visual, tactile, and olfactory markers of Christian sacred space. They replaced church steeples, stained glass windows, and the aroma of incense with jumbotron screens, stadium-style seating, and the smells of in-house coffee shops and cafeterias. In many ways, megachurches replicated the sensory experiences of shopping malls, airports, hotels, and other secular "cathedrals" of the modern world, rather than standing apart from them. "This everyday appearance of megachurches," writes Jeanne Kilde (2006: 238–9), "suggests an understanding of religion and church life that is itself 'everyday,' or a regular part of everyday life. The church is not a special destination; it is part of normal and familiar experience." New architectural designs and arrangements thus continued to give material form to the changing values of Christian congregations.

In the realm of visual art, mid-century liberal Protestant leaders embraced a distinctly modernist style, recasting aesthetic discernment as itself a form of

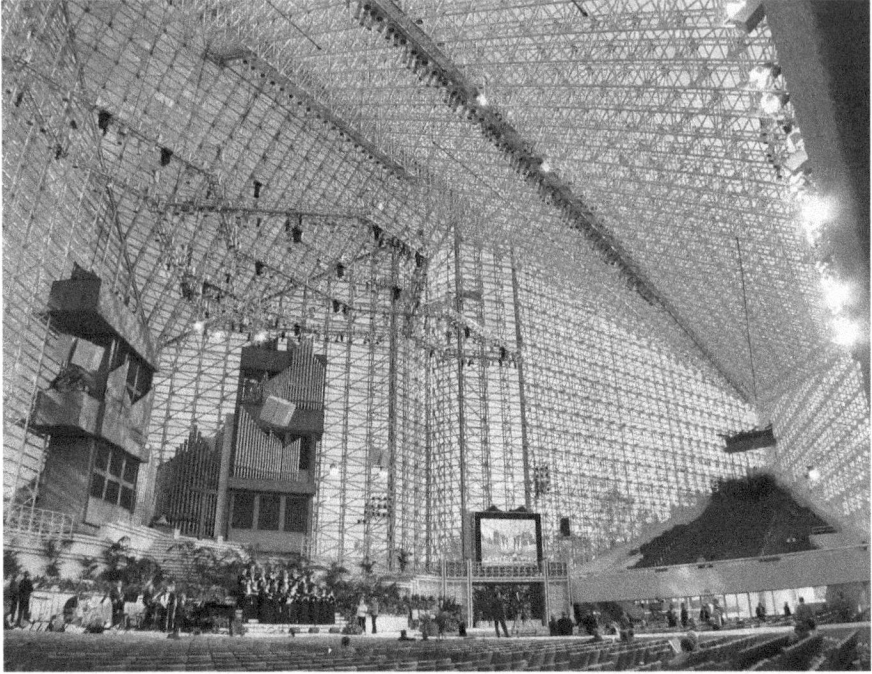

FIGURE 4.3: Amplifying the sacred in the megachurch: Crystal Cathedral, Orange County, California.

religious practice. "For the creators, promoters, and adopters of this perspective," Sally Promey (2006: 254) has argued, "the appearance of things made certain kinds of experiences and relations more or less likely; right forms would lead to right behavior and right belief, a new liberal Protestant 'orthodoxy' achieved through aesthetics. 'Good' taste would thus become a critical part of the visual and moral task of religion." This liberal Protestant aesthetic favored "high" art and abstract impressionism, railing against the "kitschy" and "effeminate" sentimentalism of mass (i.e. evangelical) culture, perhaps best exemplified by artist Warner Sallman's *Head of Christ* (1941), which had quickly become "the most recognizable face of Jesus in the world" (Blum and Harvey 2012: 208; Morgan 1996). In its place, liberal critics sought to reframe artistic activity as spiritual endeavor in and of itself, distinguished not by its content but by its celebration of freedom and pursuit of *authenticity*. "Artistically authentic art . . . is implicitly religious," the public theologian Paul Tillich wrote in 1954, "if it expresses, in whatever fashion, the artist's sensitive and honest search for ultimate meaning and significance in terms of his own contemporary culture" (Tillich and Green 1954: 9). They sought to cultivate and inculcate "good" Protestant taste in their fellow Christians by introducing new liturgical decorations for the church and new devotional images for the home, by sponsoring annual religious art festivals, and by providing new aids for Sunday school education. Although never wholly successful in their efforts, they believed that these new visual and aesthetic practices would prove essential for maintaining religion's relevance in the modern world.

An ideal of middle-class respectability infused other religious traditions at this time, as well, including the Church of Jesus Christ of Latter-day Saints. Mormon missionaries began to adopt their now familiar uniforms of white shirts and ties during the 1950s, projecting to potential converts and the surrounding world a decorous and dignified visual appearance in line with the plain truth of their theological message. They further reinforced this temperate sensibility through new styles of worship, which tended to be more formal, sedate, and "reverential" than older charismatic traditions, such as speaking in tongues. By restraining and re-training the religious senses, by carefully domesticating and disciplining them, Mormons gradually moved more fully into the "mainstream" of American society, becoming "full-fledged members of the sober American middle class" (Bowman 2012).

There were also groups who pushed back against these middle-class norms of respectability, most notably perhaps in the case of the Jehovah's Witnesses. The Witnesses dissented theologically from the teachings of mainline Protestantism, but they also dissented stylistically by refusing to abide by ecumenical standards of tolerance and civil restraint. Through the 1930s, 1940s, and 1950s, they stridently broadcast their sectarian beliefs wherever they went, insisting on the truth of God's word to all within earshot. They refused to compartmentalize or keep contained their differences, and their proselytizing techniques often seemed militant, aggressive, and obnoxious. They knocked on doors, shouted on street corners, and distributed thousands of pamphlets, magazines, and newspapers. They exploited new electro-acoustic devices, such as loudspeakers, "sound cars," and portable phonograph players. They often targeted those whom they knew would be least receptive to their message, as in one famous incident when Witnesses in Quebec drove an armor-plated sound car through a predominantly Catholic neighborhood, blasting anti-Catholic invectives over its public-address system. In these ways and others, their practices became truly sensational, in both senses of the term.

Because of the hostility they engendered, the Witnesses often fell prey to mob violence, experiencing physical assault on their corporeal—and by extension, social—bodies. In addition, city officials devised an array of legal strategies for restraining the Witnesses' practices, several of which ended up being challenged in court. In 1946, for example, police in Lockport, New York, arrested a Jehovah's Witness minister for contravening a municipal ordinance by operating loudspeakers in a public park without a permit. Municipal noise ordinances such as this one were the products of early twentieth-century progressive reform efforts that had not taken into account potential implications for religious expression. Anti-noise crusaders tended to regard religion as something to be specially protected *from* noise, as in zones of quiet that were often enforced around houses of worship, rather than as a producer of noise. Yet the Witnesses celebrated loudspeakers and sound cars as essential means for fulfilling their most fundamental religious obligation, which was to evangelize. In the Lockport case, they described noise almost as a distinct style of religious worship in itself, and contested the city's enforcement of its ordinance as an egregious violation of their religious freedom. City officials denied that their actions had anything to do with religion, however. Noise was noise, they insisted, whether religiously motivated or not, and loudspeakers offered unparalleled opportunities to dominate others with sound. They expressed concern for the rights of unwilling listeners, who had been deprived of the *choice* as to whether to listen or not. The parties to the case thus advanced competing constitutional claims, pitting a right to be heard against a right to not have to hear.

The Lockport dispute eventually made its way to the US Supreme Court, where a 5:4 majority decided in the case of *Saia v. New York* that cities could not ban loudspeakers outright, but that they could regulate the time, place, and decibel level of public expression, provided that such regulations were "neutral" with regards to content. In so ruling, the Court treated the Witnesses' preaching as no different from any other form of political or non-commercial speech. It described noise as merely incidental to religion, properly conceived, as secondary and peripheral to its theological content. The Court's decision subtly affirmed a liberal conception of religion that privileged substance over form, interior faith over external sign. Even though the Court struck down Lockport's noise ordinance in this particular case, it made clear that dissenters could be disciplined into practicing proper modes of public piety, that when religion grew too loud or too combative, it, too, could be silenced. This case made evident how the politics of sensation figured into broader contests over religion's place in the modern world. If certain types of religion could form the basis for national solidarity, then others would have to be carefully regulated. A mid-century spirit of ecumenical toleration and civic inclusion had to have its limits (Weiner 2014).

THE FRAGMENTATION OF THE 1960s AND BEYOND

The inclusionary reach of the "Judeo-Christian" tradition had other obvious limits, as well. If it subtly made space only for those religions that could be practiced in the "right" kinds of ways, then it more overtly excluded those who did not adhere to "Judeo-Christian" religions at all. It could not easily be extended to encompass followers of Islam, Buddhism, or Sikhism, for example, each of which had been practiced in North America since at least the latter part of the nineteenth century. Its imagined moral consensus also took little cognizance of racial segregation in the United States. It described an "American Way of Life" shared primarily by white Americans, implicitly excluding African-Americans and other racial minorities from its expansive embrace. In point of fact, the United States was far more divided than the rhetoric of a "tri-faith America" seemed to allow (Schultz 2011).

The religious order of mid-century America was largely overturned by the dramatic transformations of the 1960s and subsequent decades, many of which bore important implications for the religious senses. The civil rights movement, for example, worked to undo nearly a century of racially discriminatory legislation that had carefully regulated who could be seen, heard, or touched in public and in private, a system that had been expressly designed to constrain certain kinds of sensory interaction. Religious actors and communities contributed in important ways to both sides of these contentious debates, most famously, of course, in the case of the Baptist minister, Martin Luther King, Jr. Religious actors also occupied opposing sides of the sexual revolution, which loosened social and legal proscriptions governing "illicit" forms of physical contact. Competing religious values regarding human sexuality, contraception, and abortion came to figure prominently in a growing divide between liberal and conservative factions.

These liberation movements developed their own particular sensory styles. Civil rights leaders, for example, drew on African-American oratorical traditions, which included lyrical cadences of preaching and regular use of call and response. Sit-ins and other demonstrations were effective as much for the visual, auditory, and tactile experiences that they enabled as for their intellectual or cognitive content. Iconic images of Christian ministers and Jewish rabbis marching side-by-side, linked arm in arm, singing hymns drawn from a shared biblical repertoire, gave material form to their spiritual message of human equality.

The political identity-based movements of the 1960s and 1970s generated a proliferation of other visual images, as well, especially when it came to the

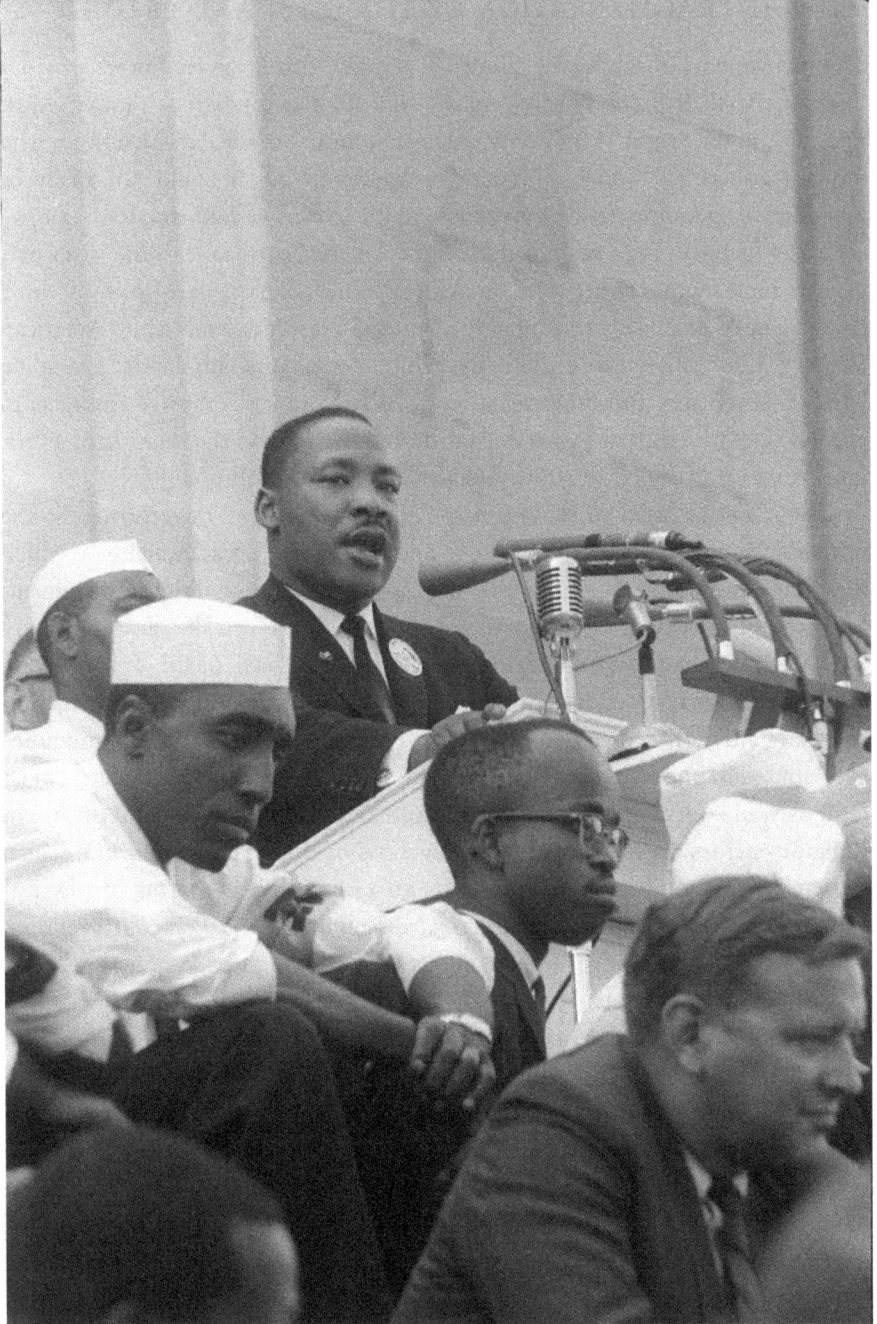

FIGURE 4.4: "I Have a Dream" speech: Martin Luther King, Jr. in Washington. Getty Images.

"color of Christ." Whereas Jesus had long been portrayed as white in Christian art and iconography, new theologies could give rise to new racial renderings. Liberation theologians of different shades and stripes re-imagined Jesus as alternately black, red, yellow, or brown. They produced arresting new images, which sought to cultivate new ways of seeing and new modes of thinking. Rather than transcend categories of race, they argued with forceful clarity that the physical body of Christ continued to matter. By re-coloring Jesus, they sought to claim him as their own, always on the side of those who were marginalized and oppressed (Blum and Harvey 2012: 215–49).

Other Christian groups also experienced profound transformations during this time, perhaps none as startling or potentially disorienting as those announced by the Roman Catholic Church at the Second Vatican Council (1962–5). In an effort to adapt the Church's teachings and traditions to modern times, Pope John XXIII introduced a wide range of theological and liturgical innovations, many of which directly impacted the everyday Catholic sensorium. Mass was no longer said in Latin, but in the vernacular, and congregations were encouraged to experiment with different types of musical styles during worship. The priest turned around to face his parishioners, rather than stand with his back to them, and he began wearing conventional trousers in place of the traditional cassock. Nuns were similarly permitted to forsake their habits and adopt modern dress. Most significantly, perhaps, the Church officially diminished the significance of its devotional culture, which involved a wide range of visual, olfactory, and tactile practices, such as lighting candles, carrying figurines, or blessing with holy water. This sensory regime had historically constituted a key point of demarcation between Catholic and Protestant Christianity, but the cumulative effect of these and other post-conciliar reforms was to lessen that divide. And while many Roman Catholics embraced these changes enthusiastically, others responded with greater ambivalence. "I suspect that the reason I despise the new liturgy is because it is mine," the Hispanic American Richard Rodriguez (1983: 113) wrote in his memoir. "It reflects and attempts to resolve the dilemma of Catholics just like me. The informal touches; the handshaking; the folk music; the insistence upon union—all these changes are aimed at serving Catholics who no longer live in a Catholic world." Vatican II did not reduce the significance of sensory practices, in other words, so much as it transformed them by accommodating them to the values and sensibilities of the outside world. For Catholics such as Rodriguez, the reforms materialized how much they had become like everyone else. "I live much of the day in a secular city where I do not measure the hours with the tolling bells of a church," he realized (1983: 116). In a society in which religious and social boundaries seemed less clearly defined, even the familiar echo of church bells came to sound differently.

The religious landscape of the 1960s and 1970s was remarkably fluid, especially for those who participated in the counterculture. Many young Americans and Europeans expressed their disillusionment with Western religions by turning to Asian or Eastern-inspired traditions, such as Buddhism, Hinduism, Hare Krishna, and Transcendental Meditation. They often encountered these traditions through mass-mediated visual representations of charismatic teachers and gurus, including D. T. Suzuki and the Maharishi Mahesh Yogi. These images played into and reinforced popular Orientalist notions that valorized the East as both hyper-spiritual and overly sensual. As American Studies scholar Jane Naomi Iwamura (2011: 7–8) has argued:

> By viewing an Oriental Monk figure in a magazine, we not only see his Asian face and manner of dress but also imagine the sound of his accent and the feel of his robes. Filmic portrayal implicates the senses even more, as we smell the wafting incense made visible in a temple shot. Prompting other sensory associations, our visually informed contact with Asian religious figures in news pictorials, television, and film generates its own stimulated environment that brings to life our often unconscious notions about the spiritual East.

"In-person" encounters with devotees of these movements were also highly mediated through the senses. Members of the International Society for Krishna Consciousness (ISKCON) chanted mantras and distributed *prasadam* (food offerings to the gods) in public places, such as parks and airports, while dressed in bright orange robes and bearing characteristically shaved heads with a queue of long hair. "It was kind of like a mystic experience," one convert described his first experience of an ISKCON communal meal, "with the smells and sights and everything" (Zeller 2012: 697). Zen Buddhism, on the other hand, which rose to prominence during the late 1950s, attracted followers not through its noise and hyper-sensoriality, but through its emphasis on silence, stillness, and contemplative breathing practices. It exerted broader influence on Western culture through the musical experimentations of composer John Cage and the poetic and literary imaginings of the Beats. In either case, Eastern spirituality proved attractive to Western audiences as much for its distinct ways of using the body and sensing the world as for its substantive theological content. These traditions seemed to offer radical visual, auditory, olfactory, and gustatory departures from the perceived drabness of the 1950s.

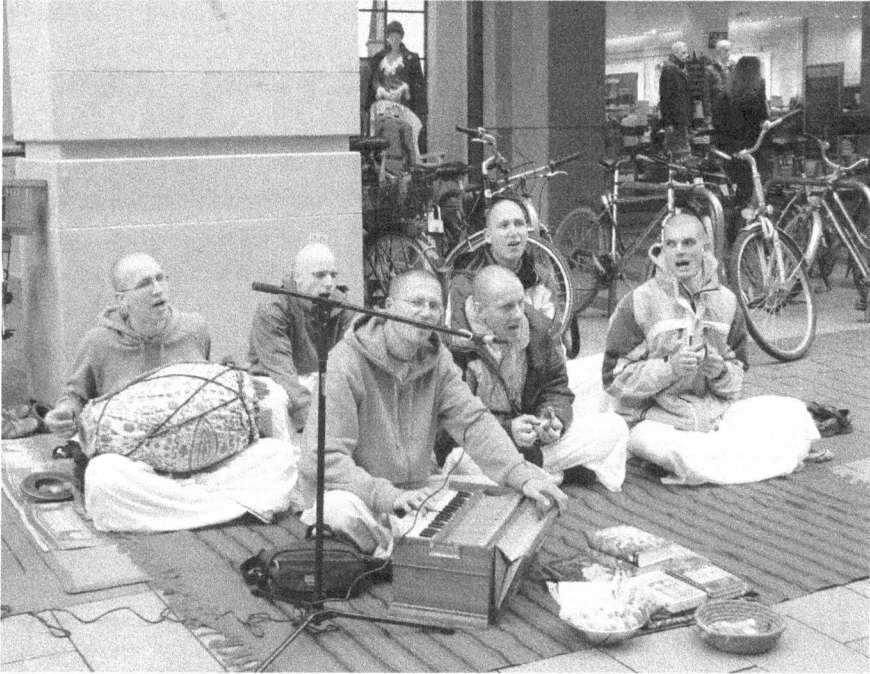

FIGURE 4.5: Krishna devotees chanting on a street corner in Leipzig, Germany. Photograph by Vaishnava 108. Public domain.

Asian religions were practiced not only by white converts, but also increasingly by transnational migrants, who brought their beliefs and rituals with them. In the United States, for example, changes in immigration laws in 1965 gradually led to greater numbers of Muslims, Hindus, Buddhists, Sikhs, Latino Catholics, and others, all of whom negotiated American society, in part, through the senses. Experiencing familiar sensations in new contexts, such as hearing the Islamic call to prayer or smelling the aroma of incense in a temple, could generate powerful feelings of continuity and belonging, connecting migrants to the homelands they had left behind, while *not* experiencing those same sensations might produce overwhelming emotions of nostalgia and regret. Observing traditional dietary laws could further reinforce a connection to the past while also functioning, in part, to minimize cultural assimilation.

Across all religions, sensorial practices have traditionally played an important part in constructing collective identity and demarcating boundaries between insiders and outsiders. They also have marked intra-group distinctions, whether between high-caste and low-caste Hindus, between women and men, or among varied regional and ethnic traditions. These practices do not remain static in new social contexts, but instead serve as a primary nexus for adaptation and change. Reformers across traditions have pushed for innovation and transformation while traditionalists have worked to defend what they perceive as most authentic or pure. Just as Catholic and Jewish immigrants during the nineteenth century debated which aspects of their traditions they should preserve in the "New World," so, too, have more recent migrants. At the Hindu Temple of Atlanta, for example, researcher Kathryn McClymond (2006) found that members continue to make offerings of fruit, milk, and other foods to the deities, as they did in India, but that they also have introduced a weekly communal vegetarian meal, akin in some ways to Catholic fish fries, as a means of adapting to American society and sustaining ethnic identity, but also as a way of upholding a religious ideal.

New communication and travel technologies have made exchanges between homeland and diaspora much more rapid and immediate, thus debates about ritual adaptation now take place transnationally, rather than merely within a given migrant community. They also transpire across disparate traditions, for negotiating religious diversity has never been solely a matter of resolving theological or doctrinal differences, but of engaging with different kinds of sensorial mediations, of making sense of new religious sights, sounds, and smells. Against the background of a global religious revival and, more recently, a global war on terror, these public expressions have grown increasingly politicized. Sensory practices have emerged as key arenas for broader debates about the place of religious minorities in pluralistic liberal democracies, especially in the case of Islam. In the United States and in Western Europe, critics have voiced opposition to the construction of new mosques and minarets, to the sounding of the call to prayer, and to the wearing of the hijab or headscarf. They have alternately complained that the public practice of Islam violates widespread secularist norms or that it stands as an affront to Western (i.e. Christian) civilization. Others have appealed to ideals of pluralism and multiculturalism to defend such practices, arguing that the public realm can and should accommodate a wide range of religious displays. Moreover, they have noted that the modernist impulse to privatize and interiorize religion has implicitly privileged those religions that place less emphasis on, or even express greater suspicion toward, the human senses (Weiner 2014).

These disputes have had the unexpected consequence of rendering many Christian practices problematic, as well. In France, for example, which is governed by strict notions of secularism (*laicité*) that restrict publicly "conspicuous" religious symbols, Muslims have questioned why headscarves seem conspicuous, but not necklaces displaying crosses or stars of David. Similar debates have transpired in the United States, as religious minorities have grown more vocal in calling attention to how the "secular" public realm has always been marked by particular forms of religious expression, rather than by none at all. As early as 1948, for example, Rabbi Mordecai Kaplan (1948: 102) pointedly asked, "Why should Jews consider it a good American practice for Christians to display Christmas trees and sing Christmas carols in public, while feeling too inhibited to display the Hanukkah lights publicly and to sing Hebrew hymns in the streets?" In more recent decades, a number of contentious legal disputes have called into question visual and auditory practices that had long been taken for granted, such as displaying Ten Commandments monuments or nativity scenes on public property or offering communal prayers in public schools. These lawsuits have hinged on how to interpret constitutional disestablishment, which distinguishes the United States from many European countries in which state churches continue to enjoy particular legal privileges. In the US, courts have tended to affirm important safeguards for private religious expression while striking down displays that seem to imply governmental approval or endorsement. Yet critics of these decisions have bemoaned what they perceive as the banishing of God and Christianity from the public sphere, a complaint that led, in part, to the rise of the Religious Right.

Other practices have become subject to political contestation, as well, often in surprising and unexpected ways. Many Native Americans, for example, have sought to reclaim their cultural and religious heritage by recovering traditional rituals, such as the Sun Dance and sweat lodge ceremonies. These same practices have often been re-appropriated by New Age enthusiasts, leading to important debates about cultural ownership and authenticity. In recent years, there has also been a growing movement to ban the practice of male circumcision, which has pitted religious and parental rights against liberal notions of bodily autonomy. These disparate examples underscore the complex politics of religious sensation in the modern world. Contentious debates about religion and public life have focused as much on embodied practices as on competing theologies. As the sights, sounds, and textures of religious life have crossed social and geographic boundaries, they have mediated contact among diverse religionists who have responded to them in different ways.

New media technologies have also continued to transform the religious sensorium, most notably with the advent of the internet at the end of the twentieth century. Online religion became a thriving concern in different forms and serving different ends. Bricks-and-mortar institutions established virtual presences, offering free "tours" that publicized their services and programs to members and non-members alike. Other popular sites encouraged visitors to pose questions directly to priests, rabbis, or Buddhist monks. Proselytizing soon flourished on the internet, and several websites even offered opportunities to perform virtual rituals, such as *pujas* (Hindu offerings) or pilgrimages. New rituals have even been created that can *only* be performed online. Critics have raised doubts about the authenticity of these cyber-rituals, often expressly because of how they transform the physical experience of performing religion. They have questioned whether it is possible to embark on a pilgrimage without "going" anywhere or to participate in a ritual without "doing" anything. Virtual religion seems only able to reproduce certain kinds of religious sensations. It tends to emphasize religion's visual and auditory dimensions, though new motion-sensing technology developed for gaming might simulate its kinesthetic components, as well. Yet it remains difficult to replicate the "lower" senses of smell, touch, and taste, all of which figure prominently in "real world" religion. Cyber-pilgrimages also seem to promote more individualized experiences, which diminish the personal sacrifice or suffering that often accompanies physical journeys. Yet online enthusiasts argue that virtual religion can connect isolated individuals to broader communities that they might not encounter in person. They suggest that visualizing rituals online can trigger the imagining of other kinds of sensations, and many sites even encourage physical re-enactment, inviting visitors to remove their shoes, light candles, turn on music, or walk in nature. Cyber-pilgrimages can serve as precursors to the "real" thing, motivating potential travelers for their trips or preparing them for what to expect. In other words, what is only seen or heard at first may later lead to other, more multisensory, experiences. Either way, religion's pervasiveness online demonstrates how its ritual components remained vitally important into the twenty-first century (Hill-Smith 2011).

Finally, we also find evidence for the continued significance of the religious senses in domains that are not as obviously "religious." Recent surveys have identified growing numbers of religious "nones" (those who do not claim any particular religious identity or affiliation) and of the "spiritual but not religious." Yet these groups often seem to believe, act, and feel in ways that resonate with traditionally religious concerns. This is evident in the ethical choices that they may make regarding food production and consumption, for example. Motivated by a range of moral, physiological, and environmental concerns, growing numbers of Americans and Europeans have promoted alternative "foodways," such as homesteading, vegetarianism, veganism, organic eating, local food (locavorism), or slow food (Finch 2010). In some cases, these decisions have been linked to particular religious traditions, as in the tendency of Euro-American converts to Buddhism to adopt vegetarian diets. In other cases, however, vegetarians or locavores may not define their choices as "religious," yet may describe them in religious terms, using language such as conversion or devotion (Zeller 2014). Religious sights, sounds, and tastes have also flowed beyond the boundaries of conventional religion when they have been commoditized, as in the development of "world music" traditions or when religious imagery has been exploited for commercial advertising. Each of these examples further reinforces how the religious senses have not been diminished in the modern world, as much as they have been transformed and re-deployed. Individuals and communities continue to invest questions about what they should properly touch or taste, see or hear, smell or feel, with deep moral and spiritual significance.

CONCLUSION

Contrary to the expectations of secularization narratives of modernity, religion did not fade away during the twentieth century, but instead grew increasingly diffuse, fragmented, and contested. The last several decades have witnessed religion's pluralization and politicization, rather than its privatization or disappearance. New media technologies and cultures of consumption have transformed the ways religion is experienced, and processes of globalization and transnationalism have multiplied occasions for contact and conflict. Debates about religion's place in pluralistic liberal democracies have grown particularly contentious in light of new migratory patterns and new national security threats. Each of these complex developments has directly affected the religious sensorium as religionists have continued to act out their beliefs, materializing them through concrete sensational forms. By cultivating particular ways of seeing, hearing, smelling, touching, and tasting, they have striven to communicate with the divine and to establish a distinct social presence. They have invested their lives with transcendent meaning, constructed personal identity, and built community, while they also have worked to articulate and negotiate their differences. Despite what many might have expected, religion continued to make a clamor in the twenty-first century, though whether this noise will be perceived as harmonious or cacophonous remains very much in question.

CHAPTER FIVE

The Senses in Philosophy and Science: From Sensation to Computation

MATTHEW NUDDS

Both philosophy and science in the twentieth century inherited a conception of perception and the senses that had remained more or less unchanged for the previous three centuries. This conception was broadly *empiricist*: each sense modality consists of a sensory receptor or sense organ that is sensitive to a particular kind of physical stimulus; this sensory receptor is connected to the brain, via bundles of nerves that function to transmit the stimulation of the sensory receptor; the effect of this stimulation on the brain is to produce an experience of certain kinds of sensations. Perception consists either in having these sensations, or results from further processes—of inference or association— that have these sensations as their starting point. At the beginning of the twentieth century, this empiricist conception of the senses constituted the framework for theorizing about the senses in physiology, philosophy, and psychology.

Within philosophy, this chapter will focus on the contribution of analytic philosophy to theorizing the senses and sense experience. The origins of this tradition may be traced to Gottlob Frege and the Logical Positivists, and to Bertrand Russell and G. E. Moore. Analytic philosophy came to be the dominant philosophical tradition in the English-speaking world over the course of the twentieth century, displacing Hegelian idealism. It is characterized by the central place it gives in philosophy to philosophical accounts of language. As Dummett puts it, analytic philosophy holds "first, that, a comprehensive account of thought can be attained through a philosophical account of language, and, second, that a comprehensive account can only be so attained" (1993: 4). More recently, philosophers studying the senses in the analytic tradition have drawn on the results of science and, in particular, on empirical psychology.

Other important streams within philosophy that engage with the senses and sense experience and that have had an impact on our understanding of science and the senses include phenomenology and feminist philosophy. Both these approaches differ from the analytic approach in the attitude they take to the natural sciences. In many ways the interests of phenomenology overlap with those of analytic philosophy of mind. Both are interested in analyzing sensory consciousness and in understanding the intentionality of the mind. But whereas philosophers working in the analytic tradition embrace the methods and results of the natural sciences and view sensory consciousness and perception as part of the natural order, phenomenologists bracket the methods and results of science, and see their approach as neutral with respect to scientific results (for a useful survey of the phenomenological approach, see Smith 2011). Feminist philosophers of science have elaborated a critical approach to the methods of the natural sciences. In particular, they argue that the distinction between "the facts" as determined by science and non-epistemic (i.e. social, moral, and political) "values" is not clear-cut—on the contrary, facts are shot through with values—and that we should not uncritically rely on the results of empirical science (for an introduction to these issues, see Potter 2006).

SENSORY PHYSIOLOGY

By the beginning of the twentieth century, developments in science had deepened the understanding of various aspects of sensory processes, in particular the physiology of the sensory receptors—the eyes, ears, nose, and so on—and of the properties and functioning of the nerves that connect the sensory receptors to the brain. In addition, a number of dedicated areas of the brain had been identified to which nerves from different sensory receptors project. But the conceptual framework within which these discoveries were made, and the conception of the mechanisms of perception of which they formed a part, remained broadly empiricist.

In particular it was thought that the stimulation of different sensory transducers—the retina, the cochlea, the tongue, the nose, the skin—produced an experience of sensations. These sensations were taken to vary along two dimensions. Firstly, the kind of sensation varied according to the kind of stimulation that produced it—stimulation of the retina produced distinctively visual sensations, stimulation of the cochlea produced auditory sensations, stimulation of the taste buds (sensory neurons in the tongue) produced sensations of taste, and so on. Secondly, the character of the particular kind of sensation produced varied according to variations in the physical properties of the particular stimulus so that, for example, brighter light produced more intense visual sensations, higher frequency sound-wave vibrations produced higher-pitch sensations, and so on.

It was supposed that there was a straightforward relationship between the stimulation of the sensory transducer and the resultant pattern of sensations produced. In the case of vision, for example, it was thought that when a retinal neuron was stimulated by light the stimulation was transmitted by a connecting nerve to the brain, where it produced a sensation. It was thought that the character of the resultant sensation was determined by the physical properties of the stimulating light: in particular, that the intensity of the sensation was determined by the brightness of the light, and the color of the sensation was determined by the wavelength of the light. Furthermore, the arrangement of nerves was thought to be such that the pattern and structure of the visual sensations produced was isomorphic with the pattern of light striking the retina. The eyes project light onto the retina to produce a retinal image of the scene in front of the perceiver; the resultant pattern of sensations was isomorphic to the retinal image; so visual experience must consist of sensations arranged in a two-dimensional image corresponding to the retinal image.

Although each of the senses was known to be sensitive to different physical stimuli, they were each taken to produce sensations that correspond to those stimuli in a similar way to vision. In each case, it was supposed that the qualities of the sensations corresponded to physical properties of the stimuli, and that in each case the pattern of sensations corresponded to the pattern of stimulation, so that there was an isomorphism between the physical stimulation of the sensory transducers and the sensations that resulted.

This picture of the operation of the senses was very compelling and *seemed* very plausible. Its seeming plausibility must explain, at least in part, why it remained the dominant conception of the senses for as long as it did. The picture also made clear what must be explained by a theory of perception. It

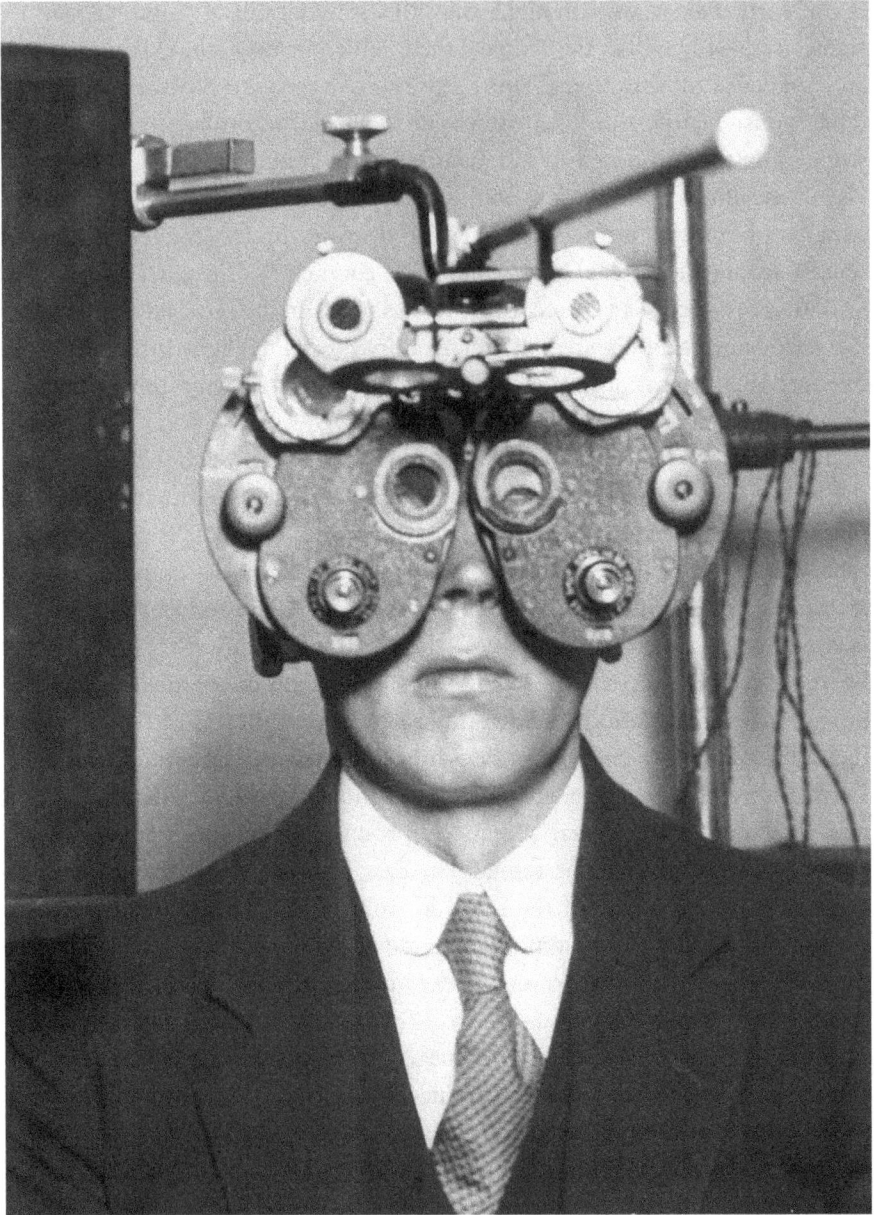

FIGURE 5.1: Eye examination. Getty Images.

must explain how we are able to perceive ordinary objects on the basis of the images and sensations produced in the mind, and it must explain in detail the physiology of the senses and how the stimulation of the sensory transducers produces images and sensations in the mind.

One focus of empirical investigations during this period was therefore the relation between stimulation of the sense organs and the sensations produced in the mind. These investigations were continuous with work done during the second half of the nineteenth century. In color perception, for example, attempts were made to discover the qualities of sensations of color—in particular what were the primary colors in terms of which sensations our experience of color should be explained—and what properties of light produced sensations with those qualities. Similarly, in the case of auditory perception, the relation between the physical properties of the stimulus and the qualities of the sensations produced was investigated.

These investigations went hand in hand with attempts to better understand the structures of the different sensory transducers. Work was done on the physiology of the ear—in particular the structure and function of the basilar membrane whose stimulation produced auditory sensations (see Boring 1942: Ch. 12). Similar investigations were carried out for taste, and it was discovered that there are four kinds of taste buds. Their function remained poorly understood during the first decades of the century: rather than thinking that each different kind of taste bud was sensitive to a different kind of stimulus—to saltiness, sourness, or sweetness—and that each produced a different kind of sensation, it was thought that the different kinds of taste bud were more or less sensitive to all flavor stimuli so produced sensations of the same kind (Boring 1942: 429ff.). Some novel senses, such as a muscle sense or a proprioceptive sense (the term was introduced by Sherrington in 1907), were postulated. These senses were taken to involve sensory transducers sensitive to a particular kind of physical stimuli and as producing distinctive sensations, and so as "new" senses in addition to the five of common sense. But since neither involved a sense organ (of the kind associated with the five senses), nor enabled the perception of things independent of the perceiver (both were taken to be a form of "inward-looking sense") they did not lead to the rejection or even revision of the conventional Western fivefold division of the sensorium.

Although some progress was made in filling in the details of the physiology of the senses and the limits of their sensitivity to stimuli, several aspects of the mechanisms of perception remained puzzling. In particular it was not known why the stimulation of nerves resulted in different kinds of sensation. The nerve fibers in different senses were thought to be functionally the same, and yet stimulation of the nerves in different senses produced different kinds of sensations. There seemed to be two possible explanations of this fact. Either the nerves themselves must have specific "energies" that resulted in different kinds of sensation, or the stimulation of the different areas of the brain to which the nerves projected produced different kinds of sensations (see Keeley 2013). Neither answer was particularly satisfactory. The problem highlighted the existence of an explanatory gap between stimulation and sensation.

SENSORY PSYCHOLOGY

Physiological and psychological investigations of the senses were not independent of one another, but whereas physiology focused on the nature of sensory transducers and of the nerves connecting them to the brain, psychology focused on the resultant sensations, in particular their relation to stimuli and how they led to the perception of everyday objects. At the turn of the century, psychology depended on introspection as a method and supposed the contents of the mind ultimately to be simple atomic impressions or sensations (of the kind physiologists supposed were produced by the stimulation of nerves). The task of psychology was twofold. First, "to discover the fundamental and introspectively unanalyzable elements of consciousness and to formulate the principles of combination whereby these elements are synthesized into the complex and familiar experiences of ordinary life" (Cummins 1983: 120). Second, to give some account of the connection between the elements of consciousness and the physiological processes that give rise to them, and in particular to find connections between the character of impressions and the external stimuli that give rise to them. There were difficulties in completing both these tasks.

The first difficulty was with the empiricist characterization of experience. When we introspect our visual experiences we are not confronted with a pattern of sensations like the spots of a pointillist painting; rather, we are aware of the ordinary material objects we take ourselves to see. If asked to introspect and describe your experience of seeing an apple, for example, the best description you could offer is in terms of what you take yourself to see—i.e., that it is an experience as of an apple. So the task of discovering the "unanalyzable elements of consciousness" was bound to fail. There was no introspective reason to think that there existed atomistic sensations involved in visual perception that could be the raw data for psychological explanation. The empiricists were not offering a neutral characterization of experience discovered through introspection; rather, their characterization was the result of a theoretical conception of the operation of senses. The raw data of experience that was supposed to be the foundation of perception was a theoretical construct. But if simple sensations could not be discovered in experience then the introspectionist project of explaining the perception of everyday objects in terms of the sensations discovered in experience was fatally undermined. The result was that no progress was made in providing an explanation of perception.

The second difficulty was methodological. In order to investigate the relation between stimulation and sensation, introspectionists conducted experiments intended to uncover law-like connections between properties of stimuli and properties of the resultant sensations. A typical experiment might involve making a noise (by, e.g., dropping a hard ball onto a hard surface) that produced a sensation in a listener; a second noise was made (by increasing the height of the drop) to produce a sensation that was just noticeably louder for the listener; a third noise was then made whose intensity was again increased to produce a just noticeably louder sensation; and so on. In this way it was possible to plot the relation between the intensity of stimulation and the intensity of sensation it caused in order to establish a law linking the two.

A problem arose if the responses of a listener in the experiment did not fit the law-like pattern. This could happen for two different reasons. The listener could either be misdescribing her sensations—failing to notice a difference, for example—or she could be psychologically idiosyncratic—her senses might not operate according to the law-like pattern. The problem was that there was no experimental way to determine which explanation was correct. In fact, it was not even possible to be sure that the responses of a subject who did fit the pattern did so because her experiences were produced in accordance with the law. The evidence was consistent with her both being psychologically idiosyncratic *and* her misdescribing her sensations. This highlighted a fundamental methodological problem with the introspectionist approach. The only access the experimenter had to a subject's sensations was inference from the nature of the stimulation, or inference from the subject's responses (in particular, her verbal reports). The first kind of inference depended on the very law that the experimenter was trying to discover. The second relied on the accuracy of the subject's introspective reports. Since there was no way to check the accuracy of the subject's reports, they could not play the required role in explanation. The problem "was enough to kill off any psychology based on introspection" (Cummins 1983: 124; see Ch. 4 for further discussion of the problem). Two different movements in psychology—Gestalt psychology on one hand and behaviorism on the other—can be seen in part as responses to the two difficulties faced by introspectionism.

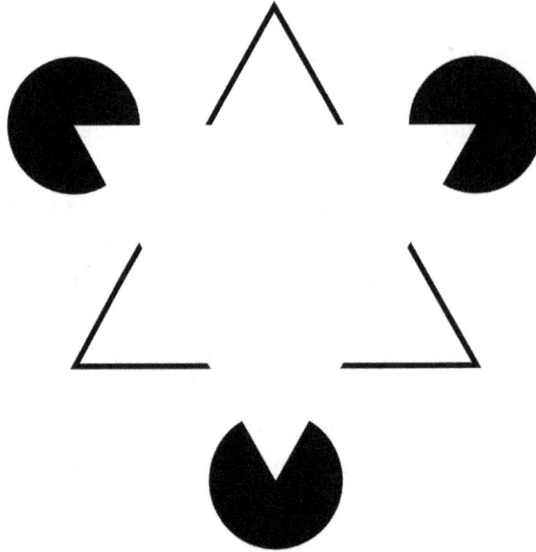

FIGURE 5.2: Kanizsa triangle. The perception of the inverted triangle is an example of the law of closure. Note also how it appears brighter. This is a perception for which there is no stimulus, and thus exemplifies the extent to which perception is an exercise in projection—*David Howes*.

Gestalt theory had its origins in Germany in the 1920s, and is most closely associated with Max Wertheimer, Wolfgang Kohler, and Kurt Koffka (the so-called "Berlin School"; for a history, see Ash 1998). Its principles were applied to a range of disciplines from biology and psychology to film theory. Gestalt psychology called into question the idea that experience was constructed out of simple or atomic sensations. Experience, the Gestalt theorists argued, was fundamentally structured or organized, and the basic units of experience were these organized wholes or "gestalten." The Gestalt theorists' project was to characterize the way perceptual experience was organized, and to describe the laws or principles that determined this organization. For example, the law of similarity says that visual elements will be grouped together if they are similar to one another; the law of proximity says that visual elements that are close to one another will tend to be perceived as a group; and the law of closure says that elements will be perceived as a complete figure even when parts are missing. They also looked for explanations for the holding of these laws in terms of the physiological organization of the brain.

Gestalt approaches offered alternative conceptions of the nature of experience, and so of the basis of perception. Rather than seeing perception as somehow the result of an experienced pattern of sensations, Gestalt theorists supposed that experience had an intrinsic organization. What was required of an explanation of our perception of ordinary objects was therefore different to that required by the empiricist conception of experience. The Gestalt theorists described a number of features of experience—figure-ground separation, the phi phenomenon—that would later figure as significant explananda in computational theories of perception, though the Gestalt theorists' own explanations were unsatisfactory. The rise to power of the Nazis led to the premature breakup of many of the institutions within which psychology was conducted in Germany. Many Jewish psychologists were dismissed from their posts, and other psychologists had their work diverted to other projects, including participating in officer selection (Ash 1998: 326). Some of those who were dismissed managed to relocate in the United States, but in any event Gestalt theory ceased to be a dominant research program in psychology.

At the same time that Gestalt psychology was developing in Germany, behaviorist psychology was emerging as the dominant paradigm in the United States. Behaviorism is the view most closely associated with J. B. Watson (1924) and B. F. Skinner (1938) and can be seen as a response to the methodological problems facing introspectionism. Those methodological problems stemmed from the problem of measuring, in any methodically acceptable way, "inner" events that take place in consciousness. Since they could not be measured, such events could play no role in scientific explanations of psychological processes. Behaviorists responded to this problem by bypassing any appeal to conscious events in their explanations. Rather than attempting to find laws linking stimulation with sensation, they looked for laws directly linking stimulation to behavioral response. The behaviorist project was to explain all animal behavior in terms of patterns of behavioral response to patterns of stimuli. Behaviorism's success was limited. The problem of explaining perception had been that of explaining perceptual experience. Behaviorism's rejection of the role of consciousness meant that it simply did not address that problem. There were other important areas of psychology that behaviorism conspicuously failed to explain, including language, as Noam Chomsky argued in his review of Skinner's *Verbal Behaviour* (Chomsky 1959).

Chomsky characterized the latter book "as a paradigm example of a futile tendency in modern speculation about language and mind" (Chomsky 1967), and his review is commonly regarded as sounding the death knell of behaviorism. The rejection of behaviorism was also made possible by the rise of the computer and computer program as a paradigm for psychological explanation, and for how "inner" events could feature in scientific explanations in a methodologically acceptable way (see below).

PHILOSOPHY OF PERCEPTION

For the first half of the twentieth century, most philosophers accepted some version of the sense datum theory—the view that perceptual experience consists in the awareness of non-material objects (sense data) that instantiate the sensory qualities that are apparent in experience (see Ayer 1940, 1956; Broad 1923, 1927; Moore 1922; Price 1932; Russell 1912, 1927). This theory was the philosophical analog of the empiricist conception of perception that dominated physiology and psychology, and a direct descendent of the empiricist theories of perception to be found in Locke and Hume. Although his terminology differs ("sense data" rather than "impression"), Russell's version of the argument from illusion is strikingly similar to Hume's published 250 years earlier; other sense datum theorists' arguments closely followed Russell's. Part of the reason for this longstanding and widespread acceptance of the theory within philosophy was the fact that it was taken to be evident, simply from reflection on experience, that when I *seem* to see something there actually exists something that is the object of my awareness. As H. H. Price puts it: "When I say 'This table appears brown to me' it is quite plain that I am acquainted with an actual instance of brownness (or equally plainly with a pair of instances when I see double). This cannot indeed be proved, but it is absolutely evident and indubitable" (Price 1932: 63). What Price takes to be absolutely evident and indubitable is that when I seem to see something brown, there exists something brown that is present in my experience and with which I am acquainted. But on some occasions my experiences of seeming to see something brown are illusory—e.g., when I see double—or hallucinatory; and on those occasions I seem to see something brown even when there is no brown material or physical object there for me to see. It follows that what I am acquainted with in experience cannot be an ordinary material object; it must be a non-material or non-physical object, a *sense datum*. Early sense datum theorists did not always take sense data to be mind-dependent, since they allowed the possibility of objects that were neither physical nor mind-dependent; later sense datum theorists, especially those few in the second half of the century, took sense data to be mind-dependent objects.

Sense datum theorists did not deny that when we see something it seems to us that we are aware of a mind-independent material object—it seems to me that the apple I see on the table in front of me is an ordinary mind-independent material object—but they viewed this as a mistake: in fact I am aware of sense data with the appearance of an apple. It doesn't follow, however, that I don't see the apple. Sense datum theorists took there to be a relation between the sense data we are aware of in experience and the ordinary material objects that we take ourselves to see such that we can correctly say that we see those ordinary objects; but we see them only indirectly, in virtue of having an experience of sense data. Sense datum theorists were therefore indirect realists (in contrast to theorists who denied that we see ordinary material objects and who were therefore idealists or phenomenalists—neither views that were widely held).

Sense datum theorists understood there to be different kinds of sense data associated with the different senses. Vision had visual sense data, hearing had auditory sense data, touch tactile sense data, and so on. These sense data differed in the sensory qualities that they were taken to instantiate. Visual sense data were taken to instantiate visual sensory qualities such as color and shape; auditory sense data were taken to instantiate auditory sensory qualities such as pitch and timbre; and so on. Accordingly, what distinguished the different senses were the different kinds of sense data that the experiences of those senses involve. Seeing is just perceiving something in virtue of having an experience involving the awareness of visual sense data. We have five different senses because we have experiences involving five different kinds of sense data. It is possible, according to this kind of view, to perceive the same material object with more than one sense—we can see and touch the same thing, for example—but in doing so we perceive the object in virtue of having experiences involving the awareness of different kinds of sense data—visual and tactile respectively.

FURTHER WORK IN PHYSIOLOGY

In the 1940s and 1950s, work in neurophysiology focused on identifying different areas of the cortex specialized for different sensory functions—for vision, touch, or hearing. Experiments were conducted (on animals) using small electrodes placed on the surface of the cortex to record brain activity; various different stimuli—flashes of light or clicks—were then used to identify the parts of the cortex responsible for visual, auditory, somatosensory, etc., activity (see Hubel and Wiesel 2004: Ch. 3).

By the mid-1950s techniques had been developed that allowed the recording of the firing rate of individual neurons within sensory pathways, in particular the activity of the neurons in the projection areas of the visual cortex of animals, and the activity of individual neurons in the retina. Early experiments were conducted using frogs (Barlow 1953), and the responses of individual retinal cells of frogs were recorded in the presence of various targets presented in the frog's visual field. The surprising discovery was made that different retinal cells responded to specific kinds of target (see Barlow 1972: 380)

What these physiological discoveries apparently showed was that the retina was not made up of receptors that responded individually to simple stimuli (i.e. to light). Rather, groups of receptors responded to particular features of the stimulus—to movement, the presence of an edge or slope, etc.—and their response indicated the presence and distribution of these features. That did not fit with the empiricist conception of vision as a system that functioned to produce patterns of simple sensations that were isomorphic with a pattern of physical stimulation of the sensory receptors. According to the empiricist, experience was made up of simple sensations whose qualities vary in such a way as to reflect the physical properties of the stimulus. However, the physiological evidence suggested that two different neurons could respond in exactly the same way, but with one responding to an edge and the other to a slope. So the *way* the neuron responded—the character of the response—did not reflect the properties of the stimulus. Rather, what appeared to matter was what the neuron's response was a response to:

> each single neuron can perform a much more complex and subtle task than had previously been thought. Neurons do not loosely and unreliably remap the luminous intensities of the visual image onto our sensorium, but instead detect pattern elements, discriminate the depth of objects, ignore irrelevant causes of variation . . . This amounts to a revolution in our outlook . . . This revolution stemmed from physiological work and makes us realise that the activity of each neuron may play a significant role in perception.
>
> Barlow 1972: 380

As well as investigating the activity of retinal neurons, it was possible to record the activity of cells in the brain. In pioneering work that eventually led to the award of a Nobel Prize, Hubel and Wiesel investigated the activity of individual neurons in the visual cortex of the cat, and discovered neurons that fired only when a particular feature—such as a line, or an edge, or a slope—stimulated a field of retinal receptors, but did not fire when individual receptors are stimulated within the same field. These neurons in the cortex acted as a kind of on/off switch that signaled the presence of the relevant feature in the retina's receptive field. They also discovered cells that responded to more elaborate stimuli (reported in a paper Hubel calls their "magnum opus"—Hubel and Wiesel 2004: 105). They called these "complex" and "hypercomplex" cells and showed that they responded to information from simpler cells. They suggested that cells in the visual cortex are organized hierarchically, and become selective for more complex properties of the retinal input at each level of the hierarchy. The "revolution in outlook" that resulted from these discoveries fundamentally undermined the empiricist conception of the physiological function of the senses. (Such experiments also contributed to the growing controversy in the twentieth century over the use of animals in scientific experimentation; see, for example, Harraway 1989.) At the same time that these physiological discoveries were being made, developments in computers and in the understanding of computation were having a significant influence on both psychology and philosophy.

COMPUTERS AND COMPUTER VISION

Developments in computing during the war led to attempts, beginning in the mid-1950s, to produce machines that could think (the beginnings of artificial intelligence are usually dated to the Dartmouth Summer Research Project on Artificial Intelligence, held in 1956 at Dartmouth College). The aim was to program computers to accomplish the tasks performed by intelligent humans, tasks such as solving problems by reasoning and deduction, and understanding language. Relatively early in the development of artificial intelligence, attempts were made to produce machines that could "see." The idea was that a video camera could be attached to a robot that would enable the robot to perceive its environment: the camera would provide visual input, and a computer program could use that input to work out what objects were in front of the camera, and how those objects were arranged. All the program had to do was to transform the two-dimensional image produced by the camera into a description or representation of the three-dimensional objects in the robot's environment—to interpret two-dimensional images in terms of three-dimensional scenes.

Initially it was supposed that writing such a program would be a relatively straightforward task. Marvin Minsky assigned it as a project for undergraduates at a summer school in 1966 (he directed students to "spend the summer linking a camera to a computer and getting the computer to describe what it sees"). The task was made easier by restricting the input to "synthetic worlds" containing variously shaped wooden blocks. The problem turned out to be far more difficult than had been anticipated. Interpreting an image of wooden blocks—identifying the objects in a scene—required first that the edges of the blocks be identified, then that different edges be grouped together as edges of a single object, then that the shape of the object be identified. This simple-sounding problem was in fact very difficult to solve. Some of what appeared to be edges of objects were in fact shadows and so should be ignored, but identifying which "edges" were shadows required first identifying the objects that cast them; working out which edges belonged together as edges of a single object was made difficult by the fact that objects occluded each other so that edges that are adjacent in an image may be edges of a single object or two distinct but overlapping objects; the shape of an object in an image varied with perspective, so to determine the shape of an object from an image required that perspective is taken into account; and so on.

The early attempts to produce machines that could think or see, although not particularly successful in the short term, were nonetheless influential. One kind of influence was on philosophy. Trying to model mental processes using a computer led to the idea that the mind should be thought of as analogous to a computer program. Computer programs are essentially rules that manipulate symbols that can be interpreted as standing for or representing things (e.g., numbers). The symbols are manipulated in such a way as to implement some function (e.g., arithmetic). If the mind is like a computer program then mental states, such as beliefs and desires, could be understood as relations between the thinker and symbolic representations (often conceived as a sentence in a language of thought). Such symbolic representations represent things (or have "semantic content"). So the belief that snow is white involves the thinker being related in a belief-like way to a symbolic representation "snow is white" (the semantic content of "snow is white" is that snow is white). Thinking could then be understood as a computational process that manipulates symbolic representations in such a way that the relations between their semantic properties are preserved. This provides a way to understand both the intentionality of thought—the content of thoughts should be understood in the same way as the semantic content of symbols—and the process of thinking—thinking should be understood as the computational manipulation of symbols. Another influence was on psychology.

FURTHER DEVELOPMENTS IN PSYCHOLOGY

Early work on computer vision treated the problem as an "artificial" one, quite separate from the theories of the operation of the physiological senses. At the same time, work in neurophysiology and neuroscience was providing new insights into how the physiological senses actually operate. In particular there was evidence, as described above, that assemblages of neurons functioned somehow to detect features. A puzzle remained as to how they did this.

David Courtney Marr (1982) applied ideas from computational theory to the problems of understanding the operation of the senses. He argued that the assemblages of neurons discovered by neurophysiologists should be viewed as implementing computational processes. The key to understanding vision, he argued, was to understand the problem that the visual system has to solve, to work out the particular computational algorithm that it uses to solve that problem, and then to show how the computation of that algorithm is implemented in neural processes in the retina and visual cortex.

Marr viewed the problem that the visual system had to solve as that of producing a representation of three-dimensional objects and their locations in space from "arrays of image intensity values as detected by the photoreceptors in the retina" (Marr 1982: 31). (This was analogous the problem faced by computer vision theorists.) He conceived of this problem as that of transforming one representation—of image intensity values—into another representation—of three-dimensional objects in space. He supposed, further, this transformation could be broken down into a series of steps, the first of which would extract abstract features of the retinal image, the second of which would produce a "2½-D sketch" that represents surfaces and their orientations, before finally producing the three-dimensional representation of objects. Each of these steps might in turn comprise a series of smaller steps. Marr drew on evidence from neurophysiology to precisely characterize the nature, for each step, of the input and output representations; and he proposed algorithms that would transform the input into the output, and so provided a computational explanation of each step.

The resultant "computational theory of vision" distinguished three different levels at which a perceptual system could be understood. At the highest level, the account describes a perceptual system in terms of what it functions to do. In the case of vision, it functions to produce a representation of objects and surfaces in the perceiver's environment on the basis of the pattern of light intensity values detected by the retina. The description at this level specifies the function that the visual system carries out—what input is transformed into what output. The top level is crucially important because "the nature of the computations that underlie perception depends more upon the computational problems to be solved than upon the particular hardware in which their solutions are implemented" (Marr 1982: 27). At the second level, the account seeks to explain *how* the function

FIGURE 5.3: David Courtney Marr: 2½-D sketch by Nicholas Wade. Nicholas Wade, *Psychologists in Word and Image*, Bradford Books, 1995. In Marr's theoretical scheme a 2½-D sketch is a description of the surface orientations of the objects with respect to the camera or observer's viewpoint. A cube, for example, would be represented as a 2-D shape with symbols indicating the orientations of the three visible faces with respect to the viewpoint. Marr is represented by pattern tokens signifying the contours of his face, rather like differences of Gaussians. His portrait is embedded in a representation of a cube; there are slight pattern differences to denote the boundaries between the three faces of the cube. These are close to the threshold of discrimination and might only become visible when the design is viewed from beyond reading distance. The cube motif also alludes to the Marroquin figure that Marr reproduces in his *Vision—Nicholas Wade.*

described at the highest level is carried out. It does so by specifying a computational algorithm that transforms—via a series of intermediate steps—the input representation into the output representation. At the lowest level, the account explains how the algorithms characterized at the second level are implemented in the brain. The focus of this level is physiological: it aims to identify the brain mechanisms responsible for carrying out the computations. What was significant about Marr's approach was that it treated the visual system as a computational system—as involving representational states that are transformed in a determinate rule-like way that can be modeled by a computational process—and provided a conceptual framework for combining the insights from physiology, psychology, and computational theory.

The computational approach to vision provides a framework within which the physiological discoveries described above can be interpreted. Those "feature detectors" can be viewed as parts of a system that functions in the way that Marr described. In particular, the neurons function to extract information about different features from the pattern of light falling on the retina; this information about features feeds into further processes that compute what objects are responsible for the features detected. To properly understand what these neurons are doing they must be understood as implementing a computational process described at the highest and intermediate levels.

Marr died aged 35, and his book *Vision* was published posthumously. His work was enormously influential, both for the particular explanations he produced of some of the early stages of visual processing and, more importantly, for the conceptual framework his approach provided that, in the decades that followed, became the dominant explanatory paradigm in vision science (the first chapter of Palmer's widely used textbook—Palmer 1999—for example, sets out Marr's framework as *the* framework within which the rest of the book should be understood). Research into the functioning of vision and the other senses gathered pace in the last two decades of the century and much of it was done within a broadly computational framework according to which sensory systems are viewed as information-processing or computational systems that transform states that carry information about the pattern of stimulation of the sensory receptors into states that represent things in the perceiver's environment.

A further important development was the emergence of connectionism as an alternative to the computational paradigm. In 1986, Jay McClelland and David Rumelhart published a two-volume book collecting together papers from the Parallel Distributed Processes research group at Stanford. These books described the methods for constructing, and applications of, connectionist networks in psychological explanation.

A connectionist network consists of a large number of elements or units connected into a network. A typical network has input units and output units, and a set of "hidden" units in between. The different units are interconnected by links of various strengths. When a pattern of activation is applied to the input units, a pattern of activation is produced by the output units in a way that depends on the strength of the connections between the units. The patterns of activation on input and output can represent different things and so the network as a whole can instantiate a function or algorithm that transforms input representations into output representations in a set way. An important feature of connectionist networks is that they can be "trained" to carry out particular functions. For example, a network might be trained to recognize male and female faces by being presented with a series of pictures of men and women. The input might be a large number of units corresponding to pixels in the pictures, and the output would be two units representing "male" and "female." During the training, the pictures are input to the network and the strength of the connections between units is adjusted to produce the correct output. After this has been repeated many times, the network will have learnt to recognize male and female faces and will generalize beyond the set of pictures it was trained with.

Connectionism networks differ from traditional computational systems in that they don't involve symbolic representations that are manipulated in a systematic way. Whereas a computer processes information serially, in a series of steps that manipulate symbols, connectionist networks do not. This goes along with the way the brain was thought to be made up of interconnected networks of neurons. Therefore, connectionism was thought by many to provide a better model of the operation of the brain than that provided by traditional computational theories. It is not clear, however, whether connectionism requires a radical revision of Marr's computational theory, or is simply an account of how computations are implemented in the brain. The issue remains unresolved.

FURTHER DEVELOPMENTS IN PHILOSOPHY

The sense datum theory fell completely out of favor in the second half of the twentieth century (in a shift that is unusual for a philosophical view, it went from orthodoxy to unconscionable in a couple of decades). It is sometimes claimed that a series of lectures delivered by J. L. Austin in the late 1940s and throughout the 1950s, and subsequently published as the book *Sense and Sensibilia*, were responsible for this shift. The lectures were an attack on a particular version of the sense datum theory espoused by A. J. Ayer, and criticized Ayer from the point of view of ordinary language philosophy. Austin described the sense datum view as "a typically scholastic view, attributable, first, to an obsession with a few particular words, the uses of which are over-simplified, not really understood or carefully studied or correctly described; and second, to an obsession with a few (and nearly always the same) half-studied 'facts'" (Austin 1962: 3).

Austin's criticism focused on the argument from illusion, the argument that (in one form or another) had been the main motivation for the sense datum view for two centuries. The argument begins with the premise that we experience visual illusions in which we seem to be visually aware of something when there is no material object present to be visually aware of; claims that we are visually aware of *something* in these cases; concludes that what we are aware of is a non-material object or *sense datum*; and, since our illusory experiences are just like our veridical experiences, generalizes from illusory experiences to visual experience in general to the conclusion that all visual experiences involve the awareness of non-material sense data. Austin attacked two steps of this argument in particular: the claim that there is something that we are aware of in illusory experiences; and the claim that what is true of illusions can be generalized to all visual experiences.

Although Austin's criticisms were trenchant, and influential on the debates that later emerged along with the renewed interest in perception towards the end of the century, the more likely explanation of the rejection of sense datum theories was that they came to be viewed as inconsistent with the naturalistic worldview articulated by science. The sense datum view was committed to the existence of non-material objects of awareness that are somehow caused to come into existence by the occurrence of events and processes in the material world (by light striking an object and entering my eyes, for example). Such casual processes were conceivable at the beginning of the twentieth century; developments in physics made them inconceivable. To maintain the sense datum theory would be to maintain that perception could be given no naturalistic or scientific explanation; few philosophers were prepared to do that.

Philosophical interest in theories of perception waned during the second half of the century as attention in philosophy shifted to the philosophy of language. The sense datum theory was viewed as clearly unattractive and false, but it was not clear what should replace it. The problem remained that of explaining the possibility of illusory and hallucinatory experiences.

Two things were influential in developing an alterative to sense datum theories. One was developments in the philosophy of language; in particular, the development of naturalistic explanations of the semantic properties of thought and language. These explanations aimed to show how thought and language could be accommodated within a scientific worldview. The other was the emerging computational or functional view of the mind. It was natural to extend the functional theory of the mind to perception; doing so meant viewing perceptual experiences as analogous to other mental states like beliefs and desires. According to the computational or functional view of the mind, mental states have intentional content—they represent the world to be a certain way: if I believe that there are sweets in the tin in front of me, my belief represents the world to be a certain way; it represents the world as such that there are sweets in the tin in front of me. The way my belief represents the world to be is the intentional content of my belief, and if the world is as I believe it to be then the content of my belief is true; if it is not then the content of my belief is false. According to naturalistic explanations of the semantics of belief, we can explain how my belief has this content in a scientifically respectable way. The intentional account of perception applies this account of the content of beliefs to perceptual experiences.

Anscombe (1965) drew attention to the fact that perception verbs are intentional in many of the ways that other mental states are (we can't infer from "Eliza is thinking about Santa Claus" that there exists something that she is thinking about; nor can we infer from "Eliza has an experience of fairies in the corner of the room" that there exists something that she is experiencing). Armstrong (1968) generalized this idea and suggested that we should think of perception *as* a form of belief. There were a number of problems with this suggestion, and the view more widely accepted was not that perception is a form of belief, but that perceptual experiences have intentional contents in the same way beliefs do. (This view was defended separately by Peacocke 1983; Searle 1983; and later Harman 1990 used it as a basis for criticizing the argument from illusion.)

According to the intentional theory of perception, perceptual experiences have intentional content that represents the world to be a certain way; if the world is as the experience represents it to be then the experience is veridical, otherwise it is illusory. When I describe my experience by saying that it looks as though there is a tin of sweets in front of me, I am describing how my experience represents the world to be, and so how the world would have to be for my experience to be veridical. In this way it was possible to accommodate the idea that it can seem that I am seeing something—a tin of sweets—even when there is nothing there for me to see, without postulating non-material sense data. It seems that I am seeing something because I am undergoing an experience that misrepresents something there. What it is for an experience to represent (or misrepresent) can be explained in semantic and functional terms.

The intentional view of perception dominated the philosophy of perception in the last two decades of the century, and was the basis for a renewed interest in the problems of perception within philosophy. (Renewed interest in the philosophy of perception dates from the time of Harman's 1990 paper; also important was a collection of conference papers published two years later— Crane 1992.) Philosophical issues that had been addressed in the context of the sense datum theory were reframed within the intentional account. Although the intentional theory seemed to offer a way to avoid the conclusion of the argument from illusion, a number of puzzles remained. One was whether the intentional theory could provide any understanding of the phenomenal or conscious character of experience. The analogy that was drawn between beliefs and experience suggested a way to explain the intentionality of experience, but beliefs don't have the phenomenology of perceptual experiences, so it was not clear that any explanation of phenomenology had been provided. One approach to this problem was to posit subjective properties of experience in addition to their representational properties (so called "qualia"), which determined their phenomenal character, but to many such qualia seemed to have the problematic features of sense data; an alternative approach emphasized that the kind of representational content that experiences had was different to that had by beliefs and that this could explain the phenomenology of experiences.

An alternative to the intentional theory of perception began to emerge in the final years of the century and was to become a significant rival in the first decade of the following century. This was the disjunctive theory of perception. The disjunctive theory rejected the claim that the intentionality of experiences should be explained in terms of their having representational content; instead the disjunctivist argued that the sense datum theorists were correct to claim that when a table appears brown to me I am acquainted with an actual instance of brownness, but were wrong to claim that I am acquainted with a sense datum: the brownness I am acquainted with is the brownness of the table—an ordinary mind-independent object. The disjunctivist avoided positing sense data by claiming that the kind of experience I have when I am perceiving the table is different to the kind of experience I have when I am hallucinating or experiencing an illusion.

One important feature of the intentional theory was that it was a naturalistic theory—it offered an account of perception that was consistent with theories in the natural sciences, in particular with psychological theories of perception. This meant that psychological evidence became relevant to debates in philosophy in a way that it had not previously been. For example, if the intentional theory claimed that experiences had representational content, and experiences were produced by sensory systems whose operation could be explained in terms of the kind of theory outlined by Marr, then the nature of the representational content of experiences in philosophical theories must be constrained by the nature of the content of experiences as it features in psychological theories. Philosophers therefore began to be far more interested in psychology than they had previously.

CONCLUSION

One theme that emerges from this survey of philosophical and scientific approaches to the senses in the twentieth century is the important role of technology in driving conceptual change. This took two forms. First, technological developments led to new tools for investigating the function of the brain. The ability to make recordings of the activity of single cells was fundamental to revising the empiricist conception of the operation of the senses. Technological developments continued, and the end of the century saw the emergence of a new kind of brain scanning—functional MRI—that has played a significant role in shaping the understanding of the functional organization of the brain in the first decades of the twenty-first century. Second, the development of the computer was hugely significant both as a model for how the mind might work and, towards the end of the century in particular, as a tool for modeling theories and for collecting and processing the data from empirical studies.

A second theme that emerges is the importance of naturalism. The success of science in providing authoritative explanations of natural phenomena in general meant that theories whose explanations were not continuous with the rest of science were no longer viewed as acceptable. This was particularly significant in philosophy where it led to the rejection of the sense datum theory, and now constitutes a constraint on philosophical theorizing about the senses.

Looking forward, at the end of the twentieth and beginning of the twenty-first century there was a greater interest than previously in the variety of sensory experience. Work on perception in the twentieth century tended to focus on vision. Towards the end of the century this changed, and work in the non-visual senses of audition, touch, and flavor perception increased, both within psychology and in philosophy. Philosophical work on perception throughout the twentieth century operated with a common-sense conception of five senses. Recent work on the non-visual senses in psychology and physiology has called

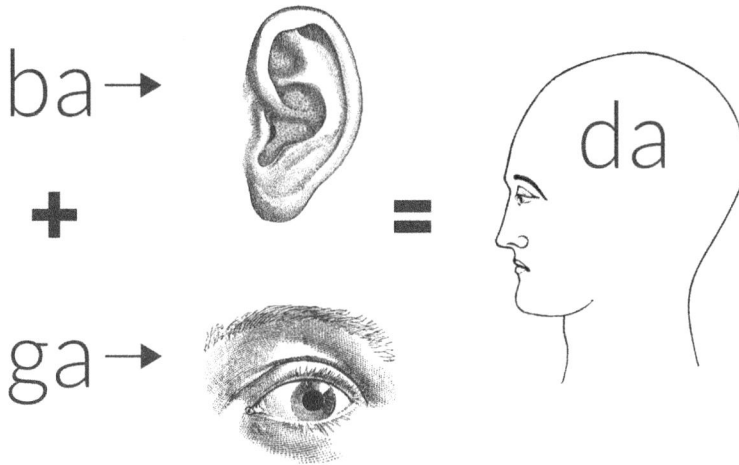

FIGURE 5.4: The McGurk Effect. Illustration by Shannon Leah Collis. The subject is shown a film of a person mouthing /ga/ /ga/ /ga/. The facial movements are synchronized with an audio track in which the person says /ba/ /ba/ /ba/. The person in the film is perceived as saying /da/ /da/ /da/. This experiment demonstrates the interaction/integration of modalities in the act of perceiving—*David Howes*.

this common-sense conception into question (see Calvert *et al.* 2004; Stein 2012). Humans appear to have more than five senses. Moreover, there are myriad forms of interaction between the different senses. An important challenge for philosophers in the twenty-first century is to accommodate these new findings within philosophical theories. Given the substantial interactions and areas of overlap among senses, philosophers might start to question whether it is legitimate to talk of different senses or experiences in different sensory modalities at all. It at least raises the question of on what grounds the number of senses possessed by any creature can be determined—and even of what makes something a sense in the first place (see Macpherson 2011).

CHAPTER SIX

Medicine and the Senses: Bodies, Technologies, and the Empowerment of the Patient

ANAMARIA IOSIF ROSS

Riding upon its wake, it is apparent that the twentieth century was one of great transformations in medicine and public health. During the last century, Western approaches to health and illness changed the way humans inhabit and experience their bodies on a global scale. Modern medicine co-mingled and co-evolved with commodity capitalism and information technologies, remodeling sensations and perceptions of bodies, moods, and behaviors, and reconfiguring the social relationships entailed in sickness, healing, and the pursuit of wellbeing.

In the twentieth century the supremacy of the visual reached new pinnacles of cyber-realism, creating hybrid sensory experiences, as technological innovation fostered diverse new forms of embodiment and healing. While patients were often positioned as objects to be penetrated by the analytical medical gaze, or as subjects of medical and pharmaceutical experimentation, they increasingly demanded greater agency in the late twentieth century, both individually and collectively, manifesting transformative potentials of illness or healing through diverse forms of participation, sensual and virtual.

The globalization of biomedicine exposed populations around the world to myriad new sensations, both trivial and profound, from the cooling sensations of antibacterial gels to the tactile and kinesthetic experience of prosthetic replacements. At the same time, the technological developments of biomedicine served to throw into relief the contrasts between rich and poor individuals and nations: those who could afford cosmetic surgery and those who could not afford life-saving surgery, those who could rent wombs for surrogate pregnancies, and those who had to sell their blood or even body parts for ready cash.

While on the one hand Western medicine strove to eradicate the ailments of the body (from disease to infertility to aging), on the other hand the globalization of Western lifestyles provoked a fresh onslaught of health problems. Globalized sensations of the period included the processed flavors of fast food, the chemical stew of urban smog, the sensory confusion (yet also ease) of urban transportation, or the spell-binding sights of television—all distinctive sensory hallmarks, as well as subjects for health concerns. With media and medical culture emphasizing personal responsibility over physical health, modern pathologies related to inactivity and over-consumption were blamed upon sensual indulgence, obscuring the role played by environmental, historical, and structural forces. The sensory malaise of the era was partially countered by fitness movements, health food trends, a rising interest in traditional and alternative medicines, and calls for the "greening" of cities through gardening, clean transport, and eco-friendly designs.

The present chapter will highlight four major ways in which sensory experience and medical practices co-evolved and mutually impacted each other in the twentieth century. These four aspects are: the transformations of perception occasioned by the technologization of medicine; the use of sensory symbols to represent health and illness; the control of sensation by the medical establishment; and the rise of complementary and alternative medicines, with their dazzling smorgasbord of sensory therapies. This examination, while not comprehensive, will bring out the extent to which twentieth-century medical practices created and employed a language of the senses to communicate social and corporeal values to their publics.

THE TECHNOLOGIZATION OF MEDICAL PERCEPTION

In 1910, a patient's medical record for a broken leg was one page and included no tests during a seven-week hospital stay. A similar patient's record in 1925 comprised eight pages, two forms, a graph, and multiple tests, including four urinalyses. This change reflects the extent to which hospitals transformed from being a refuge for patients into key medical institutions which aimed to be "actively and self-consciously based on science," using laboratory tests as routinized ways of establishing scientific truth and validating clinical impressions (Howell 1995: 2–3).Whereas the conventional medical exam of the early twentieth century still involved careful listening, smelling, touching, and viewing of diverse aspects of the patient's body, the clinical knowledge and techniques needed to perform such assessments steadily faded as the role of the laboratory and technology gained prominence, and professionals became increasingly dependent on testing for insight (Reiser 1993).

Medical education in the United States became highly formalized and standardized following the publication of the 1910 Flexner Report. This report, commissioned by the American Medical Association, exposed the eclectic and allegedly undisciplined state of medical training at the time. The exposé led to the closing of half of all US medical schools (many of them small, proprietary, heterodox institutions), and the triumph of the biomedical paradigm or "allopathic" medicine. Homeopathic, naturopathic, and other such traditions, which had flourished in the medical culture of nineteenth-century America, were decisively marginalized by the consolidation of biomedicine.

Medical training and academic medical centers, both heavily subsidized by government, were at the center of the twentieth-century expansion of the "high-tech, low-touch" system of biomedicine. The diagnostic and treatment practices promoted by this system contrasted starkly with those of previous centuries (see Classen 1998: 86–93). They also contrasted with those characteristic of many traditional medical systems, which tend to utilize multiple sensory channels for purposes of diagnosis and emphasize sensorially stimulating remedies for healing (Howes and Classen 2014: Ch. 2; Laderman and Roseman 1996; Leslie and Young 1992). Also characteristic of many traditional medical systems is the rule that the healer must have experienced a particular affliction in order to be qualified to treat it (e.g. Turner 1968). This rule promotes empathy. The main rite of passage in a biomedical education, by contrast, is the alienating and often-traumatic experience of cadaver dissection. This fosters objectification and detachment rather than empathy (Lella and Pawluch 1988; Macnaughton 2009). Byron Good (1994) and MaryJo DelVecchio Good (1995) have discussed how a biomedical education makes "doctors" out of medical students by imposing a distinctive sensory regime (with particular emphasis on the visual), instilling a set narrative style, promoting a mechanistic view of the body, and demanding significant emotional and psychological transformation on the part of the medical trainee.

While medical technology inspired confidence in modern health care, it could also provoke ambivalence, especially when its authority superseded not only that of the physician's clinical use of his or her own senses, but also that of the patient's own senses, thus disempowering and distancing patients from their caregiver and their own sensory and bodily experiences of pain or transformation.

The mechanization of birth is a prime example of the technologization of perception and the body under biomedicine. Prenatal testing and fetal monitoring, as well as epidural anesthesia became central to the process of birth in the First World over the course of the twentieth century. During the 1940s through 1960s, a birthing woman was widely viewed and represented as a machine that needed to be fixed, with the doctor as mechanic or technician (Martin 1987: 54). Hospital birth became the norm, and in the hospital it became common for a nurse or physician to authoritatively tell the birthing woman when to push (or not to push) based on a reading of electronic monitors. The absurdity of this situation inspired a well-known skit by the English comedy troupe Monty Python, called "The Machine That Goes Ping." In this skit the birthing woman is told to be quiet and stop asking about the baby, while the staff focus on the awesome pinging machine. The sensory signals of a machine are here satirized for taking precedence over those of a human being. This technologized approach to childbirth arguably equates reproduction with production and obscures the power relationships that are entailed when humans come to depend on machines to produce "products" (here: a baby), as Emily Martin observed (1987: 57) in her landmark analysis *The Woman in the Body*.

The mechanical, low-touch approach to childbirth continued with childrearing, with physicians and nurses advising mothers to bottle feed instead of breastfeed their babies, to keep them to strict feeding schedules and to avoid close physical contact (Synnott 2005). In the latter half of the century these attitudes softened somewhat. Cross-cultural research on child development pointed to the importance of physical contact between mothers and infants for healthy socialization, and spurred the evolution of attachment theory (Ainsworth 1967; Brazelton *et al.* 1974). Dr. Benjamin Spock's enormously influential *Baby and Child Care* ([1946] 2012) reassured mothers that they could kiss and hug their children without causing them the irreparable psychological damage which earlier childcare guides warned would ensue from mothers "smothering" their children with too much physical affection (Synnott 2005). Ashley Montagu's classic work *Touching* ([1971] 1986) detailed the negative health consequences of the marginalization of touch in Western medicine and society and supported a return to more nurturing, tactile modes of interaction. In the 1970s, A. Jean Ayres described the impact of sensory integration difficulties upon self-regulation and learning, laying the ground for advocacy movements and sensory therapies (such as skin brushing) for children with sensory processing disorders (Ayres 1972).

As regards childbirth, late twentieth-century hospitals began providing more "natural" and home-like options for women. These ranged from allowing family members into the birthing room to providing birthing centers predominantly staffed by nurse midwives, and promoting "unmedicated" birth. Warm showers, massage, music, aromatherapy, dimmed lights, and even birthing tubs began to be incorporated into the labor and birthing experience for women in the United States, Canada, and elsewhere. Transforming birth sensations through metaphors further placed the woman in an active role by describing birth as a dance or journey and contractions as energy rushes (Klassen 2001; Martin 1987: 158). This general progression is reflected in the way midwifery nearly disappeared in New Zealand between 1930 and the late 1970s, by which point 99 percent of all births took place in hospital, but following a decade of intense political and social activism in the 1980s, midwives were reinstated as autonomous practitioners in 1990.

SHOOTING THE BODY'S INTERIORS: ULTRASOUND AND MAGNETIC RESONANCE IMAGING

Another major way in which perceptions of the body were technologized in the twentieth century was through medical imaging. In the first decades of the century X-rays provided a dramatic new way of accessing the inside of the body without the necessity of cutting it open. The visual images of corporeal interiors provided by X-rays both fascinated and frightened the general populace. The most important thing in physicians' eyes, however, was how the use of X-rays could economize on time spent gathering information: "No more would it be necessary to spend time at the bedside meticulously percussing the chest to outline the heart, or moving the stethoscope slowly from place to place over the chest and back listening for sounds that would indicate a lesion. Instead, a swiftly written order to the X-ray department would produce the evidence needed" (Reiser 1993: 268).

A further advantage of X-rays and other laboratory tests was that the precise numerical and/or graphic information they supplied facilitated communication among medical researchers, since the latter no longer had to

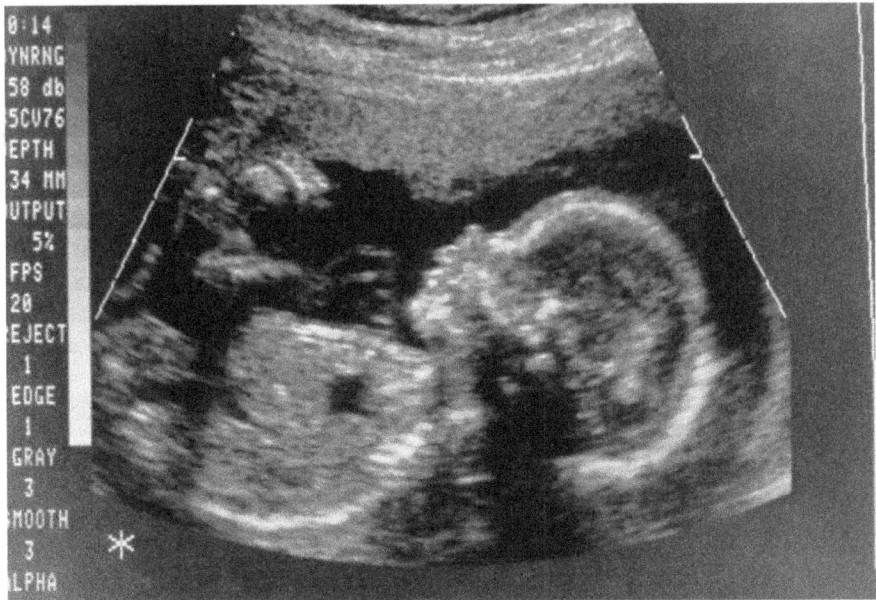

FIGURE 6.1: "Baby's first picture": ultrasound image of fetus. Public domain.

depend on their own senses to form impressions or their own linguistic skills to describe them. The epistemological benefits of this standardization of perception were extraordinary (Borell 1993).

By mid-century, X-rays had been found to have harmful effects, and their use diminished somewhat. The technology of ultrasound arose as an alternative to X-rays and entered into routine use by the 1980s, mainly as a means of screening internal organs, but most popularly as a means of revealing fetal images to future parents. When abnormalities were detected this sometimes led to parents being faced with complex moral decisions. Typically, however, the seeming view inside the womb supplied by ultrasound helped to establish the unborn baby as an independent being and provide an important attachment/ bonding experience for parents (Mitchell and Georges 1998: 105–9). At the same time, the fetal images produced by ultrasound could be seen as dissolving the bodily boundaries of the pregnant woman, rendering her invisible (see also Mentor 1998: 86).

Other imaging technologies developed during the closing decades of the century include positron emission tomography (PET scan), computerized tomography (CT scan), and magnetic resonance imaging (MRI). One research application for MRI centered on visualizing brain activity and circulatory patterns during diverse sensory experiences (from meditation to listening to music), and exploring their relationship to brain chemicals like dopamine and serotonin. Basing their findings on such imaging, scientists began to postulate complex linkages between sensory experiences, brain chemistry, and emotions (Salimpoor *et al.* 2011).

In *Magnetic Appeal*, medical sociologist Kelly A. Joyce (2008) notes how the multiplicity of "slices" of the interior of the body produced by MRI technology contrasts with the singularity of X-ray images. This slicing process presents the body as inert matter to be endlessly segmented in the pursuit of scientific facts. Another aspect of what Joyce calls "the myth of transparency" surrounding MRI has to do with the way MRI images are commonly portrayed as capturing an unmediated bodily truth (i.e. as presenting actual "pictures" of the brain and other organs) when in point of fact they involve the transformation of numerical data into visual representations, a process requiring many layers of social action, abstraction, and interpretation by medical professionals.

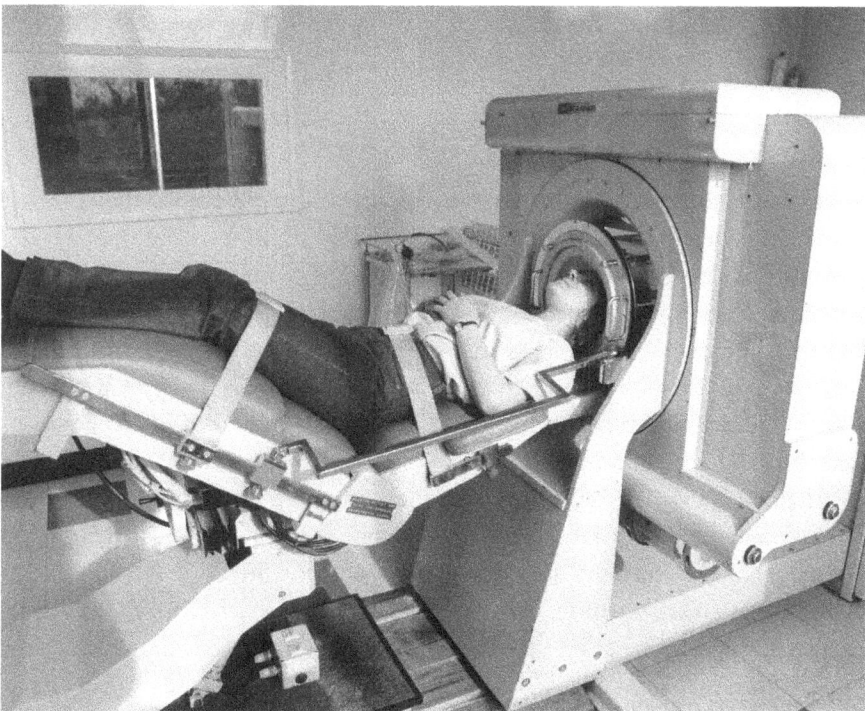

FIGURE 6.2: An early computerized tomography (CT) scanning machine. Getty Images.

Joyce relates how the sensory experience of being "imaged" through this technology was found by many of her informants to be profoundly objectifying and unsettling due to the enforced stillness and sense of enclosure from being inside the MRI chamber, compounded by the loud knocking sounds the machine emitted while in operation (Joyce 2008: 83). Immobilized inside the magnetic cocoon, subjects felt they had become "patient-objects"—completely subsumed by technology, despite the best efforts of staff to palliate the experience, albeit mainly with a view to enhancing patient docility and compliance (Joyce 2008: 84). The spread of MRI has thus contributed to the further entrenchment of the machinic model of the body. It is important to bear in mind the extent to which this model, which presents the body as an assemblage of removable, fixable, interchangeable physical components, contrasts with the holistic image of the body in most traditional medical systems. In the latter, health is normally represented as depending on a balance of elements or forces, a dynamic state in which the senses of both physician and patient have an important role to play in detecting and correcting imbalances (García *et al.* 1999).

THE SENSORY CODING OF HEALTH

Health and hygiene were widely symbolized by the color white, occasionally emblazoned by red as in the red-on-white symbol of the Red Cross. Thus, the original uniforms donned by New York City's street cleaners, "The White Wings," and other street cleaners across the US, were white, though later changed to darker colors. As a further illustration of this association, consider the mid-century public hygiene/sanitation performance depicted in a photograph from the University of Virginia Rice Collection bearing the title "Street Sanitation, Parade" (see Figure 6.3). Two white-skinned men in suits and hats lead a troupe of white-uniformed street cleaners, most of whom are people of color, wielding cleaning equipment. A sign attached to an enormous wire wastebasket reads: *Richmond, your city—help us keep it clean*, with a larger sign leaning against the basket which bears the inscription: *A clean city is everyone's job. Don't be a litter bug!* (The one woman in the picture is shown releasing balloons into the sky—ironically producing litter.)

According to convention, the white coat of the physician or lab technician represented authority, scientific rationality, and germ-free cleanliness. Classic nurses' uniforms were also white, and, in many places, included white caps. The archetypical nurse not only wore white, she *was* white. Public health images from the early twentieth century often portrayed white nurses caring

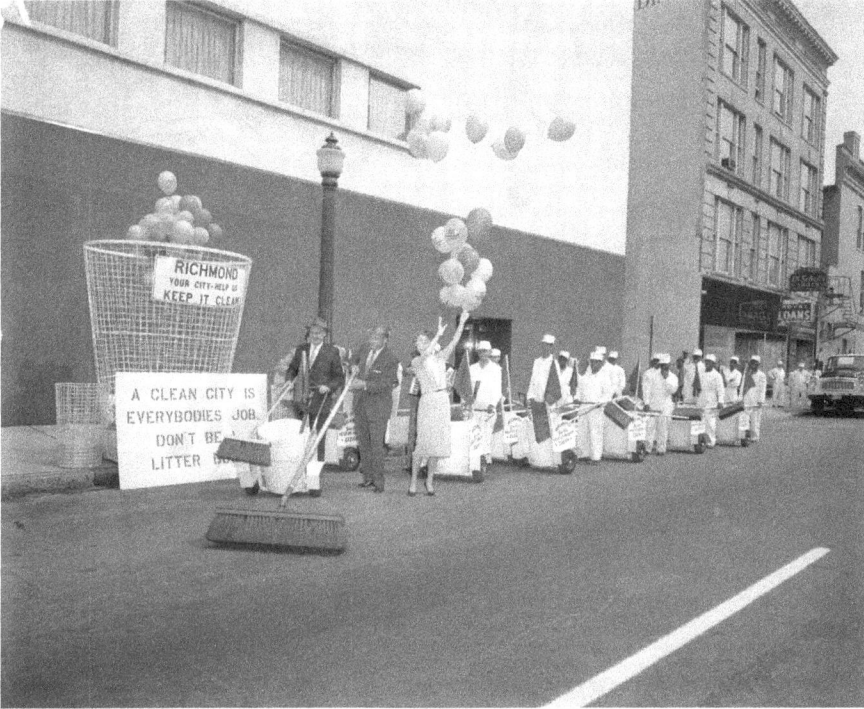

FIGURE 6.3: "Street Sanitation, Parade," Richmond, Virginia. Courtesy of The Library of Virginia.

for babies or demonstrating care to the mother, thereby supplanting (and effacing) the traditional roles of midwives, who, in the southern US, consisted mainly of African-American women (Smith 2010). It was the latter who provided most of the delivery support to both white and black women in childbirth. Patients' perceptions of nurse competency, professionalism, and caring continued to be influenced by the color and style of the nurse's appearance throughout the century.

   A forceful illustration of the association of whiteness with good health in early twentieth-century nutrition imagery is presented by a US Department of Agriculture public education poster (see Figure 6.4). The poster depicts a young blonde girl wearing a ruffled white dress and a hair bow, sitting smilingly in front of a fair-colored meal made up of milk, crackers, white bread and butter. The ad reminds parents to feed their children healthfully—"Simple Suppers Are Best"—pointing to an era in nutrition counseling when colorful foods were viewed as high in sensory appeal, but low in nutritional value. In order to

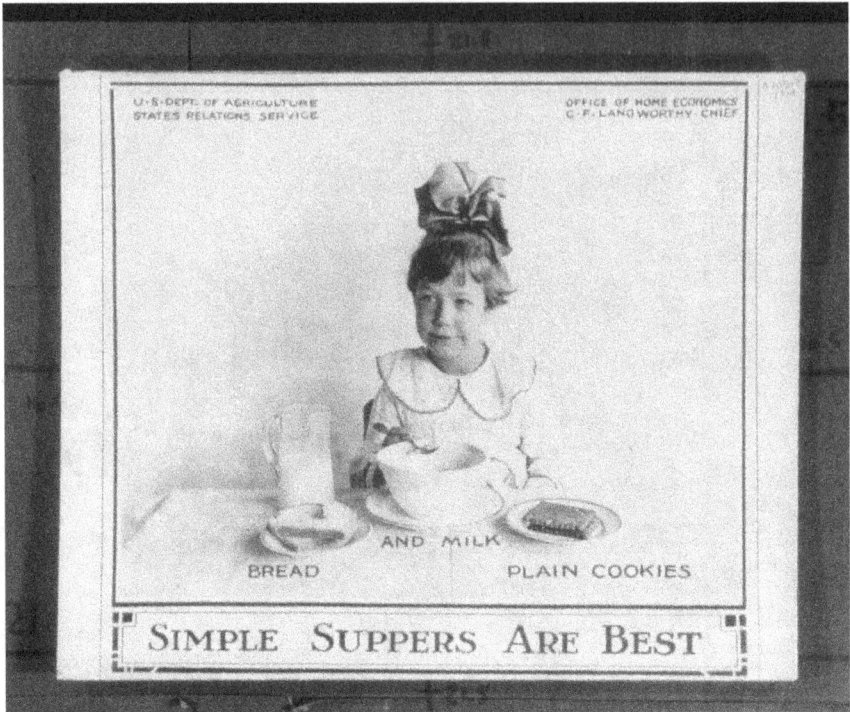

FIGURE 6.4: "Simple Suppers Are Best": US Department of Agriculture Office of Home Economics nutrition poster. National Archives and Records Administration.

produce the desired "healthy" look, the food industry devoted itself to processing grains and other foodstuffs, thus enhancing their visual appeal through whitening and "cleaning," while actually stripping key nutrients and fiber.

The color-coding of health promotion campaigns in the early twentieth century and the call for "simple suppers" for children harkened back to the Protestant ethic of monochrome clothing and minimal sensory stimulation, in addition to being informed by discourses of colonialism, which portrayed the sensuality of color as primitive and wild, a symbol of disorder and uncontrolled appetites, something to be overcome through civilization and progress. As in the ethnic/racial purity discourses of Europe's fascist movements, color was represented as a threat to uniformity, quality, modernity, and propriety.

The insistence on whiteness was, however, gradually undermined by increased popular awareness and discoveries regarding the vital role of certain food components, most notably vitamins, in health maintenance. The paucity of particular vitamins in the diet was identified as a factor in many poor health outcomes, including nervousness, irritability, and weakness, particularly among the poor and working class. These health deficiencies were blamed on the milling process, which removed important nutrients in the process of whitening. The new notion of whiteness as potentially unhealthy would later be captured in the saying "the whiter the bread the sooner you're dead." Such views led to the development of mass supplementation, whereby all kinds of processed food (even tobacco) came to have vitamins added to them so that they could be advertised as "enriched" (Apple 2007: 135–6). While some prioritized eating nutritious food and expressed skepticism about vitamin enrichment, the vitamin "craze" nevertheless helped lessen the physical and psychological impact of wartime rationing. "Taking one's vitamins" even came to be represented in popular media and advertisements as a patriotic duty. The latter development is exemplified by a red, white, and blue sign proclaiming "Vitamins for Health's Defense" which adorned drug store windows in the 1940s (Apple 2007: 144–5).

In a stunning about-face, by the late twentieth century the nutritional content of foods came to be associated with colorfulness. The public was urged to eat "all colors of food every day" for "complete nutrition." In order to combine the vivid food colors consumers now desired with the popular taste for salty or sweet convenience foods, artificial colors came into increasingly widespread use by the food industry. In this way, it became possible to eat "all colors of food every day" and yet have a nutritionally *unbalanced* diet.

The food industry did not simply make use of artificial colors to attract consumers. During the twentieth century, artificial flavors (from vanillin to saccharin) also became standard additives to processed foods (de la Peña 2010). What is more, processed foods themselves came to constitute an ever-larger proportion of the food for sale in supermarkets and convenience stores. Hence, just as the color of a food could no longer be taken as indicative of its nutritional value, nor could its flavor. Orange-colored and flavored drinks, for example, might have no trace of actual orange juice in them—though uninformed consumers might well still have thought of them as offering the health benefits of actual citrus fruit.

In the same way that the color white went from signifying "healthy" to spelling "unhealthy" as regards such foods as bread, rice, and sugar, so did certain aromas and flavors. Alongside the red, white, and blue signs of the 1940s reading "Vitamins for Health's Defense," for example, there were signs displaying the words *cigars* and *soda* (Apple 2007: 144–5). At the time, these two products might not have been thought to contradict the health imperative used to promote the consumption of vitamins, for both tobacco and soda were touted as having medicinal properties. It was not uncommon for physicians to be enlisted to promote tobacco use. In like fashion, a July 1937 issue of *Vogue* sported a full page Camel cigarette advertisement with a glamorous socialite quoted as saying that Camels taste good and "give my energy a cheering lift." The advertisement claimed that "smoking Camels speeds the natural flow of digestive fluids—alkaline digestive fluids—so indispensable to mealtime comfort." Similarly, early "soda waters" or soft drinks, including Coca-Cola, were sold in pharmacies as medicinal "elixirs."

The practice of smoking tobacco, packaged in the form of cigarettes, spread worldwide in the twentieth century. After the mid-century, however, cigarettes were increasingly recognized to be a health hazard, and one which the addictive properties of tobacco rendered particularly difficult to control. Soft drinks also became globalized over the course of the century, and likewise, although to a lesser extent, fell into disfavor with public health and medical authorities as a result of their perceived contribution to national and global spikes in obesity and diabetes rates. The smell of burning tobacco and the taste of soft drinks—both archetypical twentieth-century sensory experiences—hence lost some of their positive significations of "soothing," "refreshing," and "invigorating" and took on negative associations of unhealthiness. Such turnarounds in the perceived health effects of particular substances are not unusual in the history of medicine and public health. Many substances once considered to have medicinal uses, including alcohol, chocolate, cocaine, caffeine, and cannabis, have had similar fluctuations in fortune. Nor has the market disappeared for products offering both sensory appeal and supposed corporeal benefits. By the late twentieth century this product range included sports drinks, such as Gatorade, energy drinks, such as Red Bull, and vitamin-enhanced drinks, such as Vitamin Water.

Commodities which offered powerful sensations, such as tobacco, alcohol, and soft drinks, had a particularly strong social and health impact on working-class and indigenous populations worldwide. Among these sectors such commodities were used to temporarily mitigate the stresses of poverty, displacement, migration, and wage labor. However, the consumption of these commodities actually compounded the dependencies, inequalities, and negative health effects of rapid industrialization and urbanization, while further restricting access to fresh, nutritionally rich local foods (see Jankowiak and Bradburd 2003; Kohrman and Benson 2011; Mintz 1985).

In the late twentieth century the color green began to take on connotations of environmental health. Associated with the natural world (which was itself seen to be threatened by industrialization, urbanization, and modern warfare), the color green was used to signify a range of environmentally-friendly practices, which, in turn, were said to contribute to individual, communal, and global health. These included preserving and creating green spaces, protesting nuclear testing, protecting endangered species, recycling paper and plastics, reducing carbon emissions, using natural alternatives to allegedly toxic chemicals, creating walkable neighborhoods, and promoting vegetarian diets. The Greenpeace environmentalist organization and Green political parties helped bring this new significance of green to public prominence. While white remained the standard chromatic sign for healthcare throughout the twentieth century, as people came to view the Earth itself as being sick and in need of care, the color green arose to serve as a symbol for a broader planetary vitality and holistic wellbeing.

THE SUPPRESSION OF SENSATION

The use of anesthetics and analgesics became increasingly standard practice in the twentieth century. The idea was that the patient should not experience any pain from disease, injury, or medical intervention. This modern view of pain as an undesirable sensation to be suppressed at all costs contrasted with earlier Western views of pain as being spiritually beneficial insofar as it provided intimations of mortality and fostered empathy for fellow sufferers.

There were, however, certain notable exceptions to the twentieth-century drive to abolish pain. If, by the end of the century it was generally accepted that "pain is a universal language that can be easily understood by its vocal sounds, facial expressions, body movement [and] respiration" (Chamberlain 1998: 183), this was by no means acknowledged by the medical profession at the outset. Anesthetics, in fact, were thought unnecessary for those not deemed capable of suffering pain in the first place. Among those not thought to experience pain were babies. Many newborns underwent major surgery unanesthetized, with physicians arguing that after major surgery babies just needed to sleep. They were also subjected to extensive experimentation that would now be considered abusive. This state of affairs persisted into the 1980s (Chamberlain 1998).

Infants' reactions to (and attempted avoidance of) painful procedures were minimized by the medical profession as simple reflex actions which could not be taken as signs of actual suffering. The indifference to infant pain and physician persistence in old practices were based in the anatomical and mechanical notion that the infant brain was primitive, and the infant therefore lacked a sense of self, discrete feelings, or consciousness. This followed the same line of thinking that held that signs of pain made by animals were mechanical reflex actions and not indications of actual distress. This rationale was used to deflect criticism of the obviously painful procedures to which animals used for medical experimentation were subjected, but this argument rang increasingly hollow.

Sensation-numbing drugs, when used, were not only intended to ensure that patients and subjects felt nothing, but also that they *did* nothing. This applied both to the suppression of responses that might disturb medical procedures and experiments and to the control of socially undesirable behavior. Early sedative drugs like chloral hydrate and barbiturates were widely used to restrain patients in early twentieth-century mental asylums. Surgical procedures were also employed to control bodies which did not conform to official norms. By 1931, for example, sterilization laws existed in most of the United States, aimed mainly at the mentally ill and handicapped (Hubbard 1990: 183). Lobotomies were performed in psychiatric asylums, mostly on women, to alleviate depression and sometimes to stop masturbation and "promiscuity," for which clitoridectomy was also employed (Braslow 1997: 153, 166). Germany's 1933 eugenic-sterilization law, targeting people with hereditary blindness and deafness, epilepsy, and alcoholism, was broadened after 1935 to include euthanasia or destruction for all "lives not worth living," including disabled children and able-bodied Jewish children (Hubbard 1990: 186). In the latter half of the century, partly in response to the horror of the Holocaust (which took eugenic cleansing to its ultimate ends), the use of surgical procedures to control "bad" sensations and behaviors and prevent "unfit" persons from reproducing was significantly reduced, or prohibited.

An important finding of twentieth-century anthropological and sociological scholarship was that perceived states of health or illness, normality or abnormality, are shaped by cultural forces. The term "tyranny of the normal" was used to critique an over-emphasis on normality leading to excessive stigmatization of and interference with the minds and bodies of people who did not meet the prevailing cultural criteria of normality. While all societies recognize certain comportments as undesirable or disruptive, one of the increasingly salient characteristics of Western societies has been the degree to which presumably deviant bodies and behaviors are reconstructed as medical problems and then responded to with medical solutions.

The process of applying medical labels and medical treatments to conditions and comportments previously considered part of normal life experience was termed *medicalization* by sociologists and anthropologists studying this phenomenon (Lock 1995; Lock and Gordon 1988; Robbins and Anthony 1982). Through this process of medicalization, realms of human experience previously considered outside the domain of medicine were brought under the surveillance and control of medical professionals and recast as forms of sickness. Examples include infertility, menopause, alcoholism, attention deficit and hyperactivity disorder (ADHD), and pre-diabetes. Thus, rather than being seen as progressing through a normal life stage, a woman entering menopause and experiencing "hot flushes" and "night sweats" might well be diagnosed as having a hormone deficiency and prescribed hormone replacement therapy (which could increase her risk of strokes and cancer). The rise of ADHD diagnosis and its widespread treatment with methylphenidate (Ritalin, an amphetamine) in North America provides another example of the process of medicalization (Conrad 1975). Initially prescribed mostly to children, particularly restless boys of middle school age, by the century's end Ritalin and other similar drugs were increasingly sought out by adults to enhance mental performance.

Drug-induced transformations of sensations and behaviors became routine for many during a century which serially hailed the mass utilization of barbiturates, antipsychotics, benzodiazepines, amphetamines, and serotonin modulating anti-depressants while at the same time criminalizing recreational and traditional uses of sensory-rich psychoactive substances. This mental, sensory, and mood control through pharmaceuticals points to the growing dependence of both the medical establishment and the public on chemical remedies to physical and emotional "problems," from sleeplessness to hyperactivity. The result was a general failure to recognize or confront the social and cultural factors determining maladjustment.

MOVEMENT, TOUCH, AROMA, TASTE: COMPLEMENTARY AND ALTERNATIVE MEDICINES

Complementary and alternative health programs and practices grew in popularity worldwide during the twentieth century. Many of these practices and programs, which ranged from arts therapies to acupuncture to aromatherapy, emphasized and developed particular domains of sensory practice and experience with the understanding that these could play a key role in the maintenance of health and the treatment of illness. A selection will be described here with a view to highlighting the "return to the senses" as agents of health and healing that these globalizing movements heralded.

Over the course of the century the importance of physical exercise to good health became increasingly evident. This realization, together with the relative lack of physical activity in many modern forms of employment, led to widespread interest in fitness routines involving bodily movement. In the earlier part of the century, calisthenics were often recommended as a simple and effective means of exercising and keeping fit (Frykman 1994). In the latter part of the century, jogging and running became popular in Western countries, as did aerobics exercises and dance fitness routines, such as Zumba. These practices of movement, directed at no practical external ends (i.e. jogging was not usually employed as a means of getting from one place to another), created an awareness of corporeal motion as a means of attaining interior mental and physical states of wellbeing. Growing awareness and concern regarding the obesity "epidemic," stress, and chronic disease at the century's end further underscored the vital role of movement in healing and health maintenance.

Partly due to the new emphasis on the role of movement in health and partly due to a rising interest in Eastern religions and philosophies, Asian practices involving movement, mindful breathing, and bodily position also found increased acceptance and adoption in the West. The most prominent of these was yoga, which went from being regarded as an exotic ritual practiced by small groups of "eccentric" enthusiasts in the early twentieth century to figuring as a mainstream fitness routine offered as part of the physical education curriculum at many schools by the century's end (Syman 2010). Other examples of Asian corporeal practices which became popular in the West include various forms of meditation, martial arts, t'ai chi and qigong (Chen 2003; Kabat-Zinn 1990), cultivating diverse and enriched "somatic modes of attention" (Csordas 1993). While often dismissed by mainstream medicine, the popular interest in such alternative systems grew exponentially. Patients often turned to these slower, more sensory systems of healing after becoming disenchanted with the side-effects of Western medicines, despite the latter's general rapidity of action and overall effectiveness in the treatment of specific physical ailments.

As regards Asian health practices and therapies, questions were raised by Western researchers concerning the extent to which they were transportable across cultures. Catherine Kerr's study of qigong, for example, noted that the qigong method—which is based on the concept of *qi* or vital energy found in Chinese medicine—is deeply embedded in Chinese notions of health and the body, and Chinese interpretations of what bodily feelings mean (Kerr 2002: 437). The physiological and mental effects of such culturally-bound health practices hence could be seen as varying depending upon how notions of feelings and thoughts were embodied or "somatized" by practitioners in the receiving culture. Since the ways we inhabit our bodies are shaped by culture,

Kerr and others have argued that mimicking the motions of qigong may not necessarily duplicate the experience. Distinct somatic modes of attention and different embodiments and feelings triggered by Chinese corporeal metaphors such as "mind-in-the-belly" might therefore produce entirely different effects. While scholars pondered such issues, however, unfazed Western enthusiasts continued to adopt the practices.

A number of the complementary and alternative health practices which gained popularity in the twentieth century contained a significant tactile dimension. A prime example of this is massage, which acquired mainstream respectability in the West in the last decades of the century after being viewed with some suspicion at the outset for its seeming sensuality. Massage was employed in a variety of health routines for its relaxing and/or stimulating effects and incorporated into programs of physical therapy. In the United States a system of therapeutic touch (TT) was introduced in the 1970s by Dora Kunz and Dolores Krieger (1979) of New York University. The system consisted of practitioners using their hands to manipulate postulated "energy fields" around the patient's body, rather than directly touching the patient. TT was said to benefit a wide array of conditions, including cardiovascular problems, back problems, arthritis, depression, abuse, autoimmune dysfunctions, and stress. Alternative medical practices such as acupuncture and therapeutic touch were customarily dismissed by the biomedical establishment as without scientific foundation, but such new forms of somatic awareness were welcomed by patients who felt alienated from their bodies or bereft of a caring touch in the biomedical system (Lock and Gordon 1988).

Another sensory realm to be explored and developed by alternative and traditional medical practitioners was that of smell. Though often neglected (and sometimes tabooed) in modern medicine, or limited to the sharp odor of disinfectants, the use of aromatic treatments had a long history in both Western and non-Western cultures (Classen *et al.* 1994). Twentieth-century aromatherapists, as they came to call themselves, claimed that aromatic essential oils could regulate moods, promote relaxation, and induce sleep, among other benefits, like soothing patients at the end of life. It was argued that in this regard aromatherapy provided a valuable resource for modern health care, at the very least reducing the need for sedatives and tranquilizers with their potentially harmful side-effects, and providing delight, stimulation, and comfort for patients and their often harried caregivers (Price and Price 1999). A counterpoint to the sterile ambiance of most medical institutions, aromatherapy emerged as a particularly important element in holistic and integrative cancer treatments.

In a medical system that was perceived by many to have become depersonalized, automated, and de-sensualized as a result of technological advancements, budgetary constraints, and a dismissal of the role of the senses in healing, aromatherapy, like a number of alternative therapies, was seen as an opportunity to tap the power of our sensoria as doorways to other, more "natural" modes of wellbeing and relationality. Such sensuous therapies were seen as having the potential to engage patients bodily and mentally, and actively involve them in the process of healing (in place of remaining patient-objects), even in cases where overcoming illness was an improbable goal. While aromatherapy remained marginal to mainstream medicine in the twentieth century, it did (like therapeutic touch) enter hospital rooms through support from the nursing profession (see Price and Price 1999: 261) and the desires of patients themselves.

In certain social settings it is clear that the interest in alternative medicines did not only come as a response to personal experiences of illness and desires for wellbeing but also as a response to perceptions of societal ailments, caused by political upheaval, cultural conflicts, and economic uncertainty. In Eastern Europe, the fall of communism was marked by the rapid growth of movements and therapies addressing the manifold deprivations and pathologies that characterized the communist era, including a drought of information and a rigidly materialist approach to individual bodies, senses, and social wellbeing. During my 1998 fieldwork in Romania, I focused my attention upon alternative healing movements, competing discourses on health, illness, and the body, and their relationship to the circumstances of the Romanian "transition." I had anticipated that the rapid growth of alternative medical treatments since the fall of the Ceausescu dictatorship in 1989 represented an effort to reconfigure notions of the self, body, illness, and medical knowledge in a manner that opposed the biomedical model identified with the centralized authority of the state. I envisioned the healing that people were seeking through alternative therapies as an effort to redefine the self and the body in the face of the dictatorial authority of the communist regime and the centralized biomedical hierarchy. I also hypothesized that the restoration of balance aimed at by alternative medical practices would be analogous to and symbolic of the repair that people hoped could take place in Romanian society.

The need for social healing in the aftermath of communism was vividly illustrated in the words spoken in a February 26, 1998 interview on ProTV by Andrei Pleşu, leading Romanian writer and scholar and Minister of External Affairs at the time of my fieldwork. Pleşu affirmed: "We are ill and we are legitimately ill. For decades there were all kinds of toxins injected upon us. Sometimes the recovery lasts longer than the illness. There are convalescences that leave you more run down than the illness itself." Economic and power inequities constituted an omnipresent and painful reality in postsocialist Romania, a state of disharmony within the social body.

One healing practice that I explored was Radiant Technique, a form of Reiki which the Romanian teachers traced back to its founder, Mikao Usui, via Barbara Rey. At the most basic level, this practice involved the laying on of hands to allow vital energy to flow through the palms toward the intended body site. One member of the movement, discussing the relation of touch to wellbeing, pointed to studies carried out in orphanages, where increased tactile contact from caregivers contributed significantly to the children's development. She emphasized, in particular, the importance of the *hug*: "People have forgotten how to embrace each other. The cause of illness of our planet."

Once initiated in Radiant Technique (also called Real Reiki), the practitioner is referred to as a radiant. Radiants are "givers of light," considered to contain the same energy form as love and prayer. "Love is the essential nourishment of being, and our palms can bring it more richly into others' lives," one informant said. Students of Radiant Technique get in touch, both literally and figuratively, with new loci of individual power and meaning, and are supposed to acquire additional means to connect to others physically, spiritually, and emotionally.

Employing traditional metaphysical concepts of the body from India, Reiki teachers posited the existence of centers of vital energy (or "chakras") at different sites of the body. Each such site was associated with a color and with a musical note. The energy center near the heart was associated with the note F and the color green ("the color of healing," as one member affirmed). The chakra at the top of the head was associated with the musical note B and the color violet. It was believed possible to use the relevant musical note and color to stimulate a particular energy center for purposes of healing. In a country fragmented by the chaos of political upheaval, part of the appeal of this tactile and synaesthetic healing tradition, in which touches, sensations, and bodies correspond and unite, may well have been the vision of integrated holism it provided.

I also spent a significant amount of time with members of a Romanian dietary, social, and spiritual community called ELTA Universitate, among whose members were several medical doctors. ELTA participants ate a diet based entirely on uncooked, vegetarian foods, raw milk, and honey, stating

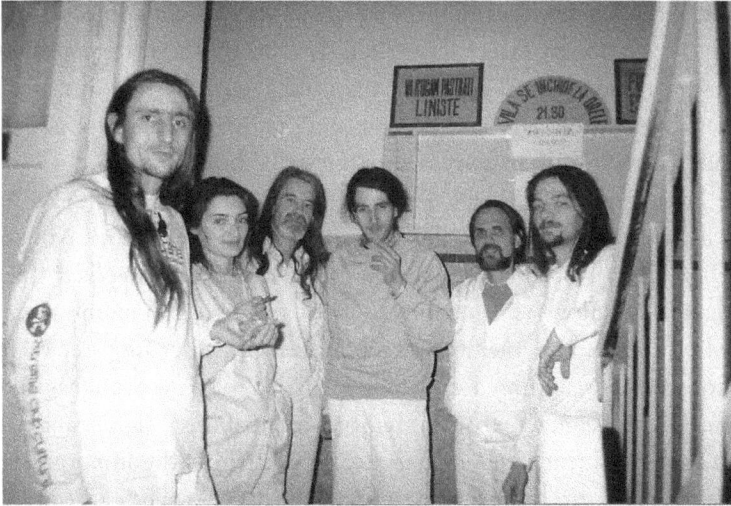

FIGURE 6.5: ELTA members on a retreat in Breaza, Romania. Photograph by the author.

that cooked foods were noxious because essential living elements of foods are destroyed by high heat. The consumption of cooked/dead/toxic food was believed to be causing a state of sensory and spiritual *anesthesia* and to constitute the basis for disease processes. It was also believed that commercially-produced food could become loaded with "negative vibrations" or harmful energy during the production process due to the profit-seeking interests of its handlers. With long flowing hair and mostly white garments, the members of this group shared in a spiritual discourse of personal enlightenment and social evolution through alternative consumption and other practices of physical and mental hygiene.

I found that such new healing practices and movements challenged the anti-spiritual materialism of the communist era while also opposing the rapid encroachment of individualism and consumerism from the West. Many ELTA members, for example, described joining the movement as a part of their life's quest for knowledge and truth, which was frustrated under the communist regime. However, ELTA also sought personal and social transformation by resisting capitalist consumption practices and centering their diets and lifestyle on home-grown produce. In some ways these postsocialist healing movements were akin to millenarian revitalization movements: for example, in their efforts to reclaim a lost or primordial state (of health, moral rectitude, and sociocultural wellbeing), in their quasi-nationalistic ethos, in their voiced suspicion of money and profit, and in their criticism of and opposition to Western individualism and materialism. From this perspective, ELTA's insistence upon the consumption of pure, raw, unprocessed food and its advocacy of a "natural" way of life for the purpose of revitalizing self and society can be seen as a reaction to the alienation brought on by the shock of transition and rapid encroachment of Western-style modernity. In such social contexts, the sensory dimensions of alternative healing programs, from the energizing touches of Radiant Healing to the vitalizing raw foods of ELTA, become a vehicle for returning to "wholeness," individual and communal.

CONCLUSION: THE SHIFTING AND BLURRING OF BOUNDARIES

"Health as an absence of disease or anxiety is long gone," writes Joseph Masco (2010: 152): "what we have instead is a negotiation of degrees of contamination, of degrees of anxious association, of degrees of escalating risk." Masco argues that there was a change in how health was experienced, beginning in the Cold War era with its looming nuclear threat. This change was ratcheted up further by the 2001 terrorist attacks in the United States, which triggered new levels of governmental and public anxiety over external threats to the social and physical wellbeing of the nation. Managing fear and having a plan became the two most essential elements in the modern survival toolkit. Indeed, as noted by Browner and Press (1995), the twentieth century came to be dominated by a preoccupation with risk in general, mitigated through technologies, such as fetal screening. Other medical interventions, such as transfusions, transplantations, and prostheses also contributed to a generalized blurring of the conventional boundaries between self and other, inside and outside, life and death, being healthy or ill.

In a further highly significant development, health-related searches on the internet increased dramatically in the 1990s, empowering patients to compare, explore and question. Boundaries between consumers and producers of information became blurred (Hardey 2002), as well as those between patients and care providers. These developments point to a not-so-distant future when patients may perform their own diagnoses. With the mapping of the human genome and the explosive development of the internet and communications in the late twentieth century, new layers of social networks and potentials have been generated, as well as new ways of being neither healthy nor sick, but "at risk," and hence vulnerable. As genomic links are identified, more medical conditions are classified as having genetic components, including adult onset diseases with no known cure. A new eugenic era is afoot in which persons and societies become enmeshed with new imaging and genomic mappings, and are called upon to decide what lives are worth living, and at what cost. The globalization of mass communication raises new fears over the porosity of the social body and its exposure to external threats. There are "viruses," both bacteriological and virtual, everywhere, it seems, spreading alongside more hopeful visions of ecological renewal, mindful living, and global health.

The distinctions and divisions among the senses themselves were increasingly challenged in the twentieth century. The dominant organ-based folk model of the five senses upon which biomedical care had been organized for centuries lost its scientific value as the sensorium was broken down and regrouped into new categories. This blurring of sensory boundaries, however, suggested possibilities for new modes of engagement and integration. At the end of the twentieth century, the Western senses emerged from under the enlightened tyranny of vision to be considered anew as agents for healing and change. The return of sensory engagement to medical therapeutics and the rise of integrative, polythetic approaches to healing can be seen as the leading edge of a new wave of medical humanism in the cybernetic era, prefiguring a new set of bioethical concerns, where minds/bodies/communities and "smart" technological creations are no longer fully distinguishable or separable from self, no longer bounded by skin and other sensory organs, no longer essentially other—a millennial crossroads for healing and renewal (Ross 2012).

In multiple ways, patients and practitioners of late twentieth-century health care found themselves slipping away from simpler dynamics of health and illness into complex configurations, straddling the boundaries of embodied and virtual sensorialities. Beyond the mind/body dualisms and holisms of the mid-twentieth century, the end of the century manifested a dissolution of bodily boundaries which could be experienced either as a negation of the self or as a potential enhancement of self through prosthetics and technology. Vivian Sobchack (1998: 313), for example, wrote of becoming a "techno-body" in highly favorable terms. She describes how she discovered prosthetic pleasure when her leg was amputated and replaced with a prosthetic limb, and how, through vigorous exercise and weight loss after the amputation, she began to feel more positive about her body in general. From prosthetic limbs to touch-screen phones, the new technological gadgets, while still potentially alienating, are no longer necessarily regarded as other, but might rather be seen as extensions and even enhancements of the postmodern self. As such they could become integral to transformative healing quests and expanded selfhood, rather than be perceived as crutches, alien components, or tools. It could just

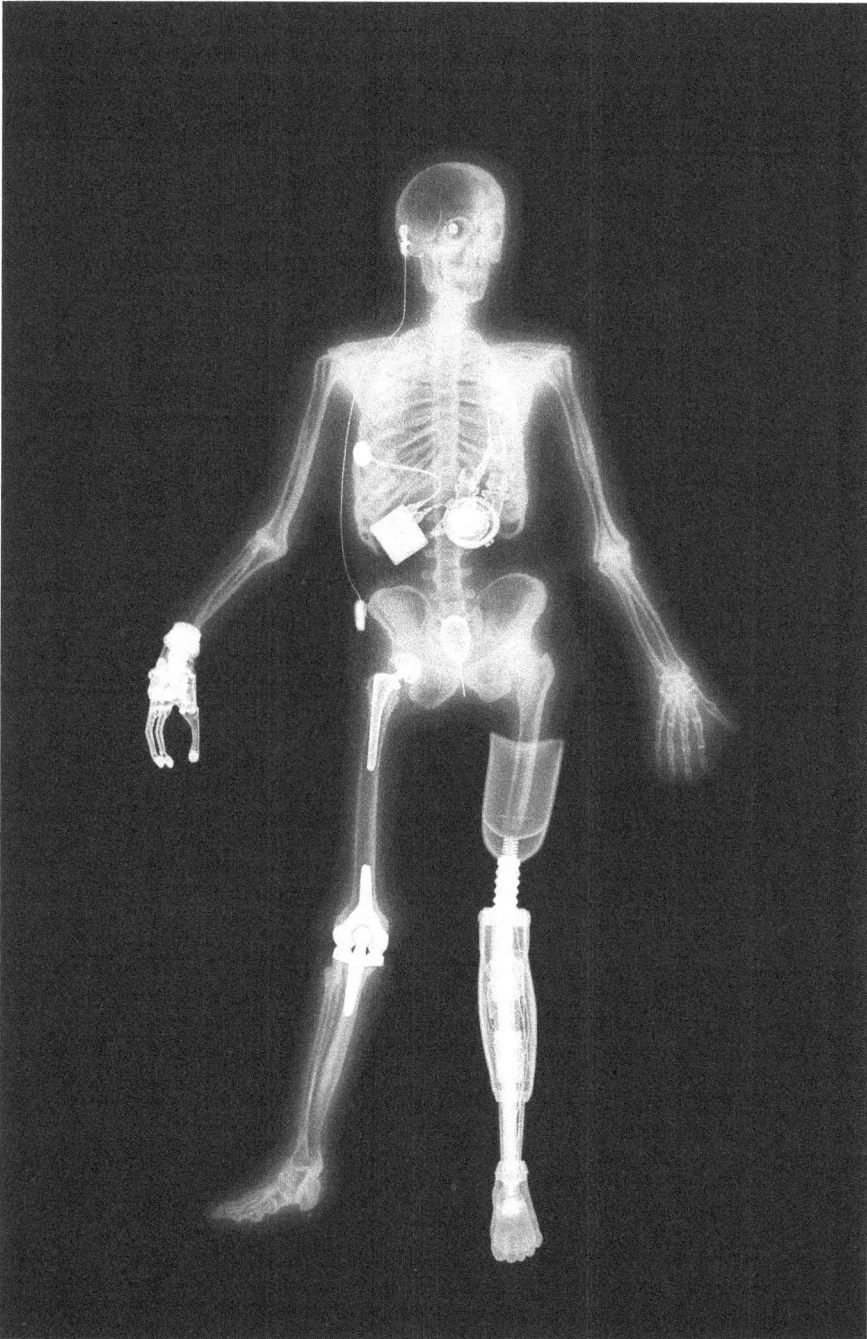

FIGURE 6.6: The body prosthetic by Cameron Slayden, from the cover of *Science* (February 8, 2002). Reprinted with permission of the American Association for the Advancement of Science.

be that these changes drive the heirs of twentieth-century medical enterprises to acknowledge and utilize formerly dormant, culturally diverse, creative capacities of the senses, and to possibly discover entirely new means, modes and maps for experiencing sensation/perception/communication—and healing.

CHAPTER SEVEN

The Senses in Literature: From the Modernist Shock of Sensation to Postcolonial and Virtual Voices

RALF HERTEL

Literature is a prime site for making visible social norms and for reflecting on their impact on sensory perception. This chapter will trace changing attitudes towards sensation, and the negotiation of these changes in literature, in three phases of twentieth-century literature: the modernist period (1920 to 1945), witnessing the impact of new means of mass communication; the postwar years (1945 to the 1970s), with their focus on traumatized bodies in pain; and the contemporary age (beginning in the 1980s), characterized by a playful, and sometimes politically charged, return of the senses and the advent of computer-generated virtual realities.

THE SHOCK OF SENSATION: MODERNIST EXPERIMENTS
(1920–45)

As Chapters 1 and 9 of the present volume demonstrate, the modern age has seen rapid technological changes that have had a profound impact on sense perception. The proliferation of new techniques of communication such as the radio, the telephone, television, and cinema directly influence the experience of the modern world. Like technical inventions in the field of medicine and the natural sciences such as the electron microscope or X-rays, the new devices of communication provide technical extensions of the senses. As Sigmund Freud, among the most prominent early commentators on the technical developments and their impact on the senses, argues, "with all his tools man improves on his own organs, both motor or sensory, or clears away the barriers to their functioning" (Freud 2002: 28). X-rays and microscopes bring into focus what is hidden from the naked eye, telephones extend the reach of hearing over continents, television allows us to perceive events that lie far beyond the reach of the human eye and ear. At the same time, tools for recording sound or sight, such as gramophones, tapes, photography, and film provide new means for storing both individuals' remembrances and the collective memory. Thus, one may argue that the modern period extends and refines sensory practices, confronting humanity with new perceptions of various kinds, sometimes perhaps even overwhelming it in a "shock of sensation" (Woolf 2000: 72, 126), to borrow a phrase from Virginia Woolf's pertinent novel *The Waves* (1931), to be discussed in the following. At the same time that these devices extend the senses, they paradoxically also impoverish them. As Western societies come to rely increasingly on prosthetic devices for sensory perception, and as the overflow of stimuli in mass culture numbs the senses, the acuteness of unaided human perception could be argued to be in decline. Thus, it has been suggested that the modern age also witnesses a "vanishing of the senses" as they are becoming increasingly dependent on, and at least partly replaced by, technological devices (Kamper and Wulf 1984a).

   Modernist literature registers, and gives expression to, these changes. Thomas Mann's novel *The Magic Mountain* (1924) provides a striking example of how the enhancement of the senses by medical apparatuses changes the protagonist's perception of the world. Set in a sanatorium in the Swiss Alps, the novel depicts the shock Hans Castorp experiences when confronted for the first time with X-rays, a comparatively new technology invented by Wilhelm Röntgen in 1895. Castorp is present when his friend's chest is exposed to this new prognostic device, and is both fascinated and intimidated by the new type of vision this image-making device offers. Aided by the prosthetic device of the X-rays, his eyes are able to see what had so far been concealed from them: life itself pulsating underneath the skin of a living human being. It is as if Castorp could see through the dress, skin, and outward bodily appearance of his friend and discern the latter's innermost being with the naked eye, as if the core of his friend's being suddenly lay exposed to view. Intrigued by this experience, Castorp has his own hand X-rayed, and again the extension of vision beneath the surface of the skin causes a titillating sensation, although now it is death rather than life that Castorp sees plainly as never before. Stripped of flesh, his X-rayed hand is an image of bones that makes Castorp realize in a flash that underneath the skin, human beings, including himself, are merely living skeletons; that hidden below clothes and skin walks death itself. Hence the new technique functions both as a *memento mori* and as a time machine of sorts, prefiguring temporarily and instantaneously the effect of death: the transformation of a human being into a mere heap of bones. Thus, the passage from Mann's novel depicts a shock of sensation brought about by new ways of seeing that could hardly be more profound: seeing through the prosthetic devices of medical invention, both life and death suddenly seem to become visible. They become a presence in the life of Mann's protagonist that he can no longer ignore.

The irritation experienced by Castorp is representative of the shock of sensation registered in much of modernist writing. A variety of other texts, too, demonstrate how new ways of perceiving the world, often brought about by technical instruments, create a sense of wonder and call into question established concepts of perception and literary representation.[1] Christopher Isherwood's *Goodbye to Berlin* (1939), for instance, emphatically defines the narrator's perspective in terms of photography: "I am a camera with its shutter open, quite passive, recording, not thinking . . . Some day, all this will have to be developed, carefully printed, fixed" (Isherwood 1986: 11). Indeed, the photographic perspective informs Isherwood's entire narration in which the young English tutor Christopher moves through pre-Second World War Berlin in a highly perceptive, yet strangely detached, mood. It is as if Isherwood wanted his protagonist to become an extension of his readers' senses, a narrative tool for tele-vision, as it were, registering in great detail the sound and sight of Berlin in the early 1930s and transporting this sensation over space and time to readers elsewhere. Of course, it might be argued that literature in general functions as an extension of the reader's perception, opening up fictional worlds at a geographical and temporal remove, yet Isherwood's explicitly photographic stance, which reduces the narrator to a dispassionate eye in the text, does much to foreground this effect. At the same time, it is representative of a literary trend devoted to the allegedly objective recording of reality which manifests itself, for instance, in a strong interest in documentary writing. This interest is shared by Isherwood and shows in his travel documentary about the Sino-Japanese War, *Journey to a War* (1939), conceived of in collaboration with W. H. Auden, who himself was strongly involved in the documentary movement.[2] It also shows in the artistic and literary movement known by its German name as *Neue Sachlichkeit* (literally "new objectivity") which formed in Germany in the 1920s and attempted to reduce to a minimum narratorial or painterly intervention in the depiction of reality. It is certainly no coincidence that Isherwood developed his objective, detached style during his Berlin years in the 1930s.

Literary products as diverse as Mann's *Magic Mountain* and Isherwood's *Goodbye to Berlin* have in common that they no longer take perception for granted. In the modern period, with its technical extensions of the senses and its overflow of stimuli, perception itself becomes the focus of literary investigation. Literature proves to be particularly well equipped to negotiate changes in sensory perception because it may not only describe sense perceptions on the level of contents but might—through the use of narrative perspective and voice—entice readers to adopt certain perspectives on the fictional world themselves and to situate them within particular consciousnesses. One of the most intriguing and far-reaching analyses of perception by means of modernist literature, and one of the most radical attempts to make the reader adopt particular perspectives on the fictional world, is Virginia Woolf's novel *The Waves*.

Sense perception forms an overwhelming presence in this experimental text, beginning with the titular waves that present a recurring leitmotif and structure the course of events, as chapters describing the flow and ebb of waves rhythmically intersect the stream of the protagonists' thoughts. Yet, they are not only the emblem of a rhythmically conceived novel—of a novel that is written "to a rhythm and not to a plot," as Woolf claims (Woolf 1978: 204)—but in their appeal to all sense they capture in a nutshell the preoccupation of the novel with sensation. Waves, Woolf's verbal evocations make clear, are a phenomenon stimulating all senses: as one sees them building up and falling, creating a heaving motion on the surface of the sea, one hears them rolling onto the shore, feels the fine spray they diffuse when they meet the shore, smells the tangy scent of sea water they transport, and might taste the saltiness they evaporate into the air. At the same time, they are, like sense perceptions, mere surface, the perceptible outside of something deeper and

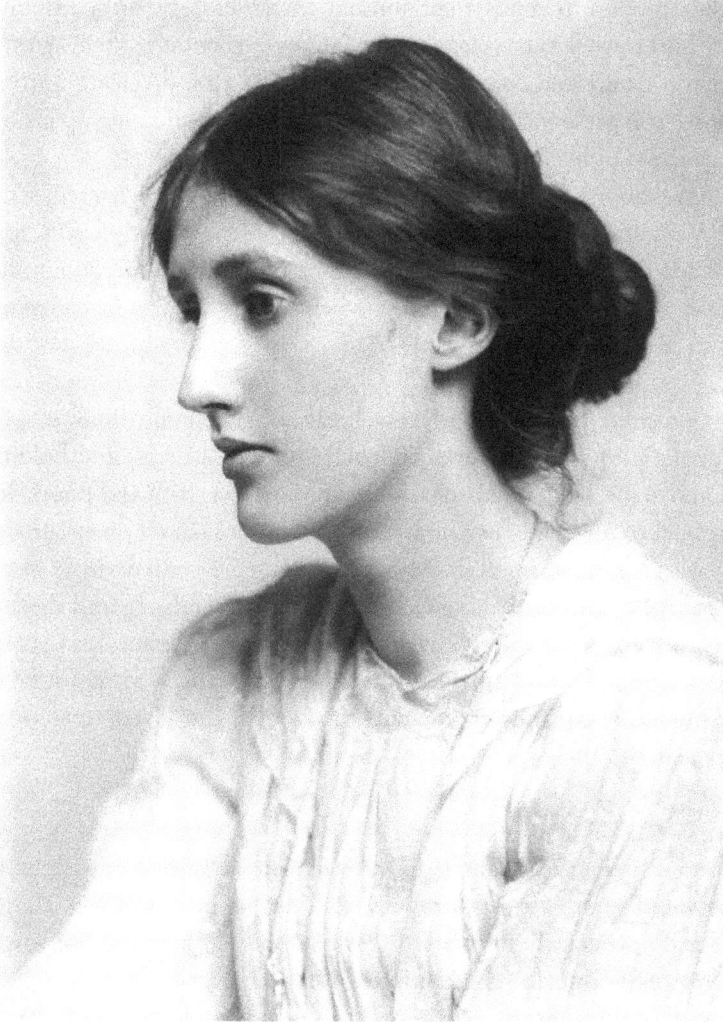

FIGURE 7.1: Portrait of Virginia Woolf by George Charles Beresford. Public domain.

more constant, just like sensory impressions present the outermost layer of personal experiences and might eventually sink in to form part of a more enduring consciousness.

Exclamations calling for sensory awareness such as "look" or "listen" literally flood the text; scents are described in great detail and the scene is repeatedly set in restaurants or banqueting halls, i.e. in places where gustatory stimuli are plentiful. Thus, we observe the six protagonists' thoughts unfold while they prepare to meet their mutual friend Perceval in a restaurant to celebrate his farewell as he is leaving for India; we encounter them again dining at Hampton Court and commemorating Perceval after his death abroad; and the final section presents us with one of the characters summing up his own life as well as those of his friends while sitting in a restaurant.

The novel abounds with instances of intense, minutely registered, sensation. Bernard's experience of being washed by Mrs Constable while at school sets the tone for this acute evocation of sensory perceptions. "Trooping upstairs like ponies . . . stamping, clattering one behind another" to be called into the bathroom, Bernard awaits his turn:

> Mrs Constable, girt in a bath-towel, takes her lemon-coloured sponge and soaks it in water; it turns chocolate-brown; it drips; and holding it high above me, shivering beneath her, she squeezes it. Water pours down the runnel of my spine. Bright arrows of sensation shoot on either side. I am covered with warm flesh. My dry crannies are wetted; my cold body is warmed; it is sluiced and gleaming. Water descends me and sheets me like an eel. Now hot towels envelop me, and their roughness, as I rub my back, makes my blood purr. Rich and heavy sensations form on the roof of my mind; down showers the day–the woods, and Elvedon; Susan and the pigeon.
>
> Woolf 2000: 13

This is an experience speaking to various senses at once, to sight (as the lemon-colored sponge turns brown), to hearing (as their feet clatter and stamp), and particularly to touch (as water "sheets" him and hot towels rub and warm his body). In its attention to "the arrows of sensation," and the minuteness of its literary evocation, this passage is representative of the novel in general, which teems with sensuous evocations of first kisses, landscapes, noisy crowds, and city life, train rides, birds in gardens, and, time and again, the sea. In fact, the entire novel seems to be about sensations minutely observed, about characters "glutted with sensations" (88) whose "senses stand erect" (98).

Woolf's concern with the minute evocation of sensory impressions is shared by some of her protagonists. In describing the attempts of Bernard, Rhoda, and Neville to pay scrupulous attention to sensation, Woolf describes her own literary program. In her essay on *Modern Fiction* (1919, extended version 1925), she had famously demanded that the modern author should "examine for a moment an ordinary mind on an ordinary day":

> The mind receives a myriad impressions—trivial, fantastic, evanescent, or engraved with the sharpness of steel. From all sides they come, an incessant shower of innumerable atoms . . . Let us record the atoms as they fall upon the mind in the order in which they fall, let us trace the pattern, however disconnected and incoherent in appearance, which each sight or incident scores upon the consciousness.
>
> Woolf 2008b: 9

In *The Waves*, Woolf herself and some of her protagonists seem to follow this modernist program as they attempt to capture the "incessant shower of innumerable atoms," the sensory impression before it is processed into meaning or abstracted into words. Time and again, the characters stress the here and now of perception, attempting to unconditionally expose themselves to the "shock of sensation" (Woolf 2000: 72, 126) and to stay on the surface of perception rather than to make meaning from the information perceived. Formulations such as "here and now" (e.g. 12, 18, 35, 70), the "present moment" (e.g. 35), and, in particular, "now" pervade the characters' thoughts like a leitmotiv. In certain passages, almost every sentence is introduced by the word "now" suggesting a lack of distance to the events perceived, an unmediated, unreflected surrender to sensation:

> All my senses stand erect. Now I feel the roughness of the fibre of the curtain through which I push; now I feel the cold iron railing and its blistered paint beneath my palm. Now the cool tide of darkness breaks its waters over me . . . I smell roses; I smell violets; I see red and blue just hidden. Now gravel is under my shoes; now grass. (98)

As they grow older, several characters adopt the sensory perception of the present moment as an artistic credo, or even as the ideal stance towards life as such. The struggle of Neville, the poet, focuses exactly on the attempt to capture the immediacy of sensory experience without distorting it through language, and reading *The Waves* one might well wonder whether Neville's dilemma is not Woolf's as well:

> "In a world which contains the present moment," said Neville, "why discriminate? Nothing should be named lest by doing so we change it. Let it exist, this bank, this beauty, and I, for one instant, steeped in pleasure. The sun is hot. I see the river. I see trees specked, and burned in the autumn sunlight. Boats float past, through the red, through the green. Far

away a bell tolls, but not for death. There are bells that ring for life. A leaf falls, from joy. Oh, I am in love with life! Look how the willow shoots its fine sprays into the air! Look how through them a boat passes, filled with indolent, with unconscious, with powerful young men. They are listening to the gramophone, eating fruit out of paper bags. They are tossing the skins of bananas, which then sink eel-like, into the river. All they do is so beautiful!" (45)

The range of sensory perceptions addressed and the exactness with which they are conveyed here is again remarkable, as is the plainness of style with its short, simple sentences. It is as if Neville—and perhaps Woolf herself—suggested that sensory impressions could only properly be registered in what Bernard terms the "little language" of simple words (135). Yet, Neville ultimately fails to achieve such a language:

I see it all. I feel it all. I am inspired. My eyes fill with tears. Yet even as I feel this, I lash my frenzy higher and higher. It foams. It becomes artificial, insincere. Words and words and words, how they gallop—how they lash their long manes and tails, but for some fault in me I cannot give myself to their backs; I cannot fly with them . . . (45)

Similarly, Bernard, when looking back at his life towards the close of the novel, attempts to return to "bare things." Bernard, who has always been a maker of stories, finally realizes that words separate us from the world rather than bring us closer to it. He has "done with phrases," preferring silence instead, rejecting his former impulse to take things or people as starting points for stories, to fashion himself and others with words: "Let me sit here for ever with bare things, this coffee-cup, this knife, this fork, things in themselves, myself being myself" (166).

This turn towards the immediacy of impressions carries several implications both crucial to the message of the novel and representative for the modernist attitude towards sensation. On the one hand, it reacts to a skeptical attitude towards language, widespread among modernists and reaching back at least to Hugo von Hofmannsthal's *The Lord Chandos Letter* (1902). In this letter addressed to Francis Bacon, Hofmannsthal has Chandos describe his desperation over words, and abstract words in particular, that never seem to capture what they denote; instead, they seem to fall apart in his mouth like decaying mushrooms, useless, disintegrating tools in the struggle with reality. What Hofmannsthal describes is an instance of the signifier and the signified falling apart—it is no coincidence that his text is contemporaneous with Ferdinand de Saussure's *Course on General Linguistics* (held between 1906 and 1911, published posthumously 1916), popularizing the idea of the signifier and the signified as distinct categories—and the realization that the former is never completely capable of conveying a sense of the latter. The decidedly simple language preferred by Neville or Bernard appears to react to such a wariness of words, and in particular of abstract words. The protagonists' attempt, and Woolf's own apparent desire, to capture sense perceptions before they are abstracted into meaning seems to respond to this verbal crisis by attempting to find a language still capable of conveying the immediacy of the world surrounding us. Theirs is a language that aims to capture "faces and things so subtle that they have smell, colour, texture, substance, but no name" (121).

The focus is on perception, not so much on meaning, and in this regard, the most prominent absence of the novel is significant, too. Perceval, who functions as a common point of reference for the characters' thoughts, has a strikingly allusive name, and even without going into the details of the mythological allusions evoked, one discerns its significance in a wider modernist context. The mere fact that through Perceval, Woolf alludes to mythology is in keeping with a prominent modernist practice; in a world experienced as changing rapidly, as falling apart and as causing a feeling of alienation, several modernists turn towards myth as the last refuge providing some sort of coherence, structure, and meaning. James Joyce's *Ulysses* (1922) bears its mythological reference in its title; William Butler Yeats's writing is characterized by a turn towards specifically Irish myths; and T. S. Eliot's conversion to Anglicanism, too, might been regarded as part of this turn towards myth as antidote to the disorientation of the modern world. Yet, in Woolf's *The Waves*, Perceval, onomastically the representative of myth and a figure providing a common focus for the various protagonists as well as meaning to some of their gatherings, not only forms a prominent absence but eventually dies. Perhaps his death might be considered a symbolic one: myth no longer provides coherence, meaning, and communion here. In the world of *The Waves*, the individual characters are increasingly reduced to themselves. And what does this imply? It means being reduced to perceptions turned into emotions, to the effect of affect, Woolf's novel appears to argue. Thus, despite the flow and overlap of the protagonists' thoughts, *The Waves* ultimately appears to be fundamentally pessimistic in tracing a sense of alienation even among close friends. It is only the turn towards the sensory experience that might temporarily reunite them in the act of sharing impressions in the same place at the same time; it is perhaps only on the surface of sensory perception that alienation might for a short time be overcome.

In demonstrating how our perception of the world crucially relies on impressions gathered by the senses, Woolf's novel prefigures later philosophical concepts such as Maurice Merleau-Ponty's notion of the embodied mind. In *Phenomenology of Perception* (1945), Merleau-Ponty discards the Cartesian separation of body and mind and the notion that the body functions merely as an instrument serving the mind. Instead he argues that our connection to the world is always in and through the body, that it is only the body which situates us in the world; that the body is in fact the very condition for us "having a world": "The body is the vehicle of being in the world, and having a body is, for a living creature, to be intervolved in a definite environment, to identify oneself with certain projects and be continually committed to them" (Merleau-Ponty 1992: 81–2). He reminds his readers that it is the body only that allows us to enter into contact with the world, and that the body, and in particular our senses, fundamentally shape this contact by filtering the impressions that reach us from the outside world. Thus, in contrast to the Cartesian view, the senses are not merely windows onto the world but crucially define what we perceive and how we do so; they are, in Woolf's own phrase, not transparent, unnoticeable windows but smeared, stained, and colored panes:

> All day, all night the body intervenes; blunts or sharpens, colours or discolours, turns to wax in the warmth of June, hardens to tallow in the murk of February. The creature within can only gaze through the pane— smudged or rosy; it cannot separate off from the body like the sheath of a knife or the pod of a pea for a single instant.
>
> Woolf 2008b: 101

Or, as Jinny phrases it in *The Waves*: "But my imagination is the bodies. I can imagine nothing beyond the circle cast by my body. My body goes before me, like a lantern down a dark lane, bringing one thing after another out of darkness into a ring of light" (Woolf 2000a: 71).

By changing perspectives and by inviting us to enter a variety of minds as they process sensory impressions in different ways, Woolf's novel reminds us of the fact that each one of us is tied to a specific affective body. In *The Waves*, the protagonists' bodies, and their sensory organs, are tools for both communion and separation: on the one hand, the body bridges intellectual, social, and gender-specific gaps as all characters alike share in the realm of the sensory; at the same time, the senses single them out, since each individual is tied to a specific body that perceives the world in a specific way and presents him or her with a unique perspective that cannot be shared since words hopelessly fall short of capturing the sensory experience. Ultimately, Woolf's obsession with the sensory thus reflects a fundamentally modernist tension between the desire to overcome a sense of alienation and the realization that all attempts to do so might be in vain, not least because the body already bars us from true communion.

Finally, Woolf's preoccupation with sensory impressions responds to her feminist concerns. If the symbolic and abstract is associated with the masculine (as it is in the concept of phallogocentricsm, a logocentricsm dominated by the phallus, first advanced by Jacques Derrida [1975] and elaborated on by feminist critics such Luce Irigaray and Julia Kristeva—see Harris 1997), the turn towards "bare things," the "things in themselves," the mere perception—in short: the pre-symbolic—might be understood as a feminist strategy of resisting the masculine order. If early twentieth-century culture is structured according to a masculine logic, the attempt to reach for impressions before they are structured and for sensations before they are integrated in, and accommodated by, social norms, might express the desire to enter a realm forgoing the symbolic order. Woolf's own style, impressionist and almost tangible in its physicality (note for instance how in sentences such as "Gradually as the sky whitened a dark line lay on the horizon dividing the sea from the sky and the grey cloth became barred with thick strokes moving, one after another, beneath the surface, following each other, pursuing each other, perpetually" Woolf imitates the rhythmic movement of the waves through the use of commas and repetitions), presents an *écriture féminine avant la lettre* and aims to convey to the reader a different perspective on the world. The perspective offered here is characterized by an immediacy and sensuousness that might be regarded as feminine perhaps rather than masculine. By asking readers to share this perspective, Woolf invites them to open up to a feminine perception of the world.

OUT OF THEIR SENSES: POSTWAR PAIN (1945–70s)

It has been argued that modernism is a period characterized by "the elevation of sight" and the "visualization of the world" (Classen 2001: 361, 362), and indeed, many modernist movements such as Impressionism, Expressionism, and Cubism take their cue from innovations in the field of vision. Literature, too, provides us with a welter of texts prominently informed by new ways of seeing. Mann's episode on technologically enhanced forms of seeing, mentioned above, comes to mind, as do Gertrude Stein's abstract writings reminiscent of a multi-perspective cubism and Woolf's novel *To the Lighthouse* (1927), centered on the painter Lilly Briscoe and deeply engaged in questions of visual representation. Prominently, the imagist movement centers its artistic credo in verbally capturing glimpses of reality, as in Pound's famous example "In the Station of a Metro" (1913), which shrinks to a two-line visual impression: "The apparition of these faces in the crowd; / Petals on a wet, black bough." Other texts respond to new visual technologies such as photography or film, either by imitating the detached, objective perspective of the camera eye (apart from Isherwood's *Goodbye to Berlin*, Vladimir Nabokov's novella *The Eye*, written in pre-Second World War Berlin comes to mind) or by integrating photography in their often semi-documentary texts (as in W. H. Auden and Isherwood's *Journey to a War* [1939] or John Steinbeck and Robert Capa's *Russian Journal* [1948]).

It appears that the dominance of vision over the proximity senses smell, taste, and touch, is the hallmark of the modern age (Classen 2001: 362; Kamper and Wulf 1984b: 12). Sight as the most detached sense, as the sense that keeps the greatest distance between stimulus and perceiving person, is often regarded as being the most rational sense, as the sense that does not demand incorporation or a physical contact between subject and object. Traditionally, it has been associated with clarity and rationality, and terms such as "enlightenment" illustrate how closely the idea of reason is interwoven with sight. At the same time, sight is sometimes also described as the most elitist sense. In contrast to the sense of smell, for instance, it allows the perceiver to stand apart from or above the perceived, to avoid intermingling, and to judge from a distance (Horkheimer and Adorno 2002: 151); it is associated with control (e.g. in terms such as to "oversee" or to "supervise"), comprehension (in cases such as "I see," where seeing is equated with understanding), and even divinatory capabilities (as in "to foresee").

If we encounter a rising interest in the other senses and a questioning of the sense of sight in the period after the Second World War, this is perhaps indicative of a turn against the elitism frequently associated with modernism. In the literature of the period after 1945, we encounter a variety of blind protagonists, such as Samuel Beckett's Hamm in *Endgame* (1957), a blinded native girl in J. M. Coetzee's *Waiting for the Barbarians* (1980), or John Berger's narrator Tsobanakos in *To the Wedding* (1995), as well as a host of texts that focus prominently on the so-called lower senses. One might think here of Beckett's often handicapped figures with their problematic digestion, smelly feet, and aching bodies, of the stench of decay in Ian McEwan's *The Cement Garden*

(1978), of Salman Rushdie, Patrick Süskind, and John Berger's olfactorily gifted protagonists in *Midnight's Children* (1981) (to which we will turn in a moment), *Perfume* (1985), and *King* (1999). This interest in the proximity senses also shows in texts focusing on the gustatory, such as Margaret Atwood's *The Edible Woman* (1969) or Italo Calvino's *Under the Jaguar Sun* (1986), as well as in the prominence of skin and touch in novels such as Coetzee's *Waiting for the Barbarians*, Jeanette Winterson's *The Passion* (1987), or Michael Ondaatje's *The English Patient* (1992). Constance Classen (2001: 356) has argued that in the Western cultural history of the senses, the ranking of the senses has often reflected social hierarchies, and that vision was repeatedly associated with the upper classes "overseeing" and guiding the lower classes, who have traditionally been linked to the lower senses. Indeed, in many of these postwar texts, the turn away from the allegedly elitist sense of sight and the turn towards the lower senses goes hand in hand with an increased interest in the lower classes and those marginalized by society, in women, ethnic outsiders, people stigmatized by diseases such as HIV/AIDS, and those of a supposedly "deviant" sexual orientation.

If postwar authors turn towards sight, it is sometimes to foreground the illusionist nature of visual perception, making the reader doubt whether the sense of sight is to be trusted at all. This is the case for example in John Banville's trilogy *Frames*, consisting of the novels *The Book of Evidence* (1989), *Ghosts* (1993), and *Athena* (1995). Here, sight often creates visual conundrums, leaving the reader to speculate about whether certain characters appearing in the novels exist at all (to the extent they can be said to exist), or whether they are merely the illusionary products of the imagination of the other characters in the novel—and of our own fancy. As sight gives way to vision, visual perception is presented as highly unreliable.

In the first decades following the Second World War, this turn away from sight forms part of a more general anti-sensual reaction, a reaction that shows perhaps most clearly in the work of Samuel Beckett. As in postwar novels such as Günter Grass' *The Tin Drum* (1959), which focuses on dwarf-like Oskar Matzerath who, at the age of three, decides to bring the growth of his body to a stop by willfully flinging himself down a flight of stairs, or his *Cat and Mouse* (1961), which centers on a protagonist with a pathologically enlarged Adam's apple, we encounter a panorama of handicapped bodies in Beckett's plays. Beckett's protagonists are plagued by an impressive list of bodily ailments: they have smelly feet as well as bad breath and suffer from incontinence, like Vladimir and Estragon in *Waiting for Godot* (1952); they are buried in the ground and thus forced to immobility like Winnie in *Happy Days* (1961); they are paralyzed

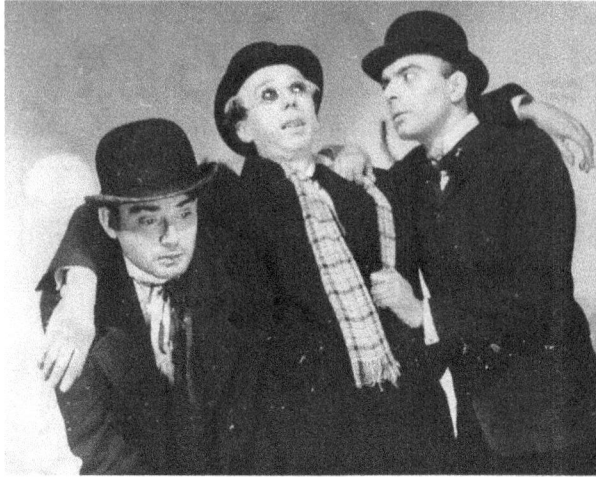

FIGURE 7.2: Performance of *Waiting for Godot* by Samuel Beckett, Buenos Aires, 1956. Public domain.

and blind like Hamm in *Endgame* or lacking legs like his parents Nagg and Nell, living like animals in rubbish bins. It appears that there is hardly a figure in Beckett's theatrical cosmos that does not have some physical impediment or other, and his prose protagonists do not fare much better; to a certain degree it appears to be precisely their handicaps that define the uniqueness of Beckett's protagonists. A short dialogue in *Endgame* sums it up acerbically:

Clov:	I can't sit.
Hamm:	True. And I can't stand.
Clov:	So it is.
Hamm:	Every man his speciality. *Pause.*

Beckett 1981: 461

More often than not, their sensory relation to the world is severely impeded as a consequence. Hamm in his blindness has to rely on his companion Clov to mount a ladder, draw back a curtain, peer through a window, and describe to him the world outside—only to be told that there is "Zero" to be seen (457). Together with Clov, Hamm is trapped inside a bare room that, with its two windows set high in the wall opposite the audience, uncoincidentally resembles the inside of a skull, suggesting that he is really caught inside himself. His inability to peer through the windows points towards his inability to communicate with the outside world. Indeed, many of Beckett's characters are trapped inside their decaying bodies, just as Winnie is stuck in the earth, increasingly unable to reach out for the outside through their failing senses—the contrast to Woolf's extremely perceptive protagonists could hardly be more pronounced. Their malfunctioning senses severely impede their contact with the world and are emblematic of a disturbed, if not ruined, relation to the world of post-Second World War subjects. A similar rationale appears to motivate Grass' use of impaired protagonists whose bodily stigmata seem to reflect the stigma of Second World War Germany (*Cat and Mouse*), or who refuse to grow up normally in a society under the growing influence of racist ideologies (*The Tin Drum*).

Simultaneously, however, focusing so obsessively on these damaged bodies with their impaired sensation is also a means of foregrounding them. The reality of Beckett's dramatic figures is quite literally a *corporeality*, a reality crucially defined by the protagonists' bodies and their perception. It is precisely by their handicaps and their impaired sensation that Beckett's protagonists are constantly reminded of their bodies and of how much they rely on the senses to make sense of the world. Thus, we witness a fundamental tension in Beckett's plays with regard to the sensuous: while sensation is often extremely unspectacular here, the plays make clear that sensation and the body are not dispensable altogether but are the very—often painful—condition for our existence.

Although in an utterly different way than Woolf's novel, Beckett's plays thus visualize Merleau-Ponty's notion of the embodied mind that exists only in and through the body and the senses. The notion of an embodied mind that Woolf's novel hints at is explored to the full in much of Beckett's work. We do not know for sure whether Beckett and Merleau-Ponty directly influenced each other, but they certainly moved in the same inter- and postwar circles in Paris and shared the same intellectual climate (Maude 2009: 4). If Merleau-Ponty is among the earliest and most original thinkers in the twentieth century, rejecting the Cartesian mind-body dualism and arguing for the interdependence of both, Beckett's stage characters render this idea tangible precisely by showing the resistance impaired bodies offer to our perception of the world. Far from vanishing, Beckett's decrepit bodies draw attention to themselves, reminding the spectator precisely by their failure to communicate that it is only through the body that contact with the world is established. If Merleau-Ponty's concept of the embodied mind can be seen as a reaction against the separation of mind and body beginning with the celebration of pure reason in the Enlightenment and prominent still in the Victorian desire to repress the body and its needs through social control, Beckett's plays popularize this return of the body on the open stage. As Ulrika Maude suggests, Beckett, however, crucially departs from Merleau-Ponty's affirmative belief that the concept of the embodied mind installs the body as a new locus of meaning; rather, Beckett's work brings to the fore a mistrust in the possibility of any transcendent knowledge (Maude 2009: 22).

In the case of Beckett's dramatic work, this tension between a reduction of the sensuous and a foregrounding of the senses characterizes the choice of medium, too. By turning to theater, Beckett chooses a medium that, unlike prose, speaks to all senses; his plays are experienced visually and acoustically, and the theater event might also be perceived in tactile or olfactory terms (in the proximity of fellow spectators, the texture of the seats the audience is seated on, etc.). Yet, Beckett's plays hardly present feasts for the senses. During the two hours a performance of *Waiting for Godot* might take, for instance, the audience sees little more than two aged bums on a nondescript countryside road, the only extra feature being a bare tree. Beckett's other plays are hardly sensual pleasures either, with their protagonists buried in the ground or trapped in wheelchairs. There is much immobility in Beckett and little color; and although drama is a medium essentially relying on the spoken word, there is often also little sound as the silence mushrooms between the sparse comments made by the protagonists. Yet, it is exactly the absence of stimuli, the silence, the dullness of setting, the minimalism of visual and auditory variation, that might make the audience come to their senses, as the minimalism of stimuli increases the attention drawn by each single perception. If Beckett's decrepit protagonists move, each movement draws attention to it; if their words pierce the silence so pervasive in his plays, each voice draws attention to itself by its bare existence; if the visual settings eventually do change, we notice these changes with particular acuity, be these changes as minimal as the sprouting of a few leaves on the bare tree of *Waiting for Godot* between its two acts. And if the protagonists do not move, and do not speak, as is often the case, the spectators are made painfully aware of how much they long for sensory input; of how much they, as *spectators*, want to see; of how much they, as members of an *audience*, want to hear. By countering the flood of stimuli of postwar mass culture for the duration of his plays, Beckett readjusts the senses, and his anti-sensual plays paradoxically sharpen the theater-goers' sense of their own senses.

COMING TO THEIR SENSES: CONTEMPORARY VOICES (1980s TO THE PRESENT)

This transition from what Dietmar Kamper and Christoph Wulf term a "Schwinden der Sinne" to a "Wiederkehr des Körpers" (i.e. from a vanishing of the senses to a return of the body), makes Beckett's work representative of postwar literature (Kamper and Wulf 1982, 1984a). This growing awareness of the crucial position of the body shows, for instance, in the philosophical concept of corporeality as advanced by Michel Foucault, who foregrounds the importance of bodily experiences such as discipline and punishment in the shaping of identity (Foucault [1975] 1979). In the realm of literature, postcolonial writing in particular has recently focused on the body and its perception. South African Nobel Prize winner J. M. Coetzee's novel *Foe* (1986), for instance, retells the story of Robinson Crusoe from the point of view of Susan Barton, who allegedly spent many years with Crusoe and Friday on the island, and discusses Friday's loss of his tongue and his inability to speak. *Waiting for the Barbarians* traces the signs of torture inscribed on the skin of a young woman in ways that may remind the reader of Franz Kafka's *In the Penal Colony* (1919), where an officer parades a machine inscribing death sentences onto the body of convicts, killing them in the process. Both novels thus bring to the fore mutilated bodies, foregrounding sensory perception as a source of pain.

This is a concern that they share with other postcolonial writings such as Michael Ondaatje's *The English Patient*, which is set against the backdrop of the Second World War and centers on a geographer who plays a dubious role as guide for the Germans and whose skin is severely burned when his plane crashes; with the Indian-born Salman Rushdie's *The Moor's Last Sigh* (1995), which is narrated by a protagonist with a misshapen fist and aging at double speed inside a body literally cracking apart; with Australian Peter Carey's *My Life as a Fake* (2003), telling the story of Bob McCorkle, a monstrous, Frankenstein-like creature; or even with Zadie Smith's Asian and Jamaican protagonists in *White Teeth* (2000), with their lack of teeth and limp arms. In the context of postcolonial writing, it makes sense that the body, and in particular the body as a source of pain, should become such a prominent topic since it often functions as a marker of frequently painfully experienced discrimination. Yet, postcolonial literature repeatedly goes beyond merely recording the pain experienced by discrimination and projecting it onto the body and the senses; in what appears to be a deliberate attempt to reject the subjugation of the body to the ideologies of racism, it frequently re-signifies the body as a source of sensuous pleasures anteceding ideological inscriptions. In these cases, the stubborn materiality of the sensuous body presents a resistance to ideologies that would reduce it to a mere sign of otherness, both by calling to mind a fundamental human oneness and by demonstrating that the body is not merely a sign or object but also an agent that in its ever-changing vivacity resists being fixed to a single meaning.

Salman Rushdie's *Midnight's Children* (1981) provides a striking example of the role sensation plays in postcolonial writing. Set in post-independence India and Pakistan, it is narrated by Saleem Sinai, a narrator noteworthy for his peculiar sensory abilities. Typically for postcolonial writing perhaps, it is not the sense of sight that makes him stand out from the rest, but hearing and smell. Born at the precise moment of India's independence—on the stroke of midnight of August 15, 1947—he is gifted with a miraculously refined sensory perception. As a boy, he is capable of telepathic hearing, and can tune in to the voices and thoughts of the 1,000 children that, like himself, were born in the first hour of India's independence—the other midnight's children. For a while he acts as a radio moderator of sorts, telepathically hosting conventions in the hope to create a better future for a country that is exactly his age, counting on the magical gifts all these children have been equipped with by the accident of their birth at this special hour.

What makes him—quite literally—stand out is his prominent nose. A "rampant cucumber" (124), "elephantine" (155), "gargantuan" (122, 353), and blooming "like a prize marrow" (154), his olfactory organ can hardly be overlooked. Not only does it enable Saleem to communicate with the other midnight's children, it also turns him into an embodiment of India as he is to learn in a painful lesson in "human geography." In front of the class Saleem's sadistic teacher takes a firm grip of the boy's nose:

> "In the face of thees ugly ape you don't see the whole map of *India*?"
> "Yes sir no sir you show us sir!"
> "See here—the Deccan peninsula hanging down!" Again ouchmynose.
> "Sir sir if that's the map of India what are the stains sir?" . . .
> And Zagallo, taking the question in his stride: "These stains", he cries, "are Pakistan! Thees birthmark on the right ear is the East Wing; and thees horribly stained left cheek, the West! Remember, stupid boys: Pakistan ees the stain on the face of India!"

At this moment, Saleem's nose stages its own revolt against the teacher's grasping fingers. Unleashing "a weapon of its own," it releases a "large blob of shining goo," prompting a classmate to shout out: "Lookit that sir! The drip from his nose, sir! Is that supposed to be *Ceylon*?" (231).

The nose, however, not only functions as a sign or index here, pointing towards Saleem's being "handcuffed to" (9) the fate of India. *Midnight's Children* is also a text crucially informed by smells as his nose is a particularly acute organ of olfaction. Cruising the streets of Karachi, Saleem not only sniffs out the "knife-sharpness of expectorated betel-nut" or the "competitive effluvia of the city's bus-drivers," but his nose distinguishes fragrances hidden from others, such as the "heady but quick-fading perfume of new love," the "sharp stink" of his grandmother's curiosity (52), or the "bitter-sweet fragrance of hope-for-marriage" (384). In other words, Saleem's olfactory organ opens up to him the nasal perception of thoughts and emotions—and of memories, too. Ending up as the pickler-in-chief of Braganza pickles, he relies on his nose to find the right mixture for the chutneys that, in turn, help him to set down his autobiography, for their smells remind him of events of the past. Thus, his novel is nasally conceived, and in its structure and language it shows characteristics that link it to olfaction. Through comic strip language, gaps, interjections, and non-verbal elements, the text imitates the emotional quality of smells. Furthermore, the immediacy with which smells overpower us is reflected in the lack of narratorial distance, the omission of conjunctions, and the rhetoric device of ellipses—changes in the story line come as suddenly and in an equally unanticipated way as smells. Finally, if smells know no clear-cut boundary, the same holds true for Rushdie's novel as subplots and even characters leak into each other like fragrances (see further Hertel 2005: 104–15).

As I have discussed elsewhere in more detail, the nose as the related sense organ functions on four different levels here: physical, symbolic, magical, and metafictional (Hertel 2005: 106; see also Crowney 2000: 138). This metafictional dimension is particularly intriguing: breaking the conventions of the nose as literary topos, Rushdie makes the nose stand not for the penis but for the pen. Indeed, smells are crucial to the protagonist's autobiographic project, for they summon up memories of his past. His olfactory organ not only noses out the right mixture of pickle and brine but also that of fact and fiction; it not only supervises the production of chutneys but also that of his story. Olfaction becomes a metafictional process as the laws of pickling apply to the laws of composing autobiographies. The thirty-one jars the protagonist produces stand for the thirty-one chapters of his tale, and if the art of pickling is to "change the flavour in degree, but not in kind" (Rushdie 1981: 416), this also holds true for the composition of his autobiography: he sticks to the flavor of truth while spicing it up to make it more palatable. Thus, Rushdie uses olfaction as a tool to reflect upon autobiographic writing. Here, the fictional world might not produce smells, but smells produce the fictional world. The reader might not experience olfactory sensations as he might experience visual ones in other novels; yet, olfaction shows a strong influence on the metaphors as well as the theme and composition of Rushdie's novel.

At the same time, Rushdie's novel is, to a certain degree, representative of a larger body of postcolonial literature. Sniffing out things, following scents, letting himself be led by the nose and entering into digression after digression as a result, Rushdie's narrator, like Rushdie the author, implicitly propagates a style of writing that lacks the logic stereotypically associated with Western post-Enlightenment rational thought but rather follows the modes of play, digression, and intuition. In other words, *Midnight's Children*, like a larger body of postcolonial writing, eschews a structure informed by a pattern of thinking that might be perceived as typically Western and hence as somewhat alien to the indigenous traditions of the colonized cultures. Instead, it seems more closely linked to the body and the senses, as the reading of the individual chapters is likened to the digestion of food (each chapter representing a different chutney) and the digressive structure as well as the sensual language employed appear to be informed by the immediacy of a sensory perception forgoing reason and abstraction. The turn towards sensation, resulting in a literature characterized by the dissolution of stable categories of genre, structure, and linguistic register, reflects on the level of form and language a crucial issue of postcolonial writing: the subversion of clear-cut, often oppositely conceived, identities, and the promotion of mixed, hybrid ones that have become an increasing reality in the globalized world of today.

At this point, it is of course impossible to predict how literature will negotiate sensation in the future. One might, for instance, only speculate on the impact of computer-generated virtual realities, and the effect these alternative worlds have on our senses. New media might not only affect the way we read but might also have an impact on the form and content of literature itself. Blogs, interlinked texts on websites, online chats, and email messages present new forms of textual expression and might reshape our relation to reality as well as its depiction in literature. An interesting example of how contemporary authors negotiate these new virtual realities is presented in Jeanette Winterson's *The PowerBook* (2000). A loose series of interlinked stories, this novel explores the world of online identity. Not only does it reflect novel forms of communication in its semantics, metaphors, and syntax—sentences are often as short and colloquial as in an internet chat—the novel in its structure also reflects the impact of computer-based realities on our perception. "What happened to the omniscient author?" the narrator is asked in an email, and replies "Gone interactive" (27). The world of *The PowerBook* is no longer the realm of all-knowing authors or narrators, of premeditated narrative structures controlled by the individual; instead, the structure of the novel is erratic, associative, and interactive as the narrator takes her cue from ideas or single words she comes across in the emails written to her by her lover. These words or thoughts function as links of sorts, prompting the narrator to invent new stories and to enter new fictional worlds. In the process, she casts herself and her addressee in various roles such as a writer in Paris, the knight Lancelot, an orphan, or a seventeenth-century messenger carrying the first tulip bulb from Turkey to the Netherlands in her underwear and initiating the Dutch tulip craze.

Demonstrating how easy it is to take on new identities in a virtual world, Winterson heightens the reader's awareness of the illusive nature of what he or she thinks is reality. In particular, she depicts the virtual reality as a world in which one is freed of the body and the biological facts apparently determining our identity in off-line reality. Here, in the virtual world, identity is not a matter of inborn essentials but of performance and self-fashioning; this is a world in which one might change sexual, political, national, or other identities within an instant. "Take off your clothes. Take off your body. Hang them up behind the door. Tonight we can go deeper than disguise" (4)—the possibility offered by computer-generated realities to escape biological determinism appears to be a tantalizing prospect for Winterson who has long experimented with literary strategies aimed to eschew biological essentialism (her earlier novel *Written on the Body* [1992] for instance, refuses to let us know the narrator's sex, and gender identities also become unstable in *The Passion* [1987]).

Perhaps there is an inherent affinity between the virtual realities generated in the computer age and the worlds created by fictional literature. If literature as a means of reproducing, interpreting, and generating reality might appear rather old-fashioned compared to the new computer-induced possibilities of simulation, it is worthwhile reminding oneself that literature has always been presenting us with similar virtual realities. Actually, much of its fascination is the direct result of this fact. All books provide us with are, strictly speaking, black letters on white pages; yet we do not experience the fictional world as an assembly of printed characters. Instead, reading is a quasi-sensuous experience, making readers see the protagonists before their inner eyes. In fiction, readers perceive a narrator's voice and hear the characters speak. Descriptions of gustatory pleasures make their mouths water; they shiver with cold at the evocation of snowy deserts and feel physically repelled by depictions of torture. As we read, we submerge ourselves in fictional worlds that no longer stay on the paper but come to life in our imagination and appear to speak to our senses. Reading turns into an out-of-body experience or, rather, an in-another-body experience, for we perceive the portrayed world not only through the protagonists' eyes but also through their ears, nose, tongue, and skin. As Henry

James remarks, we become someone else when reading; we are transported to new worlds where we lead new lives (James 1972: 93). In more up-to-date terms, we move through the literary text as if through a virtual reality (see further Hertel 2005: 191–226).

Perhaps then, literature provides us with a sixth sense of sorts, a sense of potentiality or the imaginary, opening up to our experience alternative worlds as it enables us to enter the life of literary characters and to perceive the world through their sensory organs. Seen this way, literature ultimately functions as a highly refined, and highly effective, extension of our senses. It is precisely its capacity to speak to our senses, to turn the fictive world generated by words only into a world we perceive as if through our senses, that makes literature so successful a medium for negotiating our position within the world.

CHAPTER EIGHT

Art and the Senses: The Avant-Garde Challenge to the Visual Arts

HANNAH B. HIGGINS

INTRODUCTION TO ART AND LIFE MEDIA IN TWENTIETH-CENTURY ART

If the various art movements of the twentieth century were to form a Greek chorus, the attentive listener would discern numerous competing strains limiting ambitious art to pure form, or pure expression, or pure pleasure, or pure politics, or pure experience, or institutional critique, or a sensorially-expanded awareness of life. Each voice in this rhapsodic choir would seek to drown out the rest, at times dominating and at others nearly disappearing into the din. Important differences notwithstanding, three denominations would eventually emerge: the Modernist, the Realist, and the Avant-Gardiste. To these denominations would correspond a definition of art as abstracting form, or as advocacy or propaganda, or as blurring the boundary between art and life. While they would agree on little else, the first two denominations, Modernist and Realist, would concur that art possesses visual-formal logic, although there would be no agreement as to how that logic is tethered to other art or to society, or the human spirit more broadly conceived. The Avant-Gardiste, by contrast, would bracket the question of style altogether in favor of an art deploying all senses against the mechanics of cultural hegemony, including especially the institutions promoting visual art.

This debate as to what form art should take has a history that reaches back at least to the eighteenth century. In 1766, for example, Gotthold Ephraim Lessing had argued for a division of the arts, with poetry as an art of time directed toward the ear, and painting as an art of space directed toward the eye. In his paradigmatic essay, "Laocoon: An Essay on the Limits of Painting and Poetry," Lessing argued that too much mixing of the characteristics of each led to a dangerous confusion of the arts. Depending on an artist's intention and audience, visual artists after Lessing would either seek to render the heroic narratives of history painting, which, according to Lessing, ran the risk of servility to the time-based art of literature, while, by Lessing's account, those who strove to create visual art proper would depict the space-based aspect of each medium as two- or three-dimensional, seen all at once as an image outside of sequential time. For our purposes, literary painting would tend toward the narrative, Realist function in the imaginary chorus, while painting proper would lend its voice to the Modernist. Writing on this important history of media separation, visual culture critic W. J. T. Mitchell proposes that such attempts to define and delimit artistic media be interpreted as the expression of "a dialectical struggle in which the opposed terms take on different ideological roles and relationships at different moments in history"(1986: 98).

From the 1940s into the 1960s, a version of this medium delimiting approach dominated Modernist discourse and practice in the United States. Paradigmatic Modernist critic Clement Greenberg revived Lessing's stark divisions, defining and defending Modernism in his declaration that "the purely plastic or abstract qualities of a work of art are the only ones that count" (1940: 296–310). The term "plastic" refers to a painting's flatness, color, and framing edge—that is, painting's primarily visual aspects. Greenberg's other qualifier, "abstract," refers to the work's distance from representation, meaning, that is, a painting's rejection of or departure from the so-called narrative content of images that show recognizable things existing (and therefore acting) in the world. For Modernists in the Greenbergian tradition, all non-plastic, non-abstract aspects of a painting should be systematically bracketed from the medium. Over time, it was believed, ambitious painting would become more formally pure.

Because much postmodern and contemporary art relies on representational means (photography, representational painting, everyday or real objects), Greenberg is routinely lampooned in the art world. However, Mitchell's suggestion to the effect that defining media is a dialectical struggle necessitates situating Greenberg's Modernism in the social conditions of his time. It matters, for example, that when young Greenberg was developing his visual/formal theory of artistic progress in the 1930s, the illusionistic works associated with academic painting were widely despised by progressive critics. This was in no small part due to the academic style's affiliations with government propaganda, a tie that continued in the officially sanctioned art of Stalin's Soviet Union, Hitler's Germany, and Mussolini's Italy.

Like other authoritarian regimes, the Soviets promoted a Realist art consisting of easily understood images glorifying labor and enforcing social harmony. To wit: in 1934 Andrei Zhdanov, then Secretary of the Communist Party under Stalin, proclaimed that "the artistic portrayal should be combined with *ideological remolding and education* of the toiling people in the spirit of socialism" ([1934] 1992: 410, my emphasis). The resulting industrial idylls were defended as propaganda necessary for solidifying the gains of the emerging state. Modernists saw these same images as evidence for the betrayal of the revolution, which they believed should promote an art of material innovation.

This oppositional logic found institutional expression in the 1929 founding (and 1939 permanent relocation) of the Museum of Modern Art (MoMA) in New York, launching important exhibitions from Cezanne to Picasso and, later, Abstract Expressionism. Under its Director of Collections, Alfred H. Barr, Jr., the museum promoted a history of Modernism as a progressively abstract, visual sequence. In 1983 a Canadian art historian, Serge Guilbaut, disclosed this important history, demonstrating how the type of orthodox Modernism associated with MoMA was tied to the constitution of the Board of Directors (through the Rockefeller family and the CIA) and the cultural aspirations of America's Cold War cultural machine, which promoted American abstract art abroad (1983).

Following Mitchell's logic that delimitations of media are locked in a perpetual ideological struggle with material effects, it is clear that American Modernism as an art and discourse after the Second World War ultimately conformed to the image logic of the Cold War. Accordingly, abstract or "space-based" painting signified American freedom in opposition to Soviet suppression, as embodied in Socialist Realism, with its narrative approach (Guilbaut 1983). In other words, however appealing Greenberg's advocacy for a purely visual art, free of the constraints of social functionalism was for curators, critics and artists, it does not follow that abstract art was actually free from political instrumentalization. Quite the opposite was true. Ignoring its early associations with revolutionary change, the apparent independence of abstract art from social constraints in the 1950s rendered it ideally suitable for an official ideology that equated political freedom with the free flow of capital.

The historic avant-garde and neo-avant-garde movements of the twentieth century represent a third path, rejecting the visual premises of both the Modernist and Realist practices as matters of mere style.[1] In the words of theorist Peter Bürger, "the avant-gardiste work does away with the old dichotomy between 'pure' and 'political' art" (1984: 91). Instead, Bürger argues that in avant-garde works: "Not only does reality in its concrete variety penetrate the work of art but the work no longer seals itself off from it" (1984: 91–2). The resulting works of the historic avant-garde and its progeny blurred the boundary between art and life through sensory experiments, multisensory aesthetic experiences, carefully calibrated social situations, and mass distribution. The topic is too vast to detail in this short survey, however a few benchmark works will serve to give an indication of this alternative experimental, multisensory tradition: the Dada Fair (1920); the Futurist Banquets (1930s); Happenings and Fluxus performances and objects (after 1958); and, recent relational art (1996).

THE FIRST INTERNATIONAL DADA FAIR (1920)

The Cabaret Voltaire was founded as a pacifist gathering place in Zurich in 1915. On July 28, 1916, this tiny cabaret launched Dada when one of the Cabaret's founders, Hugo Ball, read his founding Dada manifesto to a crowd. In German, the word "dada" had no fixed meaning (although it means "hobby horse" in French). The senseless term Dada stood for a principle of meaninglessness, irrationality, and post-humanism. In Ball's words: "The bankruptcy of ideas having destroyed the concept of humanity to its very innermost strata, the instincts and hereditary backgrounds are now emerging pathologically. Since no art, politics, or religious faith seems adequate to dam this torrent, there remain only the *blague* and the bleeding prose" ([1916] 1992: 246).

By this account art, politics, and faith were revealed as powerless against the destructive forces of materialism, nationalism, and corporatism that had caused the First World War. The Dadaist *blague*, which is French for practical joke or hoax, would function as an eraser of sorts, wiping clean the slate of a decadent and violent Western culture using humor, but also "bleeding prose," meaning interdisciplinary forms of literature that imply dissolving the boundaries between all media and between art and the body. Intermedia art forms linking word to music (sound poetry), word to image (collage and visual poetry), gesture to sound (performance art, modern dance), and architecture to print and sculpture (the assemblage-environment) all found expression in the Dada front against cultural complacency. In the ensuing years, Dada spread to New York, Hanover, Berlin, Cologne, Paris, and Japan. Artists making sympathetic work were co-opted by the movement, as occurred with Marcel Duchamp for his readymades and his 1917 submission of "fountain," a urinal, to the Society of Independent Artists in New York.

In postwar Berlin, the weak Weimar Republic became the target of Dada attacks. Germany after the First World War was characterized by political polarization between the radical right and left, each of whom had different ideas about how to restore the country to functionality. Making matters worse, there was an attempted coup by disgruntled military in Berlin, which was followed by a wildcat general strike and an attempt to replace the elected government with a revolutionary one. Elections were called for January 1919 and the ensuing Republic took hold in a climate of political turbulence and infighting. The political situation was, to put it bluntly, patently absurd.

Dada responded in kind. At the 1919 founding of the Weimar State Theater, Dadaist Johannes Baader threw fliers from a balcony over the crowd below. These flyers, titled *The Green Horse (Das Grüne Pferd)*, announced Baader as President of the World. Substituting the new, ineffective Weimar system with another, imaginary one, Baader proposed an anti-government of Dadaist pacifists and cultural critics whose form would parrot the Republic, with Baader as supreme leader, or "Oberdada." Coming on the heels of recent attempts by politicians to forcibly substitute one government for another through coup or revolution, Baader's antics would necessarily have seemed eerily familiar. The fliers resulted in widespread laughter, mild annoyance, and outright hostility—all of it interrupting the normal exercise of political authority.

This activist performance intervention of Dadaists Against Weimar was one of many such Baader events, which sought to erode confidence in the establishment. After quoting extensively from the *Berliner Zeitung* of January 27, 1919, *The Green Horse* declared "We shall blow Weimar sky-high. Berlin is the place . . . da . . . da." We can imagine the scene: men in formal business attire showered with sheets drifting haphazardly on the breezes in the room, some laughing, others scowling, all the while trying to avoid getting hit in the eye or being caught off guard and taking a sheet to the side of the face. Some men would be reading the proclamation and pondering in dismay their limited government options, getting the joke or not, or simply wadding the paper up in utter disgust, eager to get on with the task at hand. Similar scenes were played out in other contexts, as when, according to Dadaist Hans Richter, "Baader interrupted former Court Chaplin Dryander preaching in Berlin Cathedral, by bellowing from high up in the choir 'To hell with Christ!' or, according to another version, 'You are the ones who mock Christ, you don't give a damn about him'" (1965: 127). Like these performances, Baader's Dada collages (and works by other Dadaists) routinely depicted the tactical, even tactile, force of the scream in the form of word projectiles flung from the mouth, or from its mechanical analogue, the loudspeaker, toppling the items scattered across the rest of the page. The philosopher Walter Benjamin expressed this aspect of Dada clearly in his benchmark 1936 essay, "The Work of Art in the Age of Mechanical Reproduction." Writing about Dada's prescient anticipation of the persuasive power of the voice in non-silent film, Benjamin describes how: "From an alluring appearance or persuasive structure of sound the work of art of the Dadaists became an instrument of ballistics. It hit the spectator like a bullet, it happened to him, thus acquiring a tactile quality" (1969: 238). Sound, by this account, is fundamental to piercing through the veil of the unremarked-upon everyday "like a bullet." Loud sound is felt in the teeth and bones. The thundering "BOOM!" assaults the body, scrambling common sense.

In contrast to a nineteenth-century world, where spoken volume was limited to the acoustics of the larynx, mechanical loudspeakers had come into widespread use during the First World War. Relatedly, these sounds could now be projected over great distances through the deployment of another new invention, the radio tower. The Eiffel Tower's function as a radio tower achieved prominence during the First World War as an amplification/distance-defying piece of technology that hampered Germany's advance on Paris. By 1919, Vladimir Tatlin's model for a massive radio tower and office complex, The Monument to the Third International, had widespread acclaim in avant-garde circles.

Given his public antics and the expanding projection of sound by loudspeaker and radio tower, it comes as no surprise that the human voice, amplified sound, and radio all show up in Baader's most complex and enduring work (see Figure 8.1). This multimedia assemblage, *The Great Plasto-Dio-Dada-Drama: Germany's Greatness and Decline or The Fantastic Life of the Superdada* (*Das große Plasto-Dio-Dada-Drama: Deutschlands Grösse und Untergang oder Die phantastische Lebensgeschichte des Oberdada*) appears in many pictures of the 1920 First International Dada Fair. Raoul Hausmann's sound poems, which communicate through sounds divorced from the limited meanings attached to whole words, form the base of the work. The top

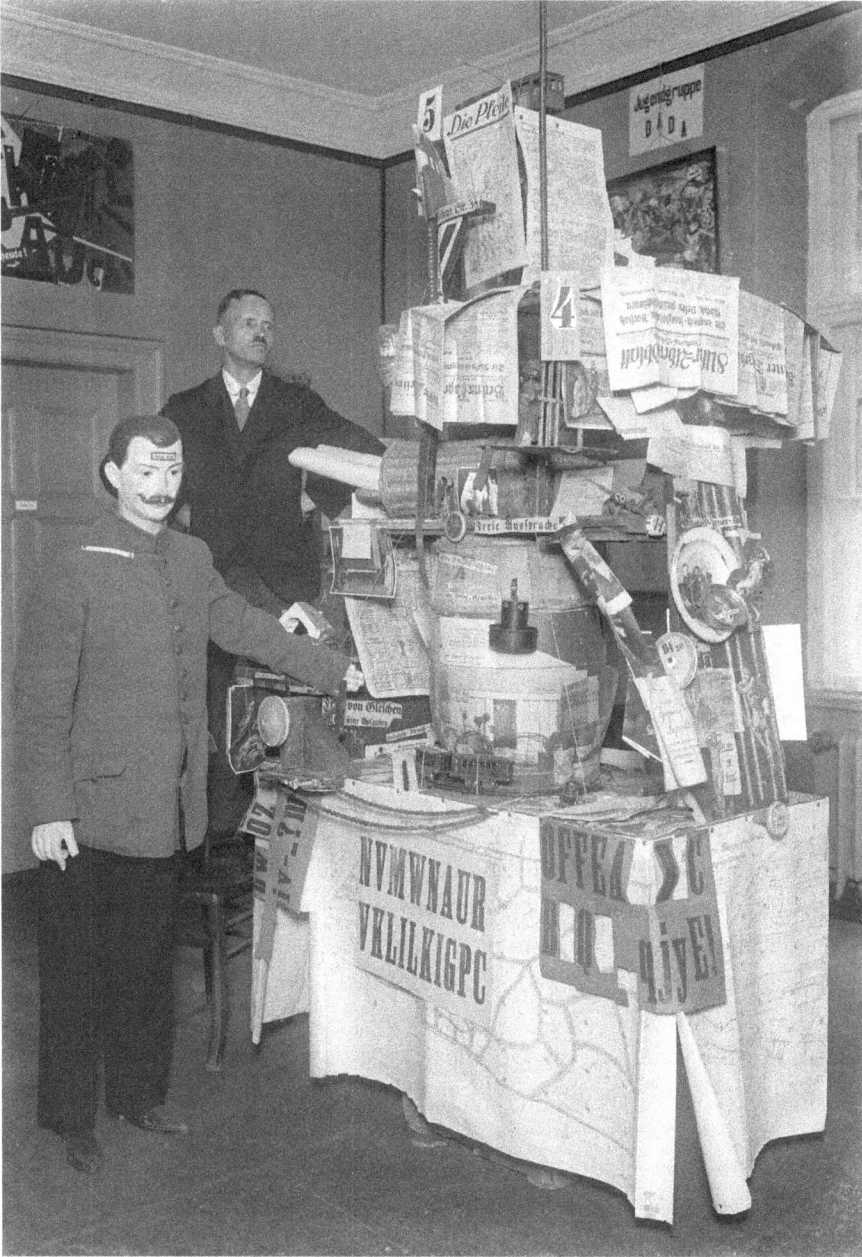

FIGURE 8.1: *The Great Plasto-Dio-Dada-Drama: Germany's Greatness and Decline or The Fantastic Life of the Superdada* (*Das große Plasto-Dio-Dada-Drama: Deutschlands Grösse und Untergang oder Die phantastische Lebensgeschichte des Oberdada*), by Johannes Baader, 1920. Object destroyed. Photographer Willy Römer. Courtesy of bpk/ Kunstbibliothek, Staatliche Museen zu Berlin, photothek Willy Römer/Willy Römer.

consisted of a cylindrical radio tower. This media-blending work, in other words, was framed by sound from top to bottom.[2]

Anticipating Kurt Schwitters's celebrated Hanover *Merzbau* (1923–33) by several years, *The Dio-Dada Drama* also blended artistic media with everyday materials: actual cloth, garbage can, rolled paper, daily newspapers, mousetrap, bird cage, cogwheel, mannequin, and toy train appear alongside Baader's collages, Hausmann's sound poems, and other Dada broadsides and montages. This first "assemblage-environment," for surely it was one even if the term did not yet exist, would be simultaneously seen, read, circumambulated, and touched. Like its mixed media materials, this work entwined a heady combination of narrative forms: world history, the history of German nationalism, fictional biography of the ascension of the monomaniacal alter ego Oberdada, and political allegory.

Trained as an architect, Baader (2001: 583–602) proposed this work as:

Dada monumental architecture in five stories, 3 parks, 1 tunnel, 2 lifts and 1 cylinder cap. The ground level or floor represents the fate determined before birth and has no other relevance. Description of the stories. 1st floor: The Preparation of the Superdada. 2nd floor: The Metaphysical Test. 3rd floor: The Inauguration. 4th floor: The World War. 5th floor: World Revolution. Penthouse: The cylinder twists into the sky and proclaims the resurrection of Germany by means of Hagendorf's lectern. Eternally.

Painstakingly mapped out by British art historian Michael White, the forms of the tower were convincingly coordinated with those aspects of Berlin's city plan associated with the aspirations of Kaiser Wilhelm I's modernization of the new German capital (2001: 583–602). In White's words:

The express train . . . can be understood as a reference to the rapid expansion of the railway network under the *Kaiserreich* . . . between the first and second story is another reference to a major Wilhelmine construction project, the "museum of masterpieces through the ages" . . . The placement of the mousetrap/mausoleum over the tunnel cleverly refers to the construction of the [five museum] *Museum-Insel* (Museum Island) in Berlin, an ambitious attempt to confirm the cultural as well as political significance of the new capital city . . . That the museum should follow the railway and Baader's assemblage is a cunning reference to Berlin topography.

2001: 589–90

If built to the urban scale imagined for it, the visitor would have ridden elevators up over the existing city. Teetering above the city, s/he would have loomed over the famed museum island, where the national treasures of Germany and its imperial booty (the *Pergamon Altar*, *Ishtar Gate*, and Ancient and Byzantine art) were displayed in five nineteenth-century museums. Around these, s/he would have seen a city in decay. At the base, a train referencing the Kaiser's enterprise of railway construction moved in a loop, around a powder keg that would eventually explode in response to the (social, economic, political, and military) friction of rapid industrialization and nationalist fervor. Instead of reading about German history as a familiar parable of the rise and fall of civilization, or seeing same parable depicted in painted images of luminescent sunrise and darkening decay, the participant would have experienced that history through transforming architectural forms, physically, even apocalyptically, in an out-scaled performance work, the Drama in the title. Remember Baader's *Green Horse* flier: "We shall blow Weimar sky-high. Berlin is the place . . . da . . . da."

As shown here in model form, dizzying rotations were threaded, so to speak, throughout *The Dio-Dada Drama* in the form of circles within collages, rolled sheets, the screw into the sky, and the train looping through the *Museuminsel*. Whether built to scale as a massive tower or circumnavigated as a sculptural environment by a Dada Fair visitor, the work would have necessitated competing circle motions by the engaged audience: up the screw, around the tracks, over the printed broadside. Kinesthetic experience, the experience associated with our sense of motion, requires the coordination of the eyes with both vestibular and joint systems. The apparently or actually rotating elements of Baader's sculpture would levy an assault on both, as the twisting parts would counter each other, sending mixed signals impacting the visitor's balance and posture by inducing a vertigo reaction, fundamentally if temporarily challenging even the most base, physical everyday experience of moving in space.

Such imaginative interventions into everyday sensation exist in less overtly destabilizing forms elsewhere in Dada and the avant-garde. Between 1918 and 1924, for example, the Russian Futurists, including Arseny Avraamov, staged city-wide concerts using extant urban sounds like sirens, ship's foghorns, artillery, and factory whistles (Davies 1994). Building on experiments associated with Futurism, Dadaist (and one-time Futurist) Yefim Golyshev worked at a more intimate scale, composing an "antisymphony" played on an orchestra of kitchen implements.[3] Golyshev created music that affected the way the listener inhabited the world outside of normative musical experience or, to borrow from Luigi Russolo's 1913 "Art of Noise" manifesto, taught the modern urban dweller to "cross a great modern capital with our ears more alert than our eyes." Dadaist Raoul Hausmann would describe Golyshev in revelatory terms: "his arhythm, his transparent notes, his mix of tones . . . which no longer want to be harmonies, is simply DADA" (Gordon 1994: 231). Reviewing the first Dada exhibition, Udo Rusker hailed Golyshev as "the most profound of all" the exhibiting Dadaists (Benson 1986: 148).

In summary, Dada rejected the official culture that unleashed the destructive force of the First World War. Its activities ranged from imaginary anarchic destruction to programmatic attempts to construct a parallel universe, to a middle ground of sensory experiments intended to change perception, and by extension, the reality perception affords us. In each case, Dada worked against the commonplace belief that art is primarily visual, deploying sensorially broad elements in staking its claims for a new reality. New sounds, objects, and forms of multi-mediated spectatorship would be orchestrated by Dada against the banality of everyday life or, perhaps, against the very "banality of evil" so poignantly described by Martin Heidegger's student, Hannah Arendt, in her explanation of the roots of Fascism in the elevation of conventional values to a mass scale (1963).

THE FUTURIST BANQUETS (1930s)

Founded in 1909, Italian Futurism endured through the 1930s as Fascism ran rampant across Europe. Deploying a machine aesthetic expressing a desire for rapid urbanization, Italian Futurism was committed to industrializing all aspects of modern life as a stimulus to economic and national development. This emphasis on modernization necessitated promoting new technologies, as well as the manufacturing and state systems that promoted rapid industrialization. Like every avant-garde, the Italian Futurists experimented across the arts: including industrial music, visual and sound poetry, visually dynamic design, industrial design, stroboscopic painting and sculpture, as well as architecture and food.[4]

The early Futurist fascination with industrial life, experimental though it was, would prove to be ideally suited to Fascist militarism, nationalism, and industrialization. Beginning in 1919, the erstwhile founder and impresario of Futurism, Filippo Tommaso Marinetti, allied himself with Mussolini and his authoritarian, nationalist cause. While he resisted Fascism's anti-Semitism as well as the German principle of modern art's "degeneracy," Marinetti remained smitten by its mobilizations of the masses, its nationalism, and its emphasis on industrial progress. Following Walter Benjamin's famous description that Fascism's mass rallies and civic programs constituted a lethal aestheticization of politics, aspects of Futurism can be likewise described as a polemical aestheticization of the everyday along precisely the same, narrow ideological lines. That its experiments in the end failed to win favor with officials matters little with regard to Marinetti's intentions.

Aesthetic interest notwithstanding, this alignment is particularly overt in Futurism's gastronomic experiments. Marinetti famously published the *Manifesto of Futurist Cooking* in *Gazzetta del Popolo* in Turin on December 28, 1930, opening his Taverna Santopalato (Holy Palate Restaurant) there in 1931 (see Figure 8.2). In both, pasta (which did not originate in Italy) appears as an impediment to industrialization. "Pasta is not beneficial to the Italians . . . Why let its massive heaviness interfere with the immense network of short long [radio] waves which Italian genius has thrown across oceans?" asks Marinetti, referring to his countryman Guglielmo Marconi's invention of the radio telegraph system (1930). Instead of spaghetti, Marinetti clamored for

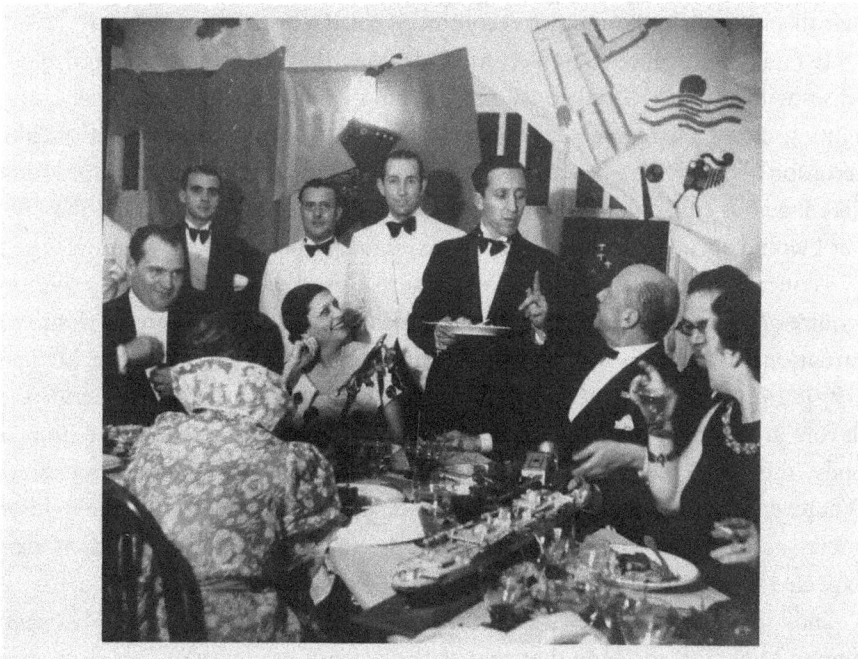

FIGURE 8.2: The Futurist table: Filippo Tommaso Marinetti and others seated at Futurist Banquet in Turin, 1931. Filippo Tommaso Marinetti Papers. General Collection, Beinecke Rare Book and Manuscript Library, Yale University, 175 × 23 cm.

"the abolition of everyday mediocrity from the pleasures of the palate" (Marinetti 1991: 56). Associating pasta with anti-industrial folk culture and the creature comforts of the age-old hearth, he wrote: "A communication to the Roman press from the painter Fillía has set the gastronomes of the capital buzzing, including those journalists particularly attached to the 'Holy Sister Happiness' school of good cooking, to the traditions of the 'spaghetti lover' and to all the other proud insignia of the true epicure" (Marinetti 1991: 65).

The new food would emphasize taste and texture, to be sure. Marinetti again: "the principal feature of the new cuisine is a rapid sequence of dishes no bigger than a mouthful or even less than a mouthful" (1991: 68). However, the Futurist table would also include carefully calibrated components of touch, sound, and environment. Nutritive content was entirely beside the point. Aerofood, for example, combined touch, sound, and scents as substitutions for the nutritive function of food. In addition to a waiter dousing the diners with scents from a large spray can, aerofood was composed of a fennel slice, an olive and a kumquat alongside which would be set a strip of velvet, silk, and sandpaper glued to cardboard. The tactile object would be used for feeling while the other hand ate. In his characteristic coy humor, Marinetti demurred that this is "a dish I would not recommend for the hungry" (1991: 84).

It could be argued that aerofood deploys the interconnectedness of all senses with regard to food consumption, since environment, touch, music, and lighting clearly shape the experience of the meal. By this logic, a dish like aerofood liberates the everyday experience of eating from mere taste, promoting (like Dada) a cultural alternative to mainstream Italian culture. That may be, but I would argue that Futurist foods' exploratory potential was compromised by a concomitant logic of sensory submission. Described by Marinetti, aerofood requires "the waiters spray the napes of the diners' necks with conporfumo of carnations" while a violent airplane motor racket comes from the kitchen (1991: 144). Since taste is tied closely to smell, the perfume would override the flavors at precisely the same time as that most vulnerable part of the human body, the neck, would be exposed to waiters and the din of the machine. Whatever sensory knowledge might be gained in the exploration of the food or circumstance of the meal, in other words, in the end the participant was expected to submit him/herself to the logic of the machine.

Individual dishes likewise demonstrate the porous boundary between human body and machine that shapes the sensory structure of Futurism. The radio tower, predictably enough, makes an appearance both in the form of a nutritive radio signal (Marinetti 1991: 67), and in Mino Rosso's *Network in the Sky*, a caramel disc topped by progressively smaller cylinders of puff pastry and meringue, and green spun sugar threads signifying, presumably, the radio waves of Italian invention (Marinetti 1991: 158). Another example, *Chicken Fiat*, is named for the Italian car manufacturer and would consist of chicken stuffed with ball bearings, the steel balls flavoring the flesh of the meat with a distinctive metallic taste and opportunity for the mouth to sort soft flesh from machine part. Finally, a proposed "aerosculptural dinner in the cockpit" of a Trimotor plane described food transubstantiated into sky: "the diners toss in the air and devour masses of fluffy whipped egg white just as the wind outside plays with the white cirrus and cumulus clouds" (Marinetti 1991: 123). As image (*Network in the Sky*), as actually combined with machine parts (*Chicken Fiat*), and as dining environment (the aerosculptural dinner in the cockpit), these dishes move the senses of taste, smell, and touch associated with eating toward a machine aesthetic.

Not all Futurist meals promoted such industrially circumscribed sensory experiments. Marinetti's sophisticated brand of racial nationalism was expressed in other meals. On the benign side, a "synthesis of Italy dinner" brought together different regional flavors and topographies in the form of geologically shaped and colored food (Marinetti 1991: 127). More vexing by far, a "dinner of white desire" attributed to Fillia, the painter, would have included ten black "Africans" serving, cooking, and eating the meal (Marinetti 1991: 136). Initially, these ten would surround a table by the sea, later to be overwhelmed (his language) by spiritual yearning and desire for the all-white meal of egg whites, mozzarella cheese, shredded coconut, white rice, whipped cream, Muscate grapes, and undiluted anise, grappa or gin. In addition to eggs filled with the scent of acacia flowers to be inhaled by the black server/cooks, this multisensory racist fantasy concludes when "The sensibilities of the Negroes feed on the white flavor colour odour of the food, while from the ceiling an incandescent globe of milky glass descends toward the table and the smell of jasmine fills the room."

This desiring by black Africans for whiteness as a color of purity is symmetrical with regard to a white person's desire for black bodies expressed in other meals, where dark, exotic foods from Africa make an appearance. The "geographic dinner," for example, prescribed a map of Africa painted on a white tunic worn by "a shapely young woman" and set in a restaurant with round windows disclosing "mysterious distant views of colonial landscapes" (Marinetti 1991: 129). Set to the sound of "loud Negro music," the guest would point at a body part on the apron based on "their touristic imagination and spirit of adventure" (Cairo = left breast = dates, or Zanzibar = right knee = chocolate, raw meat, and rum) and receive the requisite food. "In this way a gastronomic orientation inspired by continents, regions and cities, will prevail" (Marinetti 1991: 129). These would, as demonstrated in the tunic and vistas, exploit political boundaries and a highly racialized sense of nationhood as opportunistic adventure tale.

Raised in Alexandria, Egypt, Marinetti's associations with North Africa no doubt reflect genuinely fond associations with the place and its people. However, the role of Africans and African culture in the food scenarios was, to state the obvious, also tied to the political climate of Italy under Mussolini. These black and white meals clearly demonstrate white supremacy as directing a colonialist fantasy of sexual and political domination of Africa, a mystification he knew well both as a youth, but also as a traveler to Africa in the early 1930s. Within a few years (1936) Mussolini would forcibly integrate Italian Somaliland, Ethiopia, and Italian Eritrea into a unified Italian East Africa.

There are too many meals to recount here, but most share the logic of Marinetti's Fascist politics, even as it is tempting (especially given the 1930s timeframe of these works vis-à-vis the visual arts) to equate cross-sensory experimentation with political awakening of a liberal cast. That would be a mistake. As this account amply demonstrates, the art/life aspect of the avant-garde is not necessarily independent of the aspirations of official culture or totalitarian regimes, even if Futurism's antics were ultimately rejected by Mussolini and his cohorts.

THE CAGE CLASS (1958)

By the 1950s, much Dada and Futurist material had been temporarily forgotten or lost. The avant-gardes had been suppressed in Europe during the years of the Second World War and in the immediate postwar period American triumphalism dominated in the corridors of official culture, with Greenberg's formalist Modernism reigning supreme at the new center of the global art market, New York City. There were, to be sure, several notable factors countering this trend. Among these was Marcel Duchamp's presence in New York City, where he took refuge during the war and remained, apparently exchanging art for chess. Also pertinent to retrieving knowledge of the historic avant-gardes, Robert Motherwell's 1951 anthology, *The Dada Painters and Poets* put Dada imagery and manifestos back into circulation. Equally importantly, under the directorship of László Moholy Nagy, an art school opened in Chicago. This New Bauhaus (1937, closed 1938) later became the School of Design (1939) and then the Institute of Design (1944). Moholy Nagy worked to keep alive the Bauhaus commitment to visual art and design.

The Bauhaus had been central to ambitious Modernist culture in the years before its closure in 1933. This included benchmark collaborations between, for example, theater, set design, architecture, furniture design, and dance. North Carolina's Black Mountain College was also a destination for Bauhaus artists exiled by the war in 1933 and was a continuous destination for artistic experimentation until the middle of the 1950s. With the unlikely support of the Bauhaus painter Joseph Albers, Black Mountain College promoted experimentalism at the fringes of Modernist culture. At this small, rural outpost, the legacy of Dadaism blended with elements of the Bauhaus' interdisciplinary *grundkurs*, resulting in the postwar American avant-garde.

In August 1952, for example, the composer John Cage initiated a performance event, *Theater Piece No. 1* (sometimes called the first Happening) in the college dining hall. This two-hour event included simultaneous performances of Edith Piaf records, a lecture by Cage on Zen Buddhism, films, David Tudor playing a piano "prepared" with objects in the strings by Cage, dance by Merce Cunningham and several other dancers, readings by the poets M. C. Richards and Charles Olson, and a display on the ceiling of *White Paintings* by painter Robert Rauschenberg. Each element was performed independent of the others, as individual occurrences. However, the linkage of senses was clearly operative in the logic of the piece as, for example, when dancer shadows or film elements altered the all-white paintings or each other, or when a piece of recorded or performed music momentarily aligned with a dancer or poet. These unplanned "simultaneities" as they are now known, created a rhythmic sense of order and chaos that would be instrumental to the postwar American avant-gardes.

One particularly fertile cultural incubator for this interdisciplinary exchange was a course on Experimental Composition taught by Cage at the New School for Social Research in New York in 1958. Cage, who had been notorious since 1952 for his 4'33" of "silent" music, adopted a fundamentally open attitude with regard to musical composition in this course, attracting a mix of scientists, writers, poets, composers, and artists. Among the participants were several future members of the Fluxus and Happenings art movements: in addition to others, George Brecht, Al Hansen, Dick Higgins, and Allan Kaprow were in the class.

Allan Kaprow, whose benchmark *18 Happenings in Six Parts* (1958) was the first performance to be called a Happening, developed the audience participatory, multivalent style of performance associated with the term. A select few examples of works would include handling tires in an enclosed brick yard behind a gallery (*Yard*, 1961); eating apples and honey or fried bananas in a cave (*Eat*, 1964); or collaboratively constructing a closed, rectangular building of ice blocks (*Fluids*, 1967). These totally immersive, multisensory, interactive pieces required audience collaboration as laborers, assistants, and participants more generally. All senses were engaged in each Happening as tires were stacked, food was prepared and consumed, and ice blocks were carefully positioned. Kaprow's art writings were as influential as the works, establishing, as they did a framework for the "avant-garde lifelike art" of assemblage, environments, Happenings, and Fluxus (Kaprow 1983).

Chemist George Brecht also invented a new performance form in the Cage class. This radically reduced, apparently simple, form of performance instruction is called an "event" and is widely associated with Fluxus. In events, occurrences in everyday life or accidents of language are pulled from the proverbial flux of life and given attention. Brecht's event scores were later published by George Maciunas as a Fluxus edition (of about a hundred Event cards) called *Water Yam*, in 1962. At the most basic level, these Events direct the participant to perform or observe daily occurrences and thereby to frame, as special occurrences, otherwise missed dimensions of everyday life (see Figure 8.3). For example, *Solo for Violin Viola Cello or Contrabass* reads, simply:

- polishing

This would mean opening a bottle of polish, incidentally smelling it, rubbing it on the instrument, putting it away, etc. Another example, *No Smoking Event*, reads:

Arrange to observe a NO SMOKING sign.
- smoking
- no smoking

Reading, smoking, not smoking, tasting, smelling; all these play a role in Brecht's Event structures.

George Maciunas, the designer of many significant Fluxus objects, designed the *Water Yam* edition as cards placed in the box—a kind of fragmented grid of roughly a hundred frames. From its visual form, it seems obvious enough that Brecht's *Water Yam* could be placed in opposition to the progressively flat forms of modernism: the visually fractured form of the *Water Yam* cards opposing the unified field of Modernist painting's flatness. The pristine nature of these cards, with their carefully laid out texts and exquisitely crafted container, suggest however that the design is highly systematic and therefore

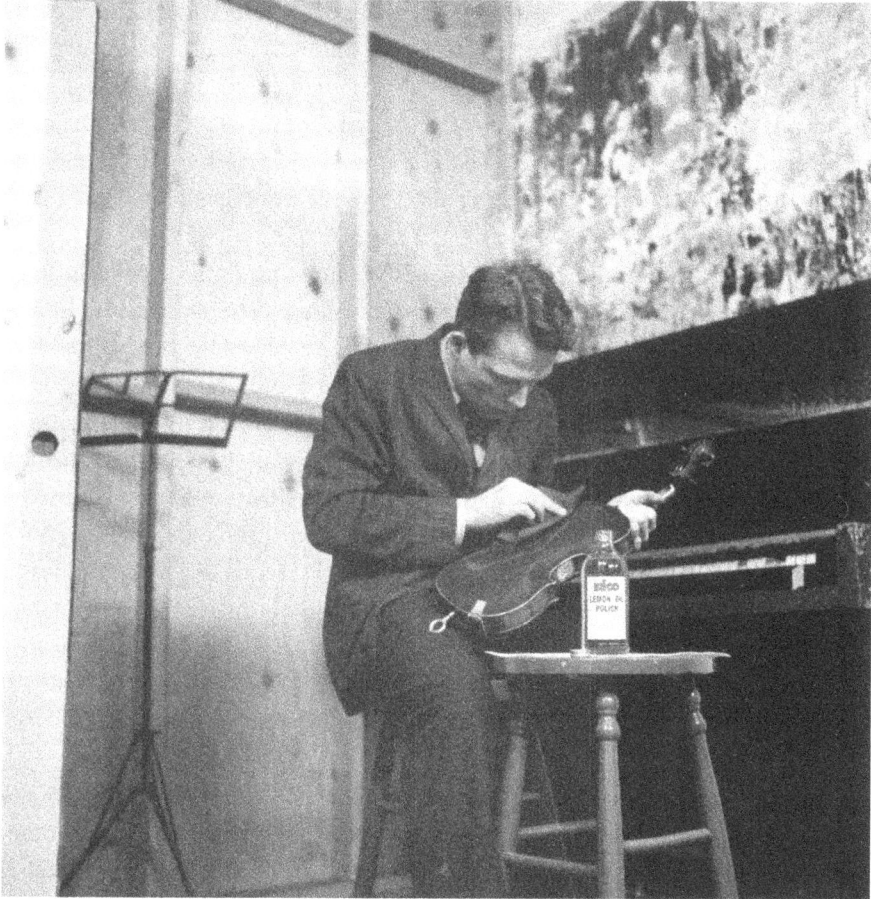

FIGURE 8.3: *Solo for Violin, Viola, Cello or Contrabass* by George Brecht, 1962. Performed at the Fluxhall, New York City, 1964. Photo by George Maciunas. Courtesy of the Gilbert and Lila Silverman Collection, Museum of Modern Art, New York.

no mere rupture in the fabric of Modernism. The Event actions and the spare form of the designed cards of *Water Yam* frame everyday life both through performance and through the visual form of the cards. Another way to state this is to suggest that, as a method of organization, the Event reflects the many interests of the chemist/artist, George Brecht, just as the visual document of the edition expresses the visual interest and skill of the designer, George Maciunas.[5]

In addition, as *scores*, both Brecht's Events and their expression in graphic form reference the simultaneously auditory and visual form of musical composition associated with his teacher/colleague, John Cage, whose notations included carefully composed verbal instructions alongside conventionally notated musical fragments. Following Cage, Fluxus Events are musical because the cards can be sequenced, and visual, because they are read for the purposes of performance. These two aspects of musical composition come together most intentionally in the experience of the performer who both reads and hears/experiences the score simultaneously. For the performer, in other words, the musical form is read and heard: it is also, however, performed, meaning that the form of composition is also felt.

When musicologist Hoene Wronsky defines music as "the corporealization of the intelligence that is sound," meaning the embodiment of sound, he has placed emphasis on the corporeal dimensions of music (Cope, quoted in Gardner 1983: 99). This corporeal aspect of music expands both the basis of its production as well as its potential for intelligible experience. When Multiple Intelligence theorist Howard Gardner cites Wronsky, his account of musicality is, understandably, based in tonality. He writes: "he [the composer] is always, somewhere near the surface of his consciousness, hearing tones, rhythms and larger musical patterns" (Gardner 1983: 101). However, he continues in terms that address specifically a bodily sensation of music: "[A]t least one central aspect of music—rhythmic organization, can exist apart from any auditory realization. It is, in fact, the rhythmic aspects of music that are cited by deaf individuals as their entry point to musical experiences" (Gardner 1983: 101).

Indeed, Cage often recalled that Arnold Schoenberg said: "In order to write music, you must have a feeling for harmony," which Cage did not. Cage retorted, "In that case I will devote my life to beating my head against that wall" (1961: 261). It is a profound description, which perhaps foreshadows the role of rhythm (embodied literally in his pounding) in Cage's explorations of meter and time that would ultimately result in his famous 4′33″ of so-called "silence." Silence was the outcome of his experimenting with increasingly long pauses in his earlier compositions. The musical aspect of the Fluxus Event, in summary, creates a curious slippage between disciplines: Fluxus work is visual (as exemplified by the cards of Water Yam), tactile, kinesthetic, gustatory, and social.

Another way to put this is to observe that with musical composition the score becomes the very mechanism for multimodal sensory experiences. The musician listens while holding, bowing, and fingering the instrument. By expanding the score from note to instructional format (the Event), the world around the artist can be performed or played in precisely the same sort of multisensory way. This description of the power of the musical format is consistent with the close association between music and experience theorized explicitly by Martin Heidegger in Being and Time. Heidegger scholar David

Michael Levin writes along these lines: "Informed by an interactive and receptive normativity, listening generates a very different episteme and ontology—a very different metaphysics," one based on "communicative rationality" (1993: 212). In contrast to visual art which is seen hung on a wall or on a pedestal, in other words, music by definition initiates a shared physical, tactile, auditory, temporal experience.

This deployment of sensory experimentation in the service of extended communality is likewise demonstrated in Fluxus Events that used food, or that establish a social space for sharing it. Alison Knowles' 1969 performance piece "The Identical Lunch" (a tuna fish sandwich on whole wheat toast with butter, no mayo and a cup of soup or buttermilk) is performed ideally for free, as when MoMA spent two months giving the lunch away in the winter of 2011, or as determined by the cost wherever a participant chooses to order one. Similarly, Knowles' Propositions instruct the preparer/performer to do something: "Make a salad" and "Make a soup."

Beginning in 1965, in part as a response to their abject poverty, Fluxus poets Robert Filliou and Emmett Williams co-invented the spaghetti sandwich, basically homemade spaghetti sauce on bread, for friends and (later) gallery visitors who sought conviviality and a community of shared food. Finally, Fluxus banquets of the 1960s and 1970s, whether rainbow food or clear, all black or all white, were only as expensive or as exotic as the dish each artist chose to contribute to the whole, meaning they lacked the domineering political framework that Futurism's admittedly similar project dragged with it.

RELATIONAL ART (1996)

Each movement described here thus far (Dada, Futurism, Happenings, Fluxus) carved out for itself unique social spaces where aspects of their programs could be presented to each other outside of the institutional confines of galleries, museums, or official art fairs, although it should be noted that each of them engaged with galleries and, to varying degrees, museums. These independent social spaces are the spaces of avant-garde conviviality and multimodal sensation. Recounting them all would require a multi-book-length study. However, even the very few works I have described move us toward the blending of art and life, or (if we limit the art to its aesthetic aspect) an expanding of the category of what Allan Kaprow famously called "pan-artistic phenomena."

In 1996, French critic Nicolas Bourriaud coined the term "relational art," which would find fuller expression in his 1998 book, *Relational Aesthetics*, where he offered a definition of work based "in the realm of human interactions and its social context, rather than the assertion of an independent and private symbolic space" (2002: 14).[6] Clearly, by this definition, relationality plays a central role in virtually every avant-garde practice relayed in this short account, since each has been based in a principle of socially interactive, art/life practice. However, as Claire Bishop has demonstrated in her critique of Bourriaud, his emphasis on high art aesthetics locates the work primarily in the realm of "spectatorship as more generally embedded within systems of display" (2012: 287), meaning the work in question took place primarily in museums, galleries, and art fairs during the 1980s and 1990s. This institutional affinity perhaps explains the pronounced blind spot to the historic avant-gardes on the part of many advocates of relational art.

Even so, the term "relational art" is extraordinarily useful as an umbrella term that describes contemporary activist, participatory, food, and sound art that originated in the late twentieth century and continues through the present. This convivial domain demonstrates the extent to which the performative aspects of avant-garde practice have, with varying degrees of success, found their way into the glass box of the modern art museum. The artists of the 1980s and 1990s associated with the term often use live bodies in various institutional settings in order to highlight (for example) issues attendant to bodily socialization, the bureaucratization of the senses, and our collective habituation to public space.

There are many examples of relational practice. A few will have to suffice as standing in for an enormous category of work. Vanessa Beecroft, for example, has used live nude or scantily clad models in identical shoes in crowded museums and other spaces, to address issues of nudity, shame, the fetish, and the narrow feminine ideal. In 1997, to name but one of many examples, she filled the ground floor of the Guggenheim Museum in New York with rows of elegant models (nude and in black string bikinis) in high heels. The interaction with both leering and uncomfortable visitors, and perhaps the hue and cry of angry feminists, constituted the artwork. Liam Gillick, another artist associated with relational art, works to expose entire social systems through publicly scaled billboards and the construction of spaces that promote social interaction. Sitting in front of one of these, talking to someone, and interacting with the passing crowd, as well as the sights and sounds of the city, forms the totality of the work. Perhaps most immersive of all, German artist Carsten Höller has worked with vestibular experience in his famous, multi-floor, corkscrew tubular slides that disorient the visitor and erase the architectural grid in an ecstasy of physical freedom.

Finally, Rirkrit Tiravanija is a Thai-born, culturally hybrid artist who lives in New York City and Chiang Mai, in Northern Thailand. Rirkrit's relational art practice specifically utilizes the socially affirmative potential of shared food and therefore resonates with the account presented here. Of particular interest is the play of food across national/cultural borders, not to reinforce them along the racially delineating lines of Futurism, but by using borders as ciphers of cultural translation and transformation. His "Flädlesoup," for example, makes note of a film, Jan Schütte's *Drachenfutter* (*Dragon Chow*, 1987). The film tells the modern story of "a Pakistani, an Afghan, and an African working in the kitchen of a German-Chinese restaurant" (Tiravanija 2010: 152). Each worker secretly flavors the Flädlesoup (a crepe cut up into broth as a pan fried noodle) to their respective taste and the customers love it. It played all day while Tiravanija cooked soup on the loading dock at the Hamburger Kunstverein in 1993.

Another example, Tiravanija's *Untitled 2001 (the magnificent seven, spaghetti western)* was installed at the Gallery Civica d'arte moderna e contemporanea, Torino (see Figure 8.4). *Untitled 2001 (the magnificent seven, spaghetti western)* consisted of "a steel floor, 7 propane gas tanks, 800 soup bowls and 800 forks, 7 cook pots, 5 stainless steel hand platters, 2 cutting boards, and four concrete walls with openings." The artwork consisted of making and serving Tom Ka Gai, a Thai coconut chicken soup. Borrowing the title from John Sturges' film *The Magnificent Seven* (which was not actually filmed in Italy and is therefore not technically a Spaghetti Western), Tiravanija describes the connection between the works. The film depicted: "a collective of bad guys trying to do good, so I had seven pots of soup for cooking the Tom Ka Gai. So the characters in the film want to help Mexican peasants protecting their village. I am certainly playing with such metaphors and double entendres" (Tiravanija 2010: 7).

Like the bad guys in the Western, Tiravanija uses his fame to feed the public, a kind of cross-cultural, relational Robin Hood. "Hunger," writes curator and Fluxus scholar, Thomas Kellein in praise of Tiravanija, "has always been a dominant force, not just today" (Tiravanija 2010: 139). By titling the piece a "Spaghetti Western" Tiravanija aligns the piece with Wild West films produced from the middle 1960s by Italian directors. The term was initially derogatory, but has come into accepted use by fans of this hybrid genre. Any number of other Tiravanija works would equally well demonstrate that, at least where this artist is concerned, the shared labor of cooking and feasting has the potential to build communities, albeit temporary ones, as artworks.

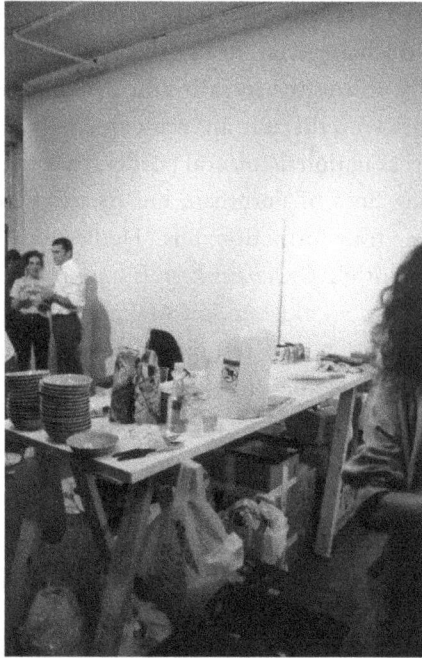

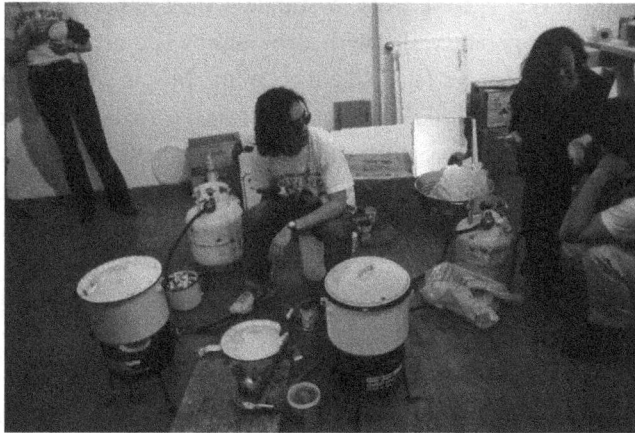

FIGURE 8.4: Performance of *Untitled (free)* at 303 Gallery, by Rirkrit Tiravanija, 1995. Photo by Larry Qualls. The exhibition consisted of serving visitors rice and Thai curry free of charge. This piece is owned for reperformance as *free/still* (including approximating the feel and size of the 303 gallery space) by the Museum of Modern Art, New York.

THE AFTERLIFE OF THE AVANT-GARDE—INTO THE TWENTY-FIRST CENTURY

As the art institutions often attacked by the avant-garde have become their archival repositories, a display version of the avant-garde has emerged whereby the works apparently congeal under the umbrella of an anti-art style, which includes yellowed avant-garde ephemera, broadsides, newsletters, and performance photographs shown in vitrines. It stands to reason that this format fails to exploit the cross-sensory and lived aspects of the work, particularly with regard to performance and food work, except arguably at the imaginary level.

Addressing the issue after nearly seven decades of ignoring the live practices of the avant-garde, in 2008 MoMA expanded its Media department to Media and Performance, effectively extending the museum's shows and programming toward relational art and the history recounted here more generally. A year later, in 2009, MoMA purchased the Gilbert and Lila Silverman Fluxus Collection and has done yeoman's work displaying Fluxus objects and inviting those few Fluxus artists that are still alive to the museum to perform.

MoMA's expanded portfolio has included blockbuster live exhibits by performance artists: most famously Marina Abromovich's 2010 retrospective, *The Artist is Present*, which consisted of reperformances of work that included, for example, the audience squeezing between two naked bodies facing each other in a doorway or, in another example, facing Abromovich across a large wooden table. Recently, the museum has been serving up food, as when Tiravanija's *free/still* (1992/5) was installed, inviting visitors to eat vegetable curry in the gallery in 2007 and 2011, the same year Knowles was brought in for a month of free-to-the-public *Identical Lunches*.

The academic art world has likewise revised itself with regard to the visual arts. In the last decade or so, a new generation of scholars has expanded research and exhibitions in ways that are open to Realism. Once marginal Soviet Socialist Realists, such as Aleksandr Deineka and Aleksandr Gerasimov, are being meaningfully recontextualized. Instead of merely shilling for their government, these artists are now understood, in more resistant terms, through their ties to the Modernist and avant-garde legacies subsequently suppressed by their leaders (Brown and Taylor 1993; Kaier 2005). The reverse is also true, as Guilbaut's project demonstrates.

This era of global pluralism, wherein Modernism, Realism, the avant-gardes and the legacies of them all easily coexist, warrants further examination. What if Mitchell's "dialectical struggle in which the opposed terms take on different ideological roles and relationships at different moments in history" (1986: 98) has concluded in an easy truce where anything goes? With regard to Realism and its arts of persuasion, we might wonder whether we have entered a new phase where ambitious art rediscovers the value of the singular story line. Might the arts of propaganda be used by other than nation states for a cause like world hunger or to denounce the wealth imbalance—as occurred around the world in 2011–12? Conversely, is it possible that even those most sensory of the exploratory, potently experiential artworks of the twentieth century actually simply paved the way for an emerging commodification of experience across all senses? Department stores and fast-food chains alike now carefully calibrate color, light, texture, sound, and aroma to create a more enticing, socially conducive atmosphere. More optimistically, we could ask whether we have entered an era of sensory liberation, where real artistic progress is possible across every sensory apparatus both within the art world and on the street.

Clearly, the cacophonous chorus that characterized most of the twentieth century has adapted itself to the newest instruments of global capital at the same time as critical culture and the arts of persuasion have become mainstays of progressive art. Even abstract art, long marginalized after its heyday in the 1950 and 1960s, is ripe for interest among emerging artists—as demonstrated by a quick pass through the contemporary art fairs that now pepper the globe each year. Are there things yet to learn, even there? Clearly questions, but no answers, abound. Suffice for the moment to prepare for a trip to the museum, gallery, or artist studio by approaching it with open eyes and ears, mouth, nose, and ready hands—as well as an open mind.

CHAPTER NINE

Sensory Media: Virtual Worlds and the Training of Perception

MICHAEL BULL

From the 1920s on, the increasing pervasiveness and influence of the media in daily life has been a subject of intense theoretical and cultural debate. An important part of this debate has centered on two issues involving the senses. One concerns the simulation of sensory environments in modern media, and the other deals with how modern media trains our senses to perceive and interact with the world in determinate ways. This chapter will consider aspects of both of these issues and how they contributed to the transformation of the very category of "experience" (Jay 2006) in the modern age.

For most of the twentieth century, the simulation of sensory environments through media involved only the senses of sight and hearing. Radio, film, and television presented worlds which, while compelling, were devoid of scents, savors, and touches. The possibility of creating more fully immersive media, however, tantalized marketers, engineers, and writers throughout the period under review here. An influential early description of such simulated sensory immersion appeared in Aldous Huxley's dystopian novel *Brave New World* ([1932] 2007). There he imagined the successor to "movies," a multisensory cinematic experience known as the "feelies":

The other night, I experienced something I never have before. Lenina took me out to The Feelies (a kind of movie theatre that incorporates the senses into a movie). Well, we got to the place and sat down in the big chairs. Soon enough, the lights went down and out of nowhere red fiery letters appeared in front of us. In order for me to get the "feely effects" Lenina told me that I had to hold on to the great metal knobs that were located on the arms of my chair. The second I took hold of those knobs I felt a strange tingly sensation on my lips. Then, the very realistic images of two people stood in front of us. It was astonishing just how actual and real the image was. It was almost as if the actors were standing right next to us. Meanwhile, something called a scent organ released a smell that tied into the film. Before I knew it, the movie was over.

Huxley [1932] 2007: 146

Huxley's description of the "feelies" anticipated a variety of later attempts to bring new sensory dimensions to the filmic experience. These involved such things as creating an illusion of three-dimensional reality through having the seats of viewers move and vibrate, and sporadic attempts to odorize cinemas. With the development of video games and virtual reality environments in the latter part of the century, the viewer was able to move from passive spectator to active participant.

The above passage from Huxley also ties in with the second theme of this chapter, for the "feelies" were not simply about providing full-bodied entertainment. Their use of immersion was intended to train citizens to conform and respond in prescribed ways to the visions of the world presented by the State, however dull or unreal these might be. In this chapter I analyze this ambivalent and dystopian view of the sensory nature of modern media as applied to the themes of technological mediation and distance, the militarization of the senses, and the resultant transformation of the moral compass of subjects who increasingly experienced much of the mediated world "as if the actors were standing right next to us"

In *The Work of Art in the Age of Mechanical Reproduction*, originally published in 1936, the Marxist cultural critic Walter Benjamin argued that "the manner in which human sense perception is organized, the medium in which it is accomplished, is determined not only by nature but by historical circumstances as well." New technologies, in particular, "subject[ed] the human sensorium to a complex kind of training," according to Benjamin (1973: 216). Subsequent writers have understood this training to involve a transformed "logistics of perception" (Virilio 1989) or to have entailed a "restructuring of perceptual experience" (Crary 1999). In the twentieth century this restructuring involved the simultaneous enhancement and restriction of the sensory experience of the world. The modern age witnessed the consolidation of a range of old and new media. The gramophone, the telephone, the radio, silent movies, sound movies (or "talkies"), and then color film and television shaped the experience of those living in the first seven decades of the century. To these were added, in the last three decades, video games and personal computers, along with diverse mobile technologies from the transistor radio to the Walkman and the mobile phone. Furthermore, the storage, transmission, and retrieval of information was revolutionized through the use of answer-phones, and later through digital libraries and the internet. These technologies augmented the senses of sight, hearing and, later, touch (or at least vibration and resistance) while screening out the so-called lower senses of smell, taste, and temperature, etc. The world, human others and the subjects' own cognitive processes were reconfigured by this transformed sensorium (Boellstorff 2008; Goggin 2011; Turkle 2011).

The German philosopher Martin Heidegger, writing in the 1940s, observed that the mediated experience of the subject in modernity had resulted in a dislocated understanding of place and space:

> The frantic abolition of all distances brings no nearness; for nearness does not consist in shortness of distance. What is least remote from us in point of distance, by virtue of its picture on film or its sound on the radio, can remain far from us. What is incalculably far from us in point of distance can be near to us.
>
> Heidegger 1972: 68

In the 1960s, Marshall McLuhan (1967: 43) famously proclaimed that the world had become a "global village" due to the seeming ability of radio and television, as "extensions of the senses," to connect distant peoples. This issue was revisited in the 1980s by Joshua Meyrowitz, who argued that: "electronic media destroy the specialness of place and time. Television, radio, and telephone turn once private places into more public ones by making them more accessible to the outside world ... Through such media, what is happening almost anywhere can be happening wherever we are. Yet when we are everywhere, we are also in no place in particular" (Meyrowitz 1985: 125).

From this transformation of mediated experience the view arose that the very nature of the relation between direct and mediated experience was challenged in the twentieth century. When the historian of technology Lewis

Mumford (2010: 217) claimed in the 1930s that social experience increasingly consisted of "the sensations of living without the direct experience of life," he was making a judgment on the nature of mediated experience in a world increasingly dominated by a wide variety of mass media. Mumford's judgment was framed by comparing "direct" experience with "mediated" experience and the assumption that direct experience was superior. In *Life on the Screen* (1995), a study of multi-user online games (or MUDs), Sherry Turkle reiterated this appeal to (and for) the direct, arguing that "we are moving toward a culture of simulation in which people are increasingly comfortable with substituting representations of reality for the real" (Turkle 1995: 23). Implicated in this loss of the phenomenal dimension of lived experience is the abolition of distance, highlighted by Heidegger, that is involved in the very nature of mediated experience. Douglas Kellner takes the discussion into the age of the internet:

> Each technology is a window to the outside world, obliterating urban boundaries and spaces to the geopolitical channels of the global world and the world of atopic cyberspace. Exposed to global culture and communication, the city loses its specificity and city life gives way to technological cyber life, an aleatory, heterogeneous and fractured space, and a world-time that enables individuals to experience events simultaneously from every time zone in the world.
>
> Kellner 1999: 107

A collective "hallucination of presence" has been seen as taking hold with the arrival of 24-hour connectivity and virtuality becoming the new normal (Cary 2013). This "hallucination of presence" was, arguably, extensively used to promote the militarization of sensory experience. This can be understood directly, as in Goodman's statement that: "From Hitler's use of the loudspeaker as a mechanism for affective mobilization during World War II, through to Bin Laden's audiotaped messages, the techniques of sonic warfare have now percolated into the everyday" (Goodman 2010: 5). However, it can also be regarded as occurring in the disciplining of the sensorium itself through technologies of warfare:

> One can notice the way in which the field of perception of war and the battlefield developed, simultaneously, at the same time. At first, the battlefield was local, and then it became worldwide and finally became global, which means satellized with the invention of video and the spy

satellites of observation of the battlefield. So at present, the development
of the battlefield corresponds to the field of perception enabled by the
telescope and wave optics, the electro-optics, video, and of course
infography, in short all the media.

Virilio 1989: 64

Mass media gave war an illusory presence in the homes of the public through
the continuous broadcast of information and images. Both the presentation
and reception of such broadcasts were, in turn, shaped by prior experiences of
cinematic spectacles. For example, it has been argued that the CNN coverage
of the 1991 Gulf War involved "coordinating all production elements—titles,
graphics, still and moving images, music, diegetic sound, narration, live
broadcasting—around the crisis to create a spectacle that tapped into the
audience's experiences with film and video games" (Deaville 2011: 114).
The increasingly saturated and scripted media environment contributed to the
transformation of the sensorium at the same time as it impacted the subject's
ability to understand and reflect upon events. The moral compass of the senses
was hence deeply affected by this immersion in mediated "reality."

Both Walter Benjamin and Theodor Adorno, in different periods, reflected
on the relationship between technological developments, the media, and
morality. At the outset of the rise of German fascism in the 1930s, Benjamin
wrote of "the gaping discrepancy between the gigantic power of technology
and the miniscule moral illumination it affords" (Benjamin 1999: 318). Adorno
noted in the 1960s that history was a narrative "leading from the slingshot to
the megaton bomb" (Adorno 1981: 320). More recently, Jonathan Crary has
observed in relation to media consumption that "the most important recent
changes concern not new machines of visualization, but the ways in which
there has been a disintegration of human abilities to see, especially of an ability
to join visual discriminations with social and ethical evaluations" (Crary 2013:
33). The ability to discriminate itself has been transformed by the speed and
volume of media messages "in which the range of responsive capacities are
frozen or neutralized" (Crary 2013: 34).

In what follows, a historically informed understanding of the mediated
sensorium and its connections to distance, sociality, militarization, and an
ethical compass is presented through a series of overlapping analyses that focus
on the visual, the auditory, the immersive, and the tactile. Embedded in this
analysis is an understanding of the ambivalent nature of sensory enhancement
and diminishment articulated through the multiple use of a wide range of
media technologies. The chapter concludes with a brief examination of the

events of September 11, 2001, also known as 9/11, which implicated all of the media technologies of the twentieth century in people's efforts to make sense of "reality."

MEDIATED MULTI-SENSORALITY I: LOOKING AND LISTENING

Prior to the First World War, the French artist Fernand Léger observed "a modern man registers a hundred times more sensory impressions than an eighteenth century artist" (cited in Blom 2010). Léger was referring to the acceleration of sensory experience that was a product of technology, the media, and urban life in general. At the time of making this observation Léger had no inkling of the impending war, and the "war on the senses" that it spelled, nor his involvement in it. Léger himself was seriously wounded and his senses overwhelmed by a mustard gas attack in the Battle of Verdun in 1916. On returning home, his vision of art and humanity was transformed—becoming "machinic," thus mirroring his wartime experience. In the early 1920s he ventured into filmmaking and produced an experimental picture entitled *Ballet Mécanique* (1924). In this film, the body was presented mechanistically by repetitively focusing in with close-ups of eyes, mouths, and legs; everyday activities were repeated endlessly from a myriad different perspectives, close up and angular. The film was played to the machinic rhythm of the music of American composer George Antheil.

The total sensory conundrum of life in the trenches, as experienced by Léger, was unimaginable to those who "covered" the war from the comforts of distant news-desks, and engaged in its propagandistic glorification. By contrast, the sensory intensity of warfare led many combatants to feel a sense of alienation whilst on leave at home, for the war seemed more real than domestic peace. It took years for combatants to articulate the trauma of their wartime experience, but articulate it they did in a host of novels, films, and memoirs that appeared in the late 1920s and early 1930s (e.g. Sassoon 1931; Williamson 1930). Embedded in the mindset of writers, artists, and intellectuals impacted by the war was the dislocation and transformation of sensory experience coupled to the propagandist potential of "experience at a distance." These themes would continue throughout the multiple conflicts of the twentieth century.

Léger's film prefigured, and provides an apt illustration of, Walter Benjamin's subsequent observation regarding the ability of film to transform what it meant to look—technologically—in the twentieth century:

By close ups of the things around us, by focusing on hidden details of familiar objects, by exploring commonplace milieus under the ingenious guidance of the camera, the film, on the one hand, extends our comprehension of the necessities which rule our lives; on the other hand, it manages to assure us of an immense and unexpected field of action . . . With the close up, space expands, with slow motion, movement is extended. The enlargement of a snapshot does not simply render more precise what in any case was visible, though unclear: it reveals entirely new structural formations of the subjects' impulses.

Benjamin 1973: 230

In the above quote, Benjamin was reflecting on the mediated proximity of the filmic look, which he interpreted as extending the sense of vision into an "optical unconscious." Picking up on Benjamin's thought, Susan Buck-Morss (1994) elaborated a theory of the cinema screen as a "prosthesis of perception," and filmic viewing as the perfect expression of a "phenomenology of looking" that bracketed out that which was exterior to the "dreams" portrayed on the screen: "Going to the movies is an 'act of pure seeing' if ever there was one. What is perceived in the cinema image is not a psychological fact, but a phenomenological one. It is 'reduced,' that is, reality is 'bracketed out'" (Buck-Morss 1994: 46). The space of the cinema, from this perspective, became the totality of the world—a dream world—wherein audiences temporarily suspended "reality" through acts of intense sensory immersion. The suspension or recession of "reality" and precession of the image was a theme taken up by Baudrillard (1994) in his theory of the simulacrum, a dystopic take on Heidegger's position, which was also supported by Virilio who, contrary to Baudrillard, mourned "the loss of the phenomenological dimension that privileges lived experience" (Kellner 1999: 119).

However, the notion of the cinematic experience as an "act of pure seeing" overlooks the non-visual correlates and accompaniments to the images on screen. Audiences that experienced Léger's film experienced it both visually and through the sound of Antheil's musical score. More generally, the experience of early cinema was an intensely multisensory one, as conveyed by the following description by Siegfried Kracauer of cinema-going in 1930s Berlin:

This total artwork of effects assaults all the senses using every possible means. Spotlights shower their beams into the auditorium, sprinkling across festive drapes or rippling through colorful, organic looking glass fixtures. The orchestra asserts itself as an independent power, its acoustic production buttressed by the responsory of the lighting. Every emotion is accorded its own acoustic expression and its color value in the spectrum—a visual and acoustic kaleidoscope that provides the setting for the physical activity on stage: pantomime and ballet. Until finally the white surface descends and the events of the three-dimensional stage blend imperceptibly into two-dimensional illusions.

Kracauer 1995: 324

Such multisensory spectacles were characteristic of early cinema. For example, when the Roxy Cinema opened in New York in 1927, it was heralded as the "Cathedral of the Motion Picture" with its luxurious décor and seating for close to 6,000 people. The film itself was merely one part of an extravagant show. The Roxy had its own 110-piece orchestra, which would play classical overtures and support ballet performances by the Martha Graham Dance Company. Films were screened at the end of the performances on a gigantic screen, thereby amplifying the distance between the everyday experience of the viewer and the "reality" of the film screen.

With the introduction of synchronized sound movies in the late 1920s, "going to the movies" became an increasingly popular leisure-time activity

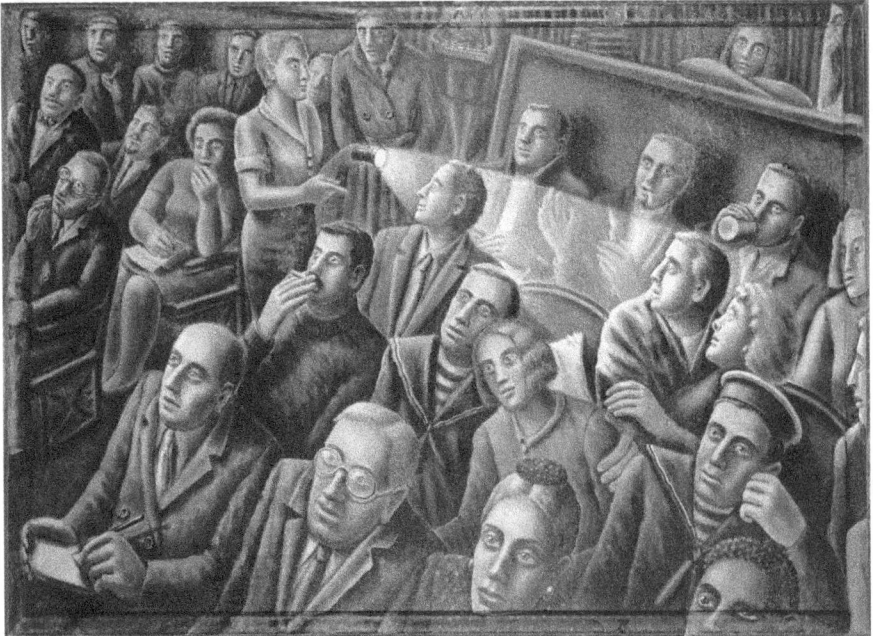

FIGURE 9.1: The cinematic experience: *Cinema* by P. J. Crook. Getty Images.

across all classes of society (Kyvig 2004: 94). It is estimated that close to 90 percent of the American populace went to the cinema weekly in 1930. The newly developed sound track of film produced an auditory training to complement Benjamin's optical training:

> Acoustic close-ups make us perceive sounds which are included in the accustomed noise of day-to-day life, but which we never heard as individual sounds because they are drowned in the general din . . . in the sound film, scarcely perceptible, intimate things can be conveyed with all the secrecy of the unnoticed eavesdropper. The general din can go on, it may even drown completely a sound like the soft piping of a mosquito, but we can get quite close to the source of the sound with the microphone and with our ear and hear it nevertheless.
>
> Balazs 2011: 176

Sound, according to this view, reconfigured "reality" in the filmic image to achieve its own version of audio-visual veracity.

Color entered the picture in the 1930s, most famously through the movie *The Wizard of Oz* (1939), though black and white film, especially in the form of newsreels, remained commonplace until much later. The use of color enhanced the verisimilitude of film, as it would that of television with the development of color TV. While the broadcast technology for color TV was invented and put in place in 1951, it would take another twenty years for the new medium to catch on, because it depended on consumers buying sets that could receive the signals.

One dominant theme that ran through early film was that of flight, from the movement of the camera to the depiction of flight itself. For example, Fritz Lang's *Frau im Mond* futuristically and realistically depicted the launch of a spaceship to the Moon. The film premiered in Berlin in 1929. It was later censored by the Nazis. As Lang recounted:

> The launching of the rocket in the film . . . was so authentic in all its technical details, as were the drawings, that the Nazis withdrew the film from distribution. Even the model of the space ship was destroyed by the Gestapo, on account of the imminence of V1 and V2 rockets on which Werner von Braun was working from 1937 onwards.
>
> Eisner 1977: 110

In fact, the first V2 rocket launched and successfully dropped on London had the *Frau im Mond* logo painted on its base. Filmic image and direct experience became fatally joined. Just prior to this, in 1927, the Roxy showed the first sound film. It depicted the American aviator Charles A. Lindbergh taking off on the first transatlantic flight to Paris recorded earlier that same day. (This reduction in the period of time between the filming of an event and its showing was itself a cinematic landmark.) Indeed, the very experience of cinema and later television was arguably aligned to the experience of flying, with its manipulation of space and depth through movement, its use of aerial and panning shots, and other such techniques (Virilio 1989).

With the coming of the Second World War, the media went into overdrive to depict scenes of war. Audiences flocked to the cinema to watch Hollywood war movies or Movietone newsreels narrated by Lowell Thomas. The connection between flight and the cinema continued through the Second World War and after with a wide range of propaganda movies such as *Casablanca*. The 1950 movie *Destination Moon* portrayed the attempt to control the world militarily by controlling the Moon, thus feeding into Cold War fears of the "communist menace." The film portrayed the crash of an early rocket prototype that would later seem hauntingly evocative of the images of the Space Shuttle *Challenger* disaster broadcast live in 1986.

Destination Moon provided the blueprint for the most popular ride in the "Tomorrowland" section of the Disneyland theme park, which opened in 1955:

> The jewel in the crown of Tomorrowland was *Rocket to the Moon,* a Hale's Tour-style ride to outer space. *Rocket to the Moon* seated riders in a theatre inside a mock rocket ship. As seats rocked and ambient sounds signaled liftoff, rocketeers could watch animation of the receding earth on a movie screen underneath the transparent floor and views of where they were headed on a movie screen directly in front of them. The ride took them around the moon and back home again . . . *Rocket to the Moon* remade the fantasy from one of visiting a destination that fulfilled the modern urbanite to the fantasy of being inside a movie . . . *Rocket to the Moon* harnessed the exhilarating sensations of kinesthesia and speed for the cinema . . . it is much easier to simulate reality when the reality being depicted is already a movie.
>
> Rabinovitz 2012: 167

Joining bodily jolts to filmic looking was a novelty. It set what Buck-Morss has called the "anaesthetized body" (i.e. the immobile body) of the cinema-goer in motion, albeit within very tight constraints, so not exactly "free." This innovation, inspired by a motion picture movie, came, however, at a time when the cultural practice of going to the movies would begin its long decline. First with televisions in the 1960s and then with personal computers in the 1980s, small domestic screens progressively replaced large public screens (see Hansen 2012: xvi). Within the small screen reality (television literally meant vision at a distance) the exceptional became juxtaposed with the domestic as viewers could watch the coronation of Queen Elizabeth II in 1953, the assassination of US President John F. Kennedy in 1963, and the moon landing in 1969 from the privacy of their homes. This was coupled with the progressive simulation of everyday life through the creation of popular serials such as *I Love Lucy* in the 1950s United States and *Coronation Street* in the 1960s UK. Television also portrayed the world's conflicts ranging from the Suez Crisis in 1956 through Vietnam, Kosovo, and Operation Desert Storm (otherwise known as the First Gulf War) in 1991. In doing so it drastically altered the relationship between the social world and the "interior psychic landscape, scrambling the relations between these two poles" (Crary 2013: 81).

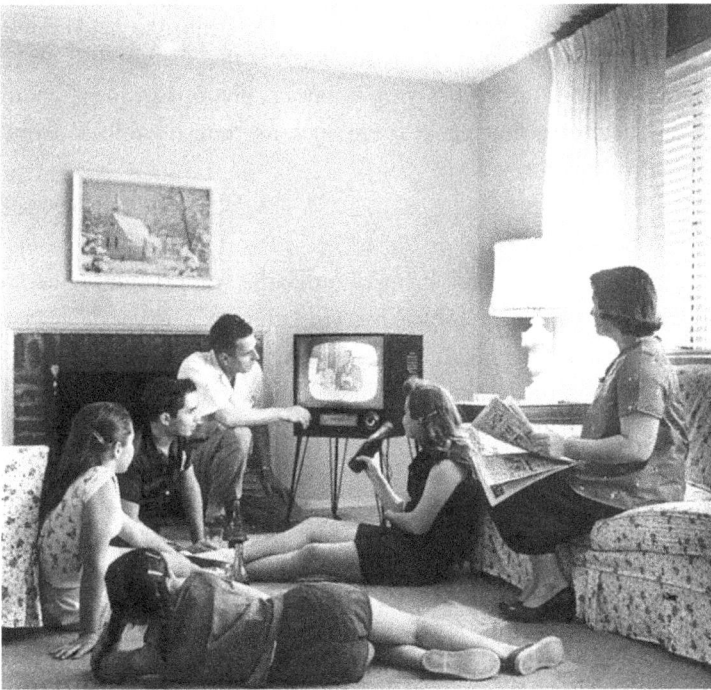

FIGURE 9.2: The electronic hearth: a family watching television. Photograph by Evert Baumgardner. National Archives and Records Administration.

Central to this new perspective was the viewing of war, which, to paraphrase Adorno, had progressed from the newsreel as embodied in Second World War reportage to the "live" 24-hour broadcast as exemplified by the coverage of Operation Desert Storm of 1991. The latter "media event" illustrated Baudrillard's theory of the advent of the age of the simulacrum to a T, as Allen Feldman brings out in the following passage:

> broadcast images [of Operation Desert Storm] functioned as electronic simulacra that were injected into the collective nervous system of the audience as antibodies that inured the viewer from realizing the human-material consequences of war. Visual mastery of the campaign pushed all other sensory dimensions outside the perceptual terms of reference. Culturally biased narrations abetted by informational technology historically molded to normative concepts of sensory truth precluded any scream of pain, any stench of corpse from visiting the American living room . . . Civilian television observation was continuous with the military optics of the fighter pilot and bombardier who were dependent on analogous prosthetic technology, and who killed at a distance with the sensory impunity and omniscient vision of the living room spectator. The combat crews who played with aggressive drives by watching pornographic videos prior to flying missions, demonstrating the uniform sensorium between viewing and violence as they up-shifted from one virtual reality to another.
>
> Feldman 1994: 92–3

William Stam attempted to bring home the moral ambiguity of this spectacularization of warfare by observing that television news flatters its "armchair imperialist viewers" into adopting a subjective position as "the audio visual masters of the world." The supposed guarantee which television offered them was the "illusionary feeling of present-ness, this constructed impression of total immediacy . . . a televisual metaphysics of presence" (quoted in Morley 2000: 185).

MEDIATED MULTI-SENSORIALITY II: LISTENING AND LOOKING

Returning to the 1930s, the lure of the cinema was increasingly challenged by another technological marvel, radio, which, while it offered no visual stimulus, could conveniently be listened to at home. Sound technologies, as distinct from more visually-based technologies, had produced their own specific relationship between the real and the virtual through their mediation of time, place, and presence. In fact, one scholar has claimed that "the succession from the 'singing wire' (telegraph), through the microphone, telephone, and phonograph to radio and allied technologies of sound marks perhaps the most radical of all sensory reorganizations in modernity" (Peters 1999: 160). Perhaps this is because sound can be characterized as "the immersive medium par excellence," offering the listener "that feeling of being here now, of experiencing oneself as engulfed, enveloped, enmeshed, in short, immersed in an environment" (Dyson 2009: 4).

Mediated sound as embodied in the gramophone and radio also created a sense of mediated "we-ness." The phrase derives from the work of Adorno (1991) who argued that the consumption of mechanically reproduced music was increasingly used as an effective substitute for the sense of connectivity that modern cultures lacked. We-ness refers to the substitution of direct experience by technologically mediated forms of experience. Sound media represented to the urban subject a utopian longing for what they desired but could not achieve, producing "an illusion of immediacy in a totally mediated world, of proximity between strangers, the warmth of those who come to feel a chill of unmitigated struggle of all against all" (Horkheimer and Adorno 1973: 46).

The understanding of what constituted sociality in a transformed media space was further influenced by the development of a range of sound technologies, such as the amplifier, the speaker, and the microphone. At first, before the advent of the loudspeaker, radio was listened to through headphones, which, paradoxically, privatized the space of listening within the household at the same time as it created a sense of connection with distant places. "Who could resist the invitation of those dainty headphones?" wrote Siegfried Kracauer, describing early domestic radio. "They gleam in living rooms and entwine themselves around the heads all by themselves . . . silent and lifeless, people sit side by side as if their souls were wandering about far away" (Kracauer 1995: 333).

Jonathan Sterne has argued that the audile individualism depicted in Kracauer's quote:

> was rooted in a practice of individuation: listeners could own their own acoustic spaces through owning the material component of a technique of producing that auditory space—the "medium" that now stands for a whole set of practices. The space of the auditory field became a form of private property, a space for the individual to inhabit alone.
>
> Sterne 2003: 160

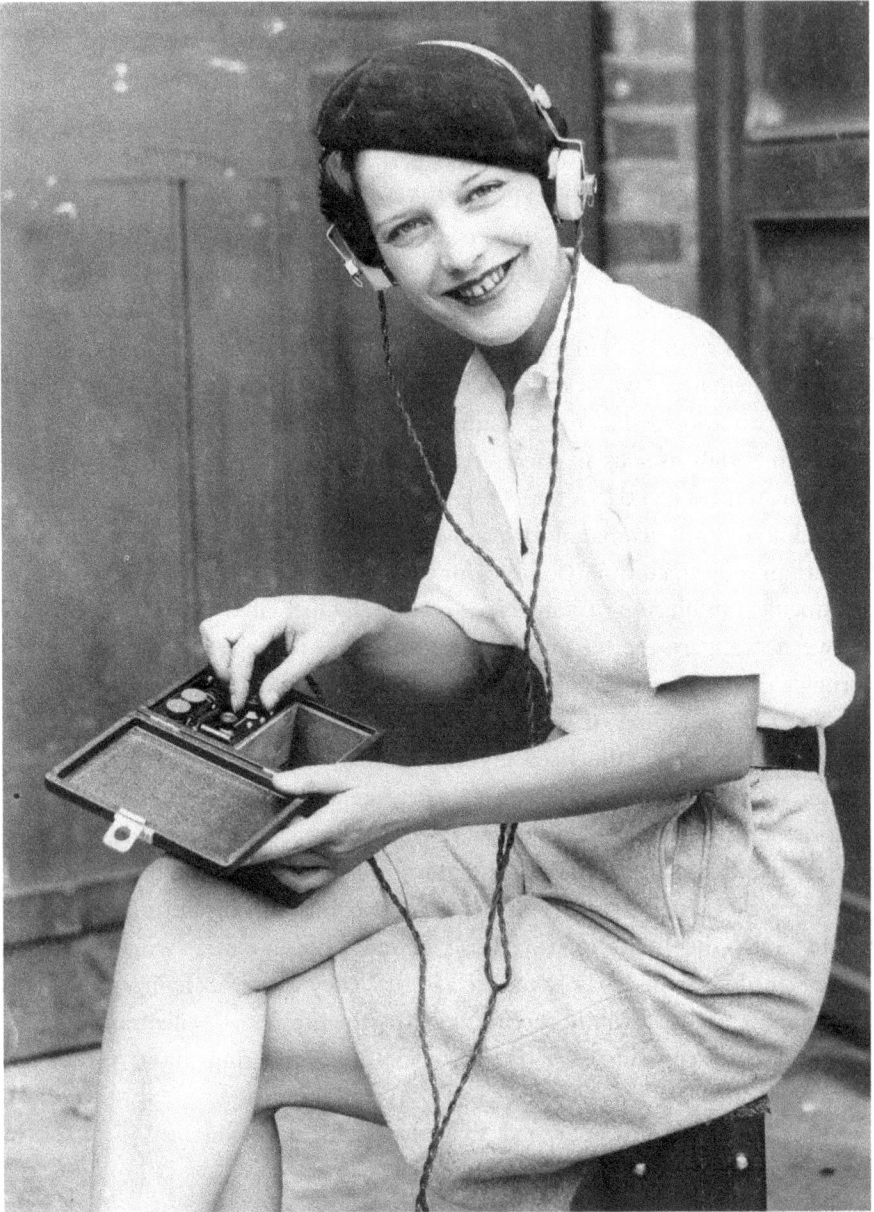

FIGURE 9.3: Early radio with headphones, London Radio-Fair, 1934. Photo by Imagno. Hulton Archive/Getty Images.

Following Benjamin, technologies and values appeared indissociably linked. From the birth of the radio through to the invention of the Walkman, a central facet of the training of perception has been the desire for immersive sonic experience, which appeared to transform both the private space of the living room and the public space of the street, often unifying or blurring the distinction between the two. Once loudspeakers were incorporated into radios, "listening to the radio" was often a shared experience. As early as the 1930s the public role of radio-listening was described in the following terms by a Chicago urbanite: "when walking home in the hot summer evenings after window shopping on Madison Street, one could follow the entire progress of *Amos 'n' Andy* from the open windows." By the 1940s, even in small towns like Honea Path, South Carolina, it was possible to "practically hear the whole of *Grand Ole Opry* as it issued out of every house on the block" (quoted in Loviglio 2005: xiv).

The power to transform space politically through the development of sound technologies was recognized by Hitler. "We should not have conquered Germany . . . without the loudspeaker," he wrote in 1938 (cited by Schafer 1994: 91). Subjects learnt how "to be" in the world by listening to the propagandist voices of Hitler in Germany, and Roosevelt and Churchill in the US and UK. This mediated world lured the subject with the very compression of its signal, which produced an aura of "objectivity." From the dulcet tones of Roosevelt's fireside chats to De Gaulle's exhortations to the French to resist the Nazi occupation during the Second World War, to the colonial sounds of "Hello, London Calling" emitted by the BBC World Service, sound both compelled and repelled. By mimicking the style of live news broadcasts, H. G. Wells' 1938 radio play *War of the Worlds* provoked panic amongst many American listeners who, suspending their knowledge of "real-time activity," fled their homes in fear of a supposed attack by aliens (Heyer 2005).

In the Soviet Union, the "Stalin Radio" was installed in all apartment blocks. This simple box, through which "The Party" advanced its political line on all things (playing only Party-approved music and presenting Party-approved dramas and variety shows), could never be turned off. This totalitarian sound world would later be replicated by certain religious cults, such as the Peoples Temple, founded by Jim Jones in the 1950s and transplanted to the interior of Guyana in the 1970s. Rebecca Layton, one of Jonestown's few survivors of the mass 1978 suicide, recounted: "In Jonestown there was a speaker system and only Jim Jones spoke on it and it went 24 hours a day, and he would tape himself so—in the middle of the night—all through the night his voice was talking to you" (Layton 1988: 86).

With the development of the Walkman in 1979, individualism once again became central to mediated listening. The Walkman, as its name implies, allowed listeners to take their private sonic world with them wherever they went. William Gibson, the science fiction writer commonly credited with coining the notion of "virtual reality," commented on the radical transformative nature of the Walkman: "the Sony Walkman has done more to change human perception than any virtual reality gadget. I can't remember any technological experience since that was quite so wonderful as being able to take music and move it through landscapes and architecture" (quoted in Bull 2000: 7). Walkman users frequently described their experience of moving through cities as "filmic" in nature. City streets would take on the quality of the music that they listened to. Users, consequently, would often choose music which they considered would "suit" the spaces they passed through, thus transforming their perceived power over the environment.

Walkman users became increasingly accustomed to experiencing not just the world but also their own cognitive states through the sounds of their machines. Sonic mediation became a form of "second nature" for many users. As one Walkman afficionado whom I interviewed for *Sounding Out the City* (2000) recounted: "I wear it all the time, like a pacemaker! A life support machine! It's like I'm a walking resource centre" (Bull 2000: 17). Control of thoughts, emotions, and desires became central to the daily management strategies of Walkman users. Listening to music permitted them to order their thoughts, feelings, and outlook towards the world—as desired. The choice of personalized music frequently set the mood of the day as users left their homes listening to their chosen music. Walkman users, in fact, created technologically mediated sanctuaries out of much of their experience, permitting them to feel "centered" wherever they might be.

The use of mobile phones furthered this privatizing impulse in twentieth-century culture. By the late 1990s mobile phones had permeated all areas of social life (Castells 2009), rearranging the meaning of, and relations between, work and home, and of sociability itself. As mobile phones became an integral tool in the management of everyday life, the nature of public space was further transformed. Steven Connor has argued that the very meaning of social space is "very largely a function of the perceived powers of the body to occupy and extend itself through its environment" (2000: 12). The sound of the voice colonized the space it inhabited, and mobile phone talk was everywhere in the 1990s. Local customs of reserve become progressively eroded as mobile phone users become more assertive in their public demonstration of conversing with absent others (Castells 2009). Urban space became decontextualized as the intimacy of the home was recreated in the public spaces of the street. This trend had relational consequences and spoke to the progressive prioritization of private space over shared social space in the modern age.

MILITARIZING THE SENSES: VISION, SOUND, AND TOUCH

In 1983, whilst on a visit to Walt Disney World in Florida to talk to children from the International Youth Initiative, the US president, Ronald Reagan, had this to say about sensory training and the media:

> Many of you already understand better than my generation ever will the possibilities of computers. In some of your homes, the computer is as available at the television set. And I recently learned something quite interesting about video games. Many young people have developed incredible hand, eye, and brain coordination in playing these games. The Air Force believes these kids will be outstanding pilots should they fly our jets. The computerized radar screen in the cockpit is not unlike the computerized video screen. Watch a 12-year-old take evasive action and score multiple hits while playing "Space Invaders," and you will appreciate the skills of tomorrow's pilot.[1]

The militarization of the senses described by Reagan became a prominent concern in late twentieth-century culture, at the same time as multisensory engagement with the world increasingly became virtual. On the one hand the development of virtual realities appeared to confirm Mumford's view of media experience as one of "the sensations of living without the experience of living." Cyber-optimists such as Howard Rheingold, however, viewed the situation more positively: "people in virtual communities do just about everything people do in real life, but we leave our bodies behind" (Rheingold 1993: 3). Similarly, in his greeting at the first IEEE Virtual Reality Annual Symposium in 1993, Tom Furness, Air Force VR pioneer, proclaimed that "advanced interfaces will provide an incredibly new mobility for the human race. We are building transportation systems for the senses ... the remarkable promise that we can be in another place or space without moving our bodies into that space" (quoted in Biocca and Levy 1995: 23). In what follows, I briefly analyze virtuality through the lens of the multisensory militarization of experience.

Walter Benjamin's analysis of the sensory transformation of sight, distance, and proximity through film and photography can be extended to video-game

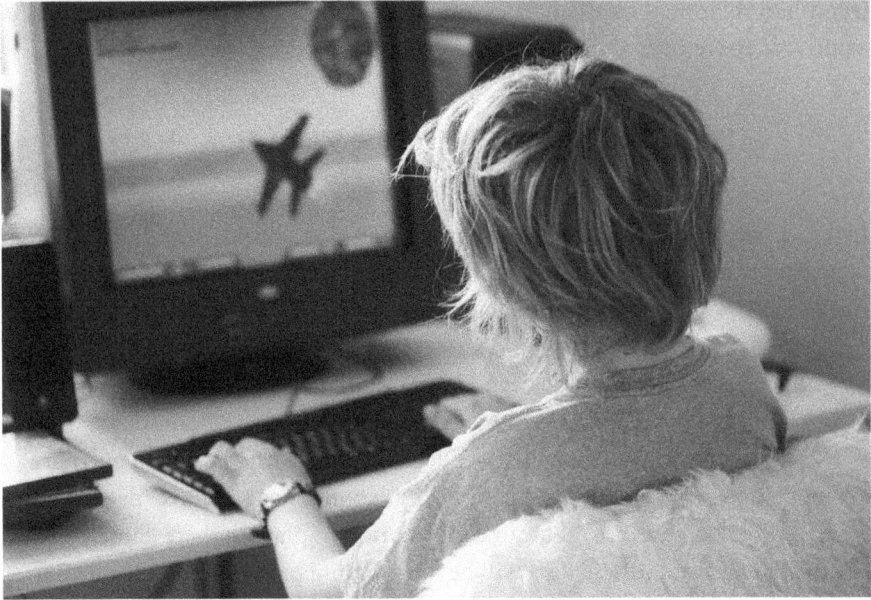

FIGURE 9.4: Young boy playing computer video game. Photo by Kennet Havgaard. Getty Images.

playing, which likewise involves an intense visual training. It has been found, for example, that video-game playing helps users "improve their spatial resolution, meaning their ability to clearly see small, closely packed together objects, such as letters . . . these games push the human visual system to the limits and the brain adapts to it" (Green and Bavelier 2007: 91). Thus a growing body of research confirms Benjamin's claim that the media "train" the subject's sensorium.

The synergetic relationship between gaming and warring alluded to by Reagan has become widely recognized. For Frederic Kittler, "media technologies discipline, mutate, and preempt the affective sensorium. Entertainment itself becomes part of the training" (cited by Goodman 2010: 34). This view echoed Theodor Adorno's earlier critique of the culture industry to the effect that amusement was merely work by other means. This critique tied the culture industry to the industrial complex—of which the military complex can be seen as an integral part (Virilio: 1989: 83).

One example of this is the development of Drone aircraft. Drone is the nickname for "unmanned aerial vehicles" (UAVs). These planes, equipped with sensors, color and black-and-white TV cameras, image intensifiers, infrared imaging for low light conditions, and lasers for targeting, are usually directed from thousands of miles away at a base camp. Operatives use the visual data proffered by the cameras on the Drone to locate targets and decide whether to attack. The use of Drone technology from the 1980s was fueled by military innovations such as The Joint Simulation System (JSIMS), which trained operatives in the use of Drone aircraft. The program itself was based on the 3D graphics used in the computer game *Wargame* and was aimed at both military personnel and the gaming public. The use of Drones themselves mirrored the development of video games dating back to the 1970s when they were used by the Israeli military to gather intelligence. They were transformed into killing machines after the 1999 NATO Kosovo campaign (Benjamin 2013). With the introduction of this technology, troops began to question the necessity to physically go to war. Thus, in 2000 the *Daily Telegraph* reported:

> The Israeli dot-com generation seems not to have the stomach for mortal combat. They have started to ask why they should risk their lives when precision weapons can reduce war to a video game. For the pony-tailed youth of Tel Aviv's night spots, the war in Lebanon was becoming their Vietnam and they would rather their government fought it by remote control.
>
> Quoted in Der Derain 2009: xxii

The rise of virtuality, the moral ambiguity of sensory distance, and the militarization of the senses were exemplified by the use of Drones. Drawing out the comparison with gaming, one operative said, "It's like playing a single game everyday but always sticking on the same level" (Darwent 2013: 52).

Even the virtual terrains in which war-game players immersed themselves were not so dissimilar to the "real" theater of war that many British and American soldiers encountered and distant "others" found themselves embroiled in at the turn of the twenty-first century:

> The construction of Arab cities as targets for US military firepower now sustains a large industry of computer gaming and simulation. Video games such as *America's Army* and the US Marine's equivalent, *Full Spectrum Warrior*, have been developed by their respective forces, with help from the corporate entertainment industries, as training ads, recruitment aids and powerful public relations exercises. Both games— which were amongst the world's most popular video game franchises in 2005—centre overwhelmingly on the military challenges allegedly involved in occupying, and pacifying, Orientalized Arab cities.
>
> Graham 2006: 265

Such games manifest a deep concern for visual and aural fidelity:

> For added realism, footsteps, bullet impacts, particle effects, grenades, and shell casings are accorded texture-specific impact noises. A flying shell casing clinks differently on concrete, wood, or metal, for instance, and the distinction is clearly heard in the game. Likewise, footsteps on dirt, mud, wood, concrete, glass, and metal are sounded correctly. The game's goal of sensory verisimilitude sets an expectation for political verisimilitude.
>
> Bogost 2007: 78

The "real" was thus rendered as a three-dimensional copy on the screens of both consumers of games and military personnel till they become virtually indistinguishable for the viewer, but not, of course, for the "target" population (speaking of the constant awareness of the presence of Drones, one Pakistani interviewed for an article in *The Atlantic* noted: "They are like a mosquito. Even when you don't see them, you can hear them, you know they are there"— Friedersdorf 2012). However, not only were and are game scenarios frequently modeled on the image of a physical environment found in Pakistan and other essentialized Middle Eastern environments, but the very representation of the local inhabitants is a contemporary example of the demonization of the "enemy" developed through propaganda techniques from the First World War onwards. In war games, employing a pseudo-Middle Eastern setting, inhabitants are typically represented "as the shadowy, subhuman, racialized Arab figure of some absolutely external 'terrorist'." As such they become "figures to be annihilated repeatedly in sanitized 'action' as entertainment or military training or both" (Graham 2006: 266). Distance dissolved through the screen does not invoke empathy. Rather, individuals become "aliens" on the screen of the army helicopter, or on the screens of the distant control center. The operators squeeze their controls—and fire.

CONCLUSION: EXPERIENCING 9/11

Susan Sontag (2004) commented some years ago that the viewing of the pain of others "at a distance" was "one of the distinguishing features of modern life." More recently Lilia Chouliariki has described the live images of the moment the second plane hit the World Trade Center on September 11, 2001, which were transmitted around the globe, as a sequence in which time itself appeared to freeze:

There is an extended sequence of the live footage, which provides us with
a long shot of the Manhattan cityscape in grey smoke. Filmed from an
Ellis Island crane, the long shot again creates an aestheticized effect,
whereby the scene of suffering appears as a spectacle to be contemplated
rather than acted upon. Confronting us with the sublime quality of
human tragedy, this management of visibility removes the urgency of the
"here and now" and opens up a space of analytical temporality, providing
us with the option for reflection on the events.

Chouliaraki 2006: 10

The events of 9/11 unfolded primarily on the world's television screens through
a mixture of studio presentation, hastily composed live shots from mobile
camera crews on the ground, and telephone interviews with New Yorkers who
were "witnessing" the events live. Spectators around the world experienced
9/11 through distant but live news footage. The studio coverage on the ABC
television network news showed the images of the burning World Trade Center
buildings on a screen that the presenters and the millions of viewers watched
simultaneously. Long shots alternated with close-ups of the exterior of the
buildings, and later the image split into a double screen with images of the
Pentagon—also aflame. Viewers listened to a voiceover in which the presenters
talked the audience through the images based on what little they themselves
knew of the event. Thus, the newscasters in the studio were viewing the same
visual frames as the audience—distant and silent—whilst simultaneously
gathering news from onlookers and others. The television audience experienced
the eerily silent and unerringly direct trajectory of the second jet aircraft to hit
the World Trade Center, and in subsequent minutes witnessed the collapse of
both Tower One and Tower Two. Hence, viewers became global immediate
witnesses. The images beamed around the world, though, were purely visual,
divorced from the blood, smell, heat, and sound of the events unfolding before
television viewers' eyes. The images were also largely devoid of bodies. When
silent images of people jumping to their deaths were briefly shown, they were
quickly removed from subsequent broadcasts. In the aftermath, many resorted
to more traditional media, such as newspapers: "people really wanted to look
at images in their own time, contemplating and absorbing the tragedy in ways
that the rush of television could not accommodate" (Zelizer 2010: 115).

In the search for meaning, many audience members turned to film as a
reference point. The unfolding events of 9/11 as presented on television
appeared to imitate Hollywood movies. The phrase "it looks just like a movie"
was one that audiences and reporters alike uttered repeatedly. For those

habituated to two-dimensional fictional representations of urban destruction
in such Hollywood films as *The Towering Inferno* (1974) and the *Die Hard*
series (1988 *et seq.*), the cultural reference point was hardly surprising. In fact,
the director of *Die Hard*, Steve de Souza, commented that the terrorist attacks
looked "like one of my movie posters" (cited by Rickli 2009: 214).

This public reception of the visual registration of the events of 9/11
contrasted with the response to the auditory record. This latter consisted of the
many telephone messages sent from the Twin Towers by those who perished.
The New York Port Authority released these tapes to the public in 2004. One
of these tapes recorded the 9/11 calls between a telephone operator and Kevin
Cosgrove, who can be heard speaking until the South Tower collapsed around
him. It is a distressing tape to listen to. However, the wife of Kevin Cosgrove
made this observation of her husband's taped conversation:

> Some people have said, you know, hearing Kevin's words made the events
> of 9/11 more human for them . . . that there were really people in there,
> that it wasn't just a building. One lady called him "the voice from the
> towers" it made it real for her—it wasn't just a news story—it seemed
> like it was just a movie but when they heard Kevin speaking realized it
> was a real thing—there were real people inside.
>
> *9/11 Phone Calls from the Towers*, Channel 4 documentary, 2009

The visual imagery of 9/11, while shocking, had something of an illusory
quality for many people. The auditory evidence, by contrast, in particular the
voices of the people who died, gave the events the "feel" of reality.

As discussed throughout this chapter, twentieth-century theorists from
Heidegger to Chouliaraki have pointed to the multisensory contraction of
space embodied in media use. Seeing and hearing the live media coverage of the
events of 9/11 inculcated in some 2 billion people around the world the sense
of just how powerful the sensory immediacy of modern media could be.

The merging of the real and the cinematic that for some characterized the
broadcasting of the events of 9/11 can be seen as part of a general trend of the
time. One major sign of this trend was the popularity of reality television, in
which the "show" consisted of the "real-life" adventures of an individual or
family or group of competitors, placed in challenging situations. Examples of
the genre include *Survivor* (1997) and *Big Brother* (1999), which enjoyed such
success that they were turned into global franchises.

In a related vein, the 1998 movie *The Truman Show* portrayed the fictional
scenario of a man who unwittingly lives his whole life as the subject of a

television show watched by millions. (Psychologists later coined the term "Truman Show Syndrome" to refer to a growing delusion suffered by individuals who believe that they too are secretly being filmed for a television show.) Such blurring of real life and televised fantasy also involved a sensory shift from the three-dimensional, multisensory world of everyday life to the two-dimensional, audio-visual "reality" of the screen. Arguably, this recounting of life as a purely audio-visual spectacle helped set the stage for the surge in emotionally compelling but sensorially limited virtual communities in the twenty-first century.

NOTES

Chapter Seven

1. For the sense of wonder in modernist fiction see Waugh (2009: esp. 135).
2. Not only did Auden write documentary texts (apart from *Journey to a War*, also *Letters from Iceland* with Louis McNeice), he also became actively engaged in documentary film productions for the General Post Office (GPO), the most prominent being *Night Mail* (1936), which depicts a train journey from London to Scotland. For Auden's involvement in the documentary movement see Bryant (1997).

Chapter Eight

1. Many in the avant-garde believed that cultural institutions were corrupt at the outset: museums by their specialist boards, galleries by their rich collectors, and national art fairs by their state support. The separation of the artwork from life in the modern period is arguably materially expressed in the bracketing off of the work from the environments that were generative for it. Modernist work is best seen in a kind of vault, the white cube without windows, hushed, timeless, and generative of a private feeling.
2. Vladimir Tatlin's famous Monument to the Third International tower was being discussed among the Dadaists at this time and references to it appear in several collages. Tatlin's tower would also function as a radio tower, setting an important precedent for Baader's.
3. Golyshev is best known for his role in the 1918 founding of the *Novembergruppe* of Expressionists whose left flank broke off in 1921 as Berlin Dada (Otto Dix, George Grosz, Yefim Golyshev, Raoul Hausmann, John Heartfield, Hannah Höch, Rudolf Schlichter, Georg Scholz). Among musicologists, he is best known for composing twelve-tone music, but he also made substantial contributions to Dadaism as

a visual artist. He worked in Assemblage, making objects using jelly jars, hair, glass, and paper lace (Gordon 1994: 230–2).

4. Albeit not Futurist per se, Marcel Duchamp's famous *Nude Descending a Staircase* (1912) likewise bears a passing resemblance to these stroboscopic images. Particularly in Duchamp's work, the space of the action appears warped as force lines turn the stable space of perspective images inside out. These are images of actions seen in the fourth dimension.

5. This is, of course, another way of thinking about Dick Higgins' "Intermedia" (Higgins 1966).

6. This criticism is fleshed out in Bishop's review of *Relational Aesthetics* (Bishop 2004).

Chapter Nine

1. Ronald Reagan, "Remarks During a Visit to Walt Disney World's EPCOT Center near Orlando, Florida, March 8, 1983," The American Presidency Project, http://www.presidency.ucsb.edu/ws/?pid=41022

BIBLIOGRAPHY

Abelson, E., 1989, *When Ladies Go A-Thieving: middle-class shoplifters in the Victorian department store*, Oxford: Oxford University Press.

Ackroyd, P., 2001, *London: the biography*, London: Random House.

Adamson, S. *et al.*, 2009, *Hidden from Public View? Racism against the UK Chinese population*, London: The Monitoring Group.

Adorno, T., 1981, *Negative Dialectics*, New York: Continuum Press.

Adorno, T., 1991, *The Culture Industry: selected essays on mass culture*, London: Routledge.

Adorno, T. W., 2002, *Essays on Music: Theodor W. Adorno*, Berkeley, CA: University of California Press.

Allitt, P., 2003, *Religion in America Since 1945: a history*, New York: Columbia University Press.

Alter, N. and Koepnick, L. (eds), 2005, *Sound Matters: essays on the acoustics of German culture*, New York: Berghahn Books.

Anderson, M., 1949, *Planning and Financing the New Church*, 2nd rev. edn, Minneapolis, MN: Augsburg.

Anjaria, J., 2012, "Is there a culture of the Indian street?", *Seminar*, 636, 21–7.

Ainsworth, M. D. Salter, 1967, *Infancy in Uganda: infant care and the growth of love*, Baltimore, MD: Johns Hopkins University Press.

Anscombe, G. E. M., 1965, "The intentionality of sensation: a grammatical feature," in R. J. Butler (ed.), *Analytical Philosophy: First Series*, Oxford: Blackwell.

Appadurai, A., 1996, *Modernity at Large: cultural dimensions of globalisation*, Minneapolis, MN: University of Minnesota Press.

Apple, R., 2007, "Vitamins win the war: nutrition, commerce, and patriotism in the United States during the Second World War," in D. S. Smith and J. Phillips (eds), *Food, Science, Policy and Regulation in the Twentieth Century, International and Comparative Perspectives*, New York: Routledge.

Apollinaire, G., 1971, *Selected Writings of Guillaume Apollinaire*, New York: New Directions.

Archer, J., 2005, *Architecture and Suburbia: from English villa to American dream house, 1690–2000*, Minneapolis, MN: University of Minnesota Press.

Arendt, H., 1963, *Eichmann in Jerusalem: the banality of evil*, London: Faber & Faber.

Armstrong, D. M., 1968, *A Materialist Theory of the Mind*, London: Routledge & Kegan Paul.

Armstrong, J., 2010, "Everyday afterlife: Walter Benjamin and the politics of abandonment in Saskatchewan, Canada," *Cultural Studies*, 25, 273–93.

Armstrong, T., 2005, "The senses and the self," in *Modernism: A Cultural History*, Cambridge: Polity Press.

Aron, C. S., 1999, *Working at Play: a history of vacations in the United States*, Oxford: Oxford University Press.

Ash, M. G., 1998, *Gestalt Psychology in German Culture, 1890–1967: holism and the quest for objectivity*, Cambridge: Cambridge University Press.

Augé, M., 1995, *Non-Places: introduction to an anthropology of supermodernity*, London: Verso.

Austin, J. L., 1962, *Sense and Sensibilia*, Oxford: Oxford University Press.

Avila, E., 2004, *Popular Culture in the Age of White Flight: fear and fantasy in suburban Los Angeles*, Berkeley, CA: University of California Press.

Ayer, A. J., 1940, *The Foundations of Empirical Knowledge*, London: Macmillan.

Ayer, A. J., 1956, *The Problem of Knowledge*, London: Macmillan.

Ayres, A. J., 1972, "Improving academic scores through sensory integration," *Journal of Learning Disabilities*, 5(6), 338–43.

Baader, J., 2001, "Johannes Baader's Plasto-Dio-Dada-Drama: The Mysticism of Mass Media," *Modernism/modernity*, 8(4), 583–602.

Babcock, M., 1930, "Hallelujah—and a percentage—Aimee Semple McPherson," *Motion Picture Classic*, 32, 30, 84.

Bacci, F., and Melcher, D. (eds), 2011, *Art and the Senses*, Oxford: Oxford University Press.

Back, L., 2007, *The Art of Listening*, London: Berg.

Balazs, B., 2011, *Early Film Theory. Visible man and the spirit of film*, London: Berghahn Books.

Ball, H., [1916] 1992, "Diary entry," in C. Harrison and P. Wood (eds), *Art in Theory: 1900–1990*, Oxford: Blackwell.

Barlow, H. B., 1953, "Summation and inhibition in the frog's retina," *Journal of Physiology*, 119, 69–88.

Barlow, H. B., 1972, "Single units and sensation: a neuron doctrine for perceptual psychology?" *Perception*, 1(4), 371–94.

Barr, J., 1970, *The Assaults on Our Senses*, London: Methuen and Co. Ltd.

Barr, W., 1928, *Baxter McLendon: a biography*, Bennettsville, SC: Bibliotheca Co.

Barthes, R., 1972, *Mythologies*, trans. A. Lavers, London: Paladin.

Bates, H. E., 1997, *Flying Bombs Over England*, Oxford: Isis Publications.

Baudrillard, J., 1994, *Simulacra and Simulation (The Body in Theory: histories of cultural materialism)*, Ann Arbor, MI: University of Michigan Press.

Baudrillard, J., 2004, *The Gulf War Did Not Take Place*, Indiana, IN: Indiana University Press.

Baxandall, R. and Ewen, E., 2000, *Picture Windows: how the suburbs happened*, New York: Basic Books.

Beckett, S., 1981, *Endgame*, in *Dramatische Dichtungen in drei Sprachen*, Frankfurt a. M.: Suhrkamp.

Belasco, W. J., 2007, *Appetite for Change: how the counterculture took on the food industry*, Ithaca, NY: Cornell University Press.

Benjamin, M., 2013, *Drone Warfare. Killing by Remote Control*, London: Routledge.

Benjamin, W., [1936] 1973, "The work of art in the age of mechanical reproduction," in *Illuminations*, London: Penguin.

Benjamin, W., 1969, *Illuminations*, New York: Schocken.

Benjamin, W., 1973, *Illuminations*, London: Penguin.

Benjamin, W., 1986, *Reflections: essays, aphorisms, autobiographical writing*, New York: Schocken Books.

Benjamin, W., 1999, *Selected Writings. Volume 2, 1927–1934*, Cambridge, MA: Harvard University Press.

Benson, T. O., 1986, *Raoul Hausmann and Berlin Dada*, Ann Arbor, MI: UMI Research Press.

Bently, L. and Flynn, L. (eds), 1996, *Law and the Senses: sensational jurisprudence*, London: Pluto Press.

Berger, J., 1972, *Ways of Seeing*, Harmondsworth: Penguin Books.

Berger, J., 1991, *About Looking*, Toronto: Random House.

Bergius, H. with Miller, N. and Riha, K. (eds), 1977, *Johannes Baader: Oberdada*, trans. from German by M. White, Gießen-Lahn: Anabas Verlag.

Berman, M., 1982, *All That is Solid Melts into Air: the experience of modernity*, London: Verso.

Best, B. W., 2004, "Dunlop, John Boyd (1840–1921)," rev. T. I. Williams, in *Oxford Dictionary of National Biography*, Oxford: Oxford University Press.

Bijsterveld, K., 2010, "Acoustic cocooning: how the car became a place to unwind," *The Senses and Society*, 5(2), 189–211.

Bilstein, R., 2003, "The airplane and the American experience," in D. Pisano (ed.), *The Airplane in American Culture*, Ann Arbor, MI: University of Michigan Press.

Biocca, F. and Levy, M. (eds), 1995, *Communication in the Age of Virtual Reality*, Hillsdale, NJ: Lawrence Erlbaum Associates.

Bishop, C., 2004, "Antagonism and relational aesthetics," *October*, 110, 51–79.

Bishop, C., 2012, *Artificial Hells*, New York: Verso.

Blom, P., 2010, *The Vertigo Years: changes and culture in the West 1900–1914*, New York: Basic Books.

Blum, E. J. and Harvey, P., 2012, *The Color of Christ: the Son of God and the saga of race in America*, Chapel Hill, NC: University of North Carolina Press.

Boddy, T., 1992, "Underground and overhead: building the analogous city," in M. Sorkin (ed.), *Variations on a Theme Park*, New York: Hill & Wang.

Boden, M., 2006, *Mind As Machine: a history of cognitive science*, Vols. I and II, New York: Oxford University Press.

Boellstorff, T., 2008, *Coming of Age in Second Life: an anthropologist explores the virtually human*, Princeton, NJ: Princeton University Press.

Bogost, I., 2007, *Persuasive Games. The expressive power of videogames*, Cambridge, MA: MIT Press.

Borden, I., 1998, "Body architecture: skateboarding and the creation of super-architectural space," in J. Hill (ed.), *Occupying Architecture: between the architect and the user*, London: Routledge.

Borell, M., 1993, "Training the senses, training the mind," in W. F. Bynum and R. Porter (eds), *Medicine and the Five Senses*, Cambridge: Cambridge University Press.

Boring, E. G., 1942, *Sensation and Perception in the History of Experimental Psychology*, New York: Appleton-Century Company, Inc.

Bottles, S. L., 1987, *Los Angeles and the Automobile: the making of the modern city*, Berkeley, CA: University of California Press.

Bourdieu, P., [1979] 1984, *Distinction: a social critique of the judgment of taste*, Cambridge, MA: Harvard University Press.

Bourriaud, N., 2002, *Relational Aesthetics*, Dijon: Presses du Réel.

Bowlby, R., 2001, *Carried Away: the invention of modern shopping*, New York: Columbia University Press.

Bowman, M., 2012, "Profits of Zion: how money has shaped Mormon Culture," *Slate.com*, October 2, http://www.slate.com/articles/life/faithbased/,2012/10/mormon_church_money_why_the_lds_church_needs_to_save_for_the_future_.html.

Braslow, J., 1997, *Mental Ills and Bodily Cures: psychiatric treatment in the first half of the twentieth century*, Berkeley, CA: University of California Press.

Brazelton, T. B., Koslowski, B., and Main, M., 1974, "The origin of reciprocity: the early mother-infant interaction," in M. Lewis and L. Rosenblum (eds), *The Effect of the Infant on its Caretaker*, New York: Wiley.

Broad, C. D., 1923, *Scientific Thought*, London: Routledge & Kegan Paul.

Broad, C. D., 1925, *The Mind and its Place in Nature*, London: Kegan Paul.

Brown, E., 1914, *The Real Billy Sunday*, Dayton, OH: Otterbein Press.

Brown, M. and Taylor, B., 1993, *Art of the Soviets: new perspectives on post-revolutionary Soviet art*, Manchester: Manchester University Press.

Browner, C. H. and Press, N. A., 1995, "The normalization of prenatal diagnostic screening," in F. D. Ginsburg and R. Rapp (eds), *Conceiving the New World Order*, Berkeley, CA: University of California Press.

Bryant, M., 1997, *Auden and Documentary in the 1930s*, Charlottesville, VA: University of Virginia Press.

Buck-Morss, S., 1994, "The cinema screen as prosthesis of perception: a historical account," in C. N. Serematakis (ed.), *The Senses Still: perception and memory as material culture in modernity*, Boulder, CO: Westview Press.

Bull, M., 2000, *Sounding Out the City: personal stereos and the management of everyday life*, Oxford: Berg.

Bull, M., Gilroy, P., Howes, D., and Kahn, D., 2006, "Introducing sensory studies," *The Senses and Society*, 1(1), 5–7.

Bürger, P., 1984, *Theory of the Avant-Garde*, Minneapolis, MN: University of Minnesota Press.

Burton, R., 2012, "Understanding farmers' aesthetic preference for tidy agricultural landscapes: a Bourdieusian perspective'," *Landscape Research*, 37(1), 51–71.

Bynum, W. F. and Porter, R. (eds), 1993, *Medicine and the Five Senses*, Cambridge: Cambridge University Press.

Cage, J., 1961, *Silence*, Middletown, CT: Wesleyan University Press.

Calvert, G., Spence, C., and Stein, B. (eds), 2004, *The Handbook of Multisensory Processes*, Cambridge, MA: MIT Press.

Carson, R., 1962, *Silent Spring*, New York: Houghton Mifflin.

Castells, M., 2009, *Mobile Communication: a global perspective*, Cambridge: MIT Press.

Castells, M., Lee G., and Yin-Wang Kwok, L., 1990, *The Shek Kip Mei Syndrome: economic development and public housing in Hong Kong and Singapore*, London: Pion.

Certeau, M. de, 1983, "The madness of vision," *Enclitic*, 7(1).

Chakrabarty, D., 1991, "Open space/public space: garbage, modernity and India," *South Asia*, 16, 15–31.

Chamberlain, D. B., 1998, "Babies don't feel pain: a century of denial in medicine," in R. Davis-Floyd and J. Dumit (eds), *Cyborg Babies: from techno-sex to techno-tots*, New York: Routledge.

Chandola, T., 2012, "Listening into others: moralising the soundscapes in Delhi," *International Development Planning Review*, 34(4), 391–408.

Chen, N., 2003, *Breathing Spaces: Qigong, psychiatry, and healing in China*, New York: Columbia University Press.

Chomsky, N., 1959, "A review of B. F. Skinner's *Verbal Behavior*," *Language*, 35(1), 26–58.

Chomsky, N., 1967, Preface to "A review of Skinner's *Verbal Behavior*," in L. A. Jakobovits and M. S. Miron (eds), *Readings in the Psychology of Language*, New York: Prentice Hall.

Chouliaraki, L., 2006, *The Spectatorship of Suffering*, London: Sage.

Clark, C. E., 1986, *The American Family Home: 1800–1960*, Durham, NC: University of North Carolina Press.

Classen, C., 1992, "The odor of the other: olfactory symbolism and cultural categories," *Ethos*, 20(2), 134–52.

Classen, C., 1993, *Worlds of Sense: exploring the senses in history and across cultures*, London: Routledge.

Classen, C., 1997, "Foundations for an anthropology of the senses," *International Social Science Journal*, 49, 401–12.

Classen, C., 1998, *The Color of Angels: cosmology, gender and the aesthetic imagination*, London: Routledge.

Classen, C., 2001, "The senses," in P. N. Stearns (ed.), *Encyclopedia of European Social History: from 1350 to 2000*, New York: Charles Scribner's Sons.

Classen, C., 2005, "The witch's senses: sensory ideologies and transgressive femininities from the Renaissance to modernity," in D. Howes (ed.), *Empire of the Senses: the sensual culture reader*, Oxford: Berg.

Classen, C., 2012, *The Deepest Sense: a cultural history of touch*, Urbana, IL: University of Illinois Press.

Classen, C., 2013, "Green pleasures," in B. L. Ong (ed.), *Beyond Environmental Comfort*, Oxford: Routledge

Classen, C., Howes, D., and Synnott, A., 1994, *Aroma: the cultural history of smell*, London and New York: Routledge.

Claude, A., 1935, Electric Gaseous Discharge Device, US Patent Office.

Cloke, P., 2006, "Rurality and racialised others: out of place in the countryside?" in P. Cloke, T. Marsden, and P. Mooney (eds), *Handbook of Rural Studies*, London: Sage.

Cloke, P. and Perkins, P., 1998, "'Cracking the canyon with the awesome foursome': representations of adventure tourism in New Zealand," *Environment and Planning D: Society and Space*, 16, 185–218.

Cohen, E. and Avieli, N., 2004, "Food in tourism: attraction and impediment," *Annals of Tourism Research*, 31(4), 755–78.

Cohen, L., 1996, "From town center to shopping center: the reconfiguration of community marketplaces in postwar America," *American Historical Review*, 101(4), 1050–81.

Cohen, L., 2003, *A Consumers' Republic: the politics of mass consumption in postwar America*, New York: Vintage.

Cohen, S. and Taylor, L. 1992. *Escape Attempts*, London: Routledge.

Collins, J. and Jervis, J., 2008, "Introduction," in J. Collins and J. Jervis (eds), *Uncanny Modernity: cultural theories, modern anxieties*, Basingstoke: Palgrave.

Connor, S., 2000, *Dumbstruck. A cultural history of ventriloquism*, Oxford: Oxford University Press.

Conrad, P., 1975, "The discovery of hyperkinesis: notes on the medicalization of deviant behavior," *Social Problems*, 23(1), 12–21.

Corbin, A., [1982] 1986, *The Foul and the Fragrant: odor and the French social imagination*, trans. M. L. Kochan, R. Porter, and C. Prendergast, Cambridge, MA: Harvard University Press.

Corbin, A., 1990, "Histoire et anthropologie sensorielle," *Anthropologie et Sociétés*, 20(2).

Corbin, A., [1994] 1998, *Village Bells: sound and meaning in the 19th-century French countryside*, New York: Columbia University Press.

Corbin, A., 2005, "Charting the cultural history of the senses," in D. Howes (ed.), *Empire of the Senses: the sensual culture reader*, Oxford: Berg.

Corbin, A., and Heuré, G., 2000, *Alain Corbin: historien du sensible. Entretiens avec Gilles Heuré*, Paris: Editions la Découverte.

Corn, J. J., 1983, *The Winged Gospel: America's romance with aviation*, Oxford: Oxford University Press.

Crane, T., 1992, *The Contents of Experience: essays on perception*, Cambridge: Cambridge University Press.

Crary, J., 1999, *Suspension of Perception: attention, spectacle, and modern culture*, Cambridge, MA: MIT Press.

Crary, J., 2013, *24/7, Late Capitalism and the End of Sleep*, London: Verso.

Creadick, A. G., 2010, *Perfectly Average: the pursuit of normality in postwar America*, Amherst, MA: University of Massachusetts Press.

Crowley, D. and Reid, S., 2002, *Socialist Spaces: sites of everyday life in the Eastern Bloc*, London: Berg.

Crowney, M., 2000, "The nose of India. The representation of the nose in *Midnight's Children*," in V. de Rijke *et al.* (eds), *Nose Book: representations of the nose in literature and the arts*, London: Middlesex University Press.

Csordas, T., 1993, "Somatic modes of attention," *Cultural Anthropology*, 8(2), 135–56.

Cummins, R., 1983, *The Nature of Psychological Explanation*, Cambridge, MA: MIT Press.

Danius, S., 2002, *The Senses of Modernism: technology, perception and aesthetics*, Ithaca, NY: Cornell University Press.

Darwent, C., 2013, "How truth and fiction become blurred," *The Independent on Sunday*, August 25.

Davies, H., 1994, "The sound world: instruments and music of Luigi Russolo," *Resonance Magazine*, 2(2), http://www.resonancemag.com/.

De Grazia, V., 2005, *Irresistible Empire: America's advance through twentieth-century Europe*, Cambridge, MA: Harvard University Press.

de la Peña, C., 2010, *Empty Pleasures: the story of artificial sweeteners from saccharin to Splenda*, Charlotte, NC: University of North Carolina Press.

Deaville, J., 2011, *Music in Television. Channels of listening*, London: Routledge.

Degen, M. 2008. *Sensing Cities: regenerating public life in Barcelona and Manchester*, London: Routledge.

Degen, M., Desilvey, C. and Rose, G., 2008, "Experiencing visualities in designed urban environments: learning from Milton Keynes," *Environment and Planning A*, 40, 1901–20.

DeGrandpre, R., 1999, *Ritalin Nation: rapid-fire culture and the transformation of human consciousness*, New York: W. W. Norton & Co, Inc.

Der Derian, J., 2009, *Virtuous War: mapping the military-industrial media-entertainment network*, London: Routledge.

Derrida, J., 1975, "The purveyor of truth," trans. W. Domingo *et al.*, *Yale French Studies*, 52, 31–113.

DeSilvey, C., 2006, "Observed decay: telling stories with mutable things," *Journal of Material Culture*, 11(3), 317–37.

Deutsch, C. H., 1992, "Luring crowds—and buyers—with fun and games," *New York Times*, September 27.

Deutsch, T., 2002, "Untangling alliances: social tensions surrounding independent grocery stores and the rise of modern retailing," in W. Belasco and P. Scranton (eds), *Food Nations: Selling Taste in Consumer Societies*, New York: Routledge.

Deutsch, T., 2010, *Building a Housewife's Paradise: gender, politics, and American grocery stores in the twentieth century*, Chapel Hill, NC: University of North Carolina Press.

Douglas, G. H., 1996, *Skyscrapers: a social history of the very tall building in America*, Jefferson, NC: McFarland & Company.

Douglas, M., 2002, *Purity and Danger*, London: Routledge.

Drobnick, J., 2002, "Toposmia: art, scent and interrogations of spatiality," *Angelaki*, 7(1), 31–46.

Drobnick, J., 2005, "Volatile effects: olfactory dimensions of art and architecture," in D. Howes (ed.), *Empire of the Senses: the sensual culture reader*, Oxford: Berg.

Dummett, D., 1993, *The Origins of Analytical Philosophy*, London: Duckworth.

Dyer, S., 2002, "Markets in the meadows: department stores and shopping centers in the decentralization of Philadelphia, 1920–1980," *Enterprise & Society*, 3, 606–12.

Dyson, F., 2009, *Sounding New Media: immersion and embodiment in arts and culture*, Berkeley, CA: University of California Press.

Edensor, T., 1998, *Tourists at the Taj*, London: Routledge.

Edensor, T., 2000a, "Moving through the city," in D. Bell and A. Haddour (eds), *City Visions*, London: Prentice Hall.

Edensor, T., 2000b, "Walking in the British countryside," *Body and Society*, 6(3–4), 81–106.

Edensor, T., 2001, "Performing tourism, staging tourism: (re)producing tourist space and practice," *Tourist Studies*, 1, 59–82.

Edensor, T., 2005, 'The ghosts of industrial ruins: ordering and disordering memory in excessive space," *Environment and Planning D: Society and Space*, 23(6), 829–49.

Edensor, T., 2006, "Sensing tourism," in C. Minca and T. Oakes (eds), *Travels in Paradox*, London: Rowman & Littlefield.

Edensor, T., 2007, "Sensing the ruin," *The Senses and Society*, 2(2), 217–32.

Edensor, T., 2012, "Illuminated atmospheres: anticipating and reproducing the flow of affective experience in Blackpool," in *Environment and Planning D: Society and Space*, 30, 1103–22.

Edensor, T., 2013, "The gloomy city: rethinking the relation between light and dark," special issue on "Geographies of Urban Nights," *Urban Studies*.

Edensor, T. and Falconer, E., 2011, "The sensuous geographies of tourism," in J. Wilson (ed.), *New Perspectives in Tourism Geographies*, London: Routledge.

Edensor, T. and Millington, S., 2009, "Illuminations, class identities and the contested landscapes of Christmas," *Sociology*, 43(1), 103–21.

Eisner, L., 1977, *Fritz Lang*, Oxford: Oxford University Press.

Euchner, C., 2010, *Nobody Turn Me Around: a people's history of the 1963 march on Washington*, Boston, MA: Beacon Press.

Ewen, S., 1988, *All-Consuming Images: the politics of style in contemporary culture*, Boston, MA: Basic Books.

Featherstone, M., 1991, *Consumer Culture and Postmodernism*, London: Sage.

Febvre, L., [1942] 1982, *The Problem of Unbelief in the Sixteenth Century: the religion of Rabelais*, trans. B. Gottlieb, Cambridge, MA: Harvard University Press.

Feldman, A., 1994, "From Desert Storm to Rodney King via ex-Yugoslavia: on cultural anaesthesia," in C. N. Serematakis (ed.), *The Senses Still: perception and memory as material culture in modernity*, Boulder, CO: Westview Press.

Finch, M. L., 2010, "Food, taste, and American religions," *Religion Compass*, 4(1), 39–50.

Firth, R. 1965, "Sense-data and the percept theory," in R. Swartz (ed.), *Perceiving, Sensing and Knowing*, Berkeley, CA: University of California Press.

Flexner, J. (ed.), 1933, *City Noise II* [manuscript], Department of Health, Administration/ Subject Files, Box: 1933, "Mi–N" (07-025962), folder: "Noise," New York City Municipal Archives.

Foucault, M., [1963] 1973, *The Birth of the Clinic: an archaeology of medical perception*, trans. A. M. Sheridan Smith, New York: Random House.

Foucault, M., [1975] 1979, *Discipline and Punish: the birth of the prison*, trans. A. Sheridan, New York: Vintage Books.

Foucault, M., 1980, *Power/Knowledge: selected interviews and other writings, 1972– 1977*, New York: Knopf/Doubleday Publishing Group.

Foxell, S., 2011, *Mapping London: making sense of the city*, London: Black Dog Publishing Limited.

Francis, A., 2010, *Finest Hour*, Episode 4, "The Excitement of the Dogfights," BBC, http://www.bbc.co.uk/programmes/p0095vpp.

Franklin, A., 2003, *Tourism: an introduction*, London: Sage.

Freud, S., 2002, *Civilization and Its Discontents*, trans. D. McLintock, London: Penguin.

Friedan, B., 1963, *The Feminine Mystique*, New York: Norton.

Friedersdorf, C., 2012, "Every person is afraid of the drones: the strikes' effect on life in Pakistan," *The Atlantic* (September).

Friend, D., 2007, *Watching the World Change: the stories behind the images of 9/11*, London: I. B. Tauris.

Frykman, J., 1994, "On the move: the struggle for the body in Sweden in the 1930s," in C. N. Seremetakis (ed.), *The Senses Still: perception and memory as material culture in modernity*, Boulder, CO: Westview Press.

García, H., Sierra, A., and Balám, B., 1999, *Wind in the Blood: Mayan healing and Chinese medicine*, trans. J. Conant, Berkeley, CA: North Atlantic Books.

Gardner, H., 1983, *Frames of Mind: the theory of multiple intelligences*, New York: Basic Books.

Garrett, B., 2011, "Assaying history: creating temporal junctions through urban exploration," *Environment and Planning D: Society and Space*, 29(6), 1048–67.

Gartman, D., 2012, *From Autos to Architecture: Fordism and architectural aesthetics in the twentieth century*, San Francisco, CA: Chronicle Books.

Gassner, G., 2010, "Skylines and the whole city," in S. Hall, M. Fernandez, and C. Dinardi (eds), *Writing Cities*, London: London School of Economics.

Ginsberg, A., 1959, *Howl, and Other Poems*, San Francisco: City Lights Books.

Giordano, R. G., 2008, *Satan in the Dance Hall: Rev. John Roach Straton, social dancing, and morality in 1920s New York City*, New York: Scarecrow Press.

Giucci, G., 2012, *The Cultural Life of the Automobile: roads to modernity*, trans. A. Mayagoitia and D. Nagao, Austin, TX: University of Texas Press.

Goatcher, J. and Brunsden, V., 2011, "Chernobyl and the sublime tourist," *Tourist Studies*, 11(2), 115–38.

Goggin, G., 2011, *Global Mobile Media*, London: Routledge.

Good, B. J., 1994, *Medicine, Rationality, and Experience: an anthropological perspective*, Cambridge: Cambridge University Press.

Good, M. D., 1995, *American Medicine: the quest for competence*, Berkeley, CA: University of California Press.

Goodman, S., 2010, *Sonic Warfare: sound, affect, and the ecology of fear*, Cambridge, MA: MIT Press.

Gordon, M., 1994, "Songs from the museum of the future: Russian Sound Creation 1910–1930," in D. Kahn and G. Whitehead (eds), *Wireless Imagination: sound, radio and the avant-garde*, Cambridge, MA: MIT Press.

Gottdiener, M., 1997, *The Theming of America*, Oxford: Westview Press.

Graham, S., 2006, "Cities and the 'War on Terror'," *International Journal of Urban and Regional Research*, 30(2), 255–76.

Green, C. S. and Bavelier, D., 2007, "Action-video-game experience alters the spatial resolution of vision," *Psychological Science*, 18, 88–94.

Greenberg, C., 1940, "Towards a newer Laocoon," *Partisan Review*, VII(4), 296–310.

Griffin, J. H., 2004, *Black Like Me*, San Antonio, TX: Wings Press.

Guilbaut, S., 1983, *How New York Stole the Idea of Modern Art*, trans. A. Goldhammer, Chicago, IL: University of Chicago Press.

Hall, S. and Back, L., 2009, "At home and not at home: Stuart Hall in conversation with Les Back," *Cultural Studies*, 23(4), 658–87.

Hall, S. *et al.*, 1978, *Policing the Crisis: mugging, the state and law and order*, London: Palgrave Macmillan.

Hammarén, N., 2010, "See you in the suburbs if you dare," in H. Holgersson, C. Thörn, and M. Wahlström (eds), *(Re)searching Gothenberg: essays on a changing city*, Gothenberg: Glänta.

Hangen, T. J., 2002, *Redeeming the Dial: Radio, Religion, & Popular Culture in America*, Chapel Hill, NC: University of North Carolina Press.

Hansen, M., 2012, *Cinema and Experience: Siegfried Kracauer, Walter Benjamin, and Theodor W. Adorno*, Berkeley, CA: University of California Press.

Hardey, M., 2002, "Health for sale: quackery, consumerism, and the internet," in W. Ernst (ed.), *Plural Medicine, Tradition and Modernity, 1800–2000*, New York: Routledge.

Harman, G., 1990, "The intrinsic quality of experience," in J. Tomberlin (ed.), *Philosophical Perspectives*, Atascadero: Ridgeview.

Harraway, D., 1989, *Primate Visions: gender, race and nature in the world of modern science*, London: Routledge.

Harris, A. L., 1997, "'Bare things': returning to the senses in Virginia Woolf's *The Waves*," *LIT*, 7, 339–50.

Hausmann, R., [1971] 1994, "Am Anfang war Dada," in D. Kahn and G. Whitehead (eds), *Wireless Imagination: sound, radio and the avant-garde*, Cambridge, MA: MIT Press.

Heidegger, M., 1972, *Poetry, Language, Thought*, London: Joanna Coter Books.

Hein, L. and Selden, M., 1997, "Commemoration and silence: fifty years of remembering the bomb in America and Japan," in L. Hein and M. Selden (eds), *Living With the Bomb: American and Japanese cultural conflicts in the nuclear age*, New York: East Gate.

Heitmann, J., 2009, *The Automobile and American Life*, Jefferson, NC: McFarland & Company.

Herberg, W., [1955] 1983, *Protestant Catholic Jew: an essay in American religious sociology*, Chicago: University of Chicago Press.

Hertel, R., 2005, *Making Sense: sense perception in the British novel of the 1980s and 1990s*, Amsterdam: Rodopi.

Heyer, P., 2005, *The Medium and the Magician. Orson Welles, the radio years, 1934–1952*, Oxford: Rowman & Littlefield.

Higgins, D., 1966, "Intermedia," *Something Else Newsletter*, 1(1).

Hill, G., 1955. "A world Walt Disney created," *New York Times*, July 31.

Hill, G., 1958, "Disneyland reports on its first ten million," *New York Times*, February 2.

Hill, G., 1959, "The Never-Never Land Khrushchev never saw," *New York Times*, October 4.

Hill-Smith, C., 2011, "Cyberpilgrimage: the (virtual) reality of online pilgrimage experience," *Religion Compass*, 5(6), 236–46.

Hirsch, J., 2000, "It's the most profitable unit after all," *Los Angeles Times*, July 22.

Hkaprow, A., 1983, *Essays on the Blurring of Art and Life*. Berkeley, CA: University of California Press.

Horkheimer, M. and Adorno, T., 1973, *The Dialectic of Enlightenment*, London: Penguin.

Horkheimer, M. and Adorno, T., 2002, *Dialectic of Enlightenment: philosophical fragments*, ed. G. Schmid Noerr, trans. E. Jephcott, Stanford, CA: Stanford University Press.

Howell, J. D., 1995, *Technology in the Hospital: transforming patient care in the early twentieth century*, Baltimore, MD: Johns Hopkins University Press.

Howes, D. (ed.), 1991, *The Varieties of Sensory Experience*, Toronto: University of Toronto Press.

Howes, D., 2003, *Sensual Relations: engaging the senses in culture and social theory*, Ann Arbor, MI: University of Michigan Press.

Howes, D., 2005a, "Skinscapes: embodiment, culture and environment," in C. Classen (ed.), *The Book of Touch*, Oxford: Berg.

Howes, D., 2005b, "Hyperesthesia, or, the sensual logic of late capitalism," in D. Howes (ed.), *Empire of the Senses: the sensual culture reader*, Oxford: Berg.

Howes, D. (ed.), 2009, *The Sixth Sense Reader*, Oxford: Berg.

Howes, D., 2010, "Oh bungalow," in G. Borasi (ed.), *Journeys: how travelling fruit, ideas and buildings rearrange our environment*, Montreal and Barcelona: Canadian Centre for Architecture in association with Actar.

Howes, D. and Classen, C., 2014, *Ways of Sensing: understanding the senses in society*, Oxford and New York: Routledge.

Hubbard, R., 1990, *The Politics of Women's Biology*, New Brunswick, NJ: Rutgers University Press.

Hubel, D. and Wiesel, T. N., 2004, *Brain and Visual Perception: the story of a 25-year collaboration*, New York: Oxford University Press.

Huxley, A., [1932] 2007, *Brave New World*, London: Vintage Classics.

Huxley, A., 1954, *The Doors of Perception*, London: Chatto & Windus.

Ingrassia, P. and White, J. B., 1994, *Comeback: the fall and rise of the American automobile industry*, New York: Touchstone.

Isherwood, C., 1986, *Goodbye to Berlin*, London: Triad/Panther Books.

Iwamura, J. N., 2011, *Virtual Orientalism: Asian religions and American popular culture*, New York: Oxford University Press.

Jackson, F., 1977, *Perception: a representative theory*, Cambridge: Cambridge University Press.

Jackson, K. T., 1985, *Crabgrass Frontier: the suburbanization of the United States*, Oxford: Oxford University Press.

Jacobs, J., 1989, *The Death and Life of Great American Cities*, New York: Vintage Books.

Jacobs, J., 1996, *Edge of Empire: postcolonialism and the city*, London and New York: Routledge.

Jakle, J., 2001, *City Lights: illuminating the American night*, Baltimore, MD: Johns Hopkins University Press

James, H., 1972, *Theory of Fiction*, ed. J. E. Miller, Jr, Lincoln, NE: University of Nebraska Press.

Jankowiak, W. and Bradburd, D. (eds), 2003, *Drugs, Labor, and Colonial Expansion*, Tucson, AZ: University of Arizona Press.

Jay, M., 1993, *Downcast Eyes: the denigration of vision in contemporary French thought*, Berkeley, CA: University of California Press.

Jay, M., 2006, *Songs of Experience: modern American and European variations on a universal theme*, Berkeley, CA: University of California Press.

Jordan, F. and Aitchison, C., 2008, "Tourism and the sexualisation of the gaze: solo female tourists' experiences of gendered power, surveillance and embodiment," *Leisure Studies*, 27(3), 329–49.

Jorgensen, A. and Keenan, R., 2011, *Urban Wildscapes*, London: Routledge.

Joyce, K. A., 2008, *Magnetic Appeal: MRI and the myth of transparency*, Ithaca, NY: Cornell University Press.

Jütte, R., 2005, *A History of the Senses: from antiquity to cyberspace*, Cambridge: Polity Press.

Kabat-Zinn, J., 1990, *Full Catastrophe Living: using the wisdom of your body and mind to face stress, pain, and illness*, New York: Delta.

Kaier, C., 2005, "Was socialist realism forced labor? The case of Aleksandr Deineka in the 1930s," *The Oxford Art Journal*, 28(3), 321–45.

Kalekin-Fishman, D. and Low, K. (eds), 2010, *Everyday Life in Asia: social perspectives on the senses*, Farnham: Ashgate.

Kamper, D. and Wulf, C. (eds), 1982, *Die Wiederkehr des Körpers*, Frankfurt a. M.: Suhrkamp.

Kamper, D. and Wulf, C. (eds), 1984a, *Das Schwinden der Sinne*, Frankfurt a. M.: Suhrkamp.

Kamper, D. and Wulf, C., 1984b, "Blickwende. Die Sinne des Körpers im Konkurs der Geschichte," in D. Kamper and C. Wulf (eds.), *Das Schwinden der Sinne*, Frankfurt a. M.: Suhrkamp.

Kaplan, M., 1948, "Living in two civilizations calls for a redefinition of religion," in *The Future of the American Jew*, New York: Macmillan.

Karasov, D. and Martin, J. A., 1993, "The mall of them all," *Design Quarterly*, 159, 18–27.

Kasson, J., 1978, *Amusing the Million: Coney Island at the turn of the century*, New York: Hill & Wang.

Keats, J., 1957, *The Crack in the Picture Window*, Boston, MA: Houghton Mifflin.

Keeley, B., 2013, "The role of neurobiology in differentiating the senses," in J. Bickle (ed.), *Oxford Handbook of Philosophy and Neuroscience*, Oxford: Oxford University Press, pp. 226–50.

Keith, M., 2005, *After the Cosmopolitan? Multicultural cities and the future of racism*, London: Routledge.

Kellner, D., 1999, "Virilio, war, and technology: some critical reflections," *Theory, Culture and Society*, 16(5–6), 103–5.

Kenzari, B., 2011, *Architecture and Violence*, Barcelona: ACTAR Publishers.

Kerr, C., 2002, "Translating 'Mind-in-Body': two models of patient experience underlying a randomized controlled trial of Qigong," *Culture, Medicine and Psychiatry*, 26, 419–47.

Kihlstedt, F. T., 1983, "The automobile and the transformation of the American house," in D. Lanier Lewis and L. Goldstein (eds), *The Automobile and American Culture*, Ann Arbor, MI: University of Michigan Press.

Kilde, J. H., 2006, "Reading megachurches: investigating the religious and cultural work of church architecture," in L. P. Nelson (ed.), *American Sanctuary: understanding sacred space*, Bloomington, IN: Indiana University Press.

King, A. D., 1984, *The Bungalow: the production of a global culture*, London: Routledge & Kegan Paul.

Kirsner, S., 1998, "Hack the magic," *Wired* (March).

Kittler, F., 1999, *Gramophone, Film, Typewriter*, Stanford, CA: Stanford University Press.

Klassen, P. E., 2001, *Blessed Events: religion and home birth in America*, Princeton, NJ: Princeton University Press.

Kohrman, M. and Benson, P., 2011, "Tobacco," *Annual Review of Anthropology*, 40, 329–44.

Korsmeyer, C., 1999, *Making Sense of Taste: food and philosophy*, Ithaca, NY: Cornell University Press.

Koslofsky, C., 2011, *Evening's Empire: a history of the night in Early Modern Europe*, Cambridge: Cambridge University Press.

Kracauer, S., 1995, *The Mass Ornament: Weimar essays*, Cambridge, MA: Harvard University Press.

Kramer, M. J., 2013, *The Republic of Rock: music and citizenship in the sixties counterculture*, Oxford: Oxford University Press.

Krieger, D., 1979, *The Therapeutic Touch: how to use your hands to help or to heal*, Englewood Cliffs, NJ: Prentice Hall.

Kyvig, D. E., 2004, *Daily Life in the United States, 1920–1940*, Chicago: Ivan R. Dee.

Laderman, C. and Roseman, M. (eds), 1996, *The Performance of Healing*, New York: Routledge.

Lahiri, S., 2011, "Remembering the city: translocality and the senses," *Social and Cultural Geography*, 12(8), 855–69.

Lappé, F. M., 1971, *Diet for a Small Planet*, New York: Ballantine.

Lash, S., 1999, *Another Modernity: a different rationality*, Oxford: Blackwell.

Lawler, S., 1999, "'Getting out and getting away': women's narratives of class mobility," *Feminist Review*, 63, 3–24.

Layton, D., 1988, *Seductive Poison. A Jonestown survivor's story of life and death in the Peoples Temple*, New York: Random House.

Le Corbusier, 1933, *The Radiant City*, New York: The Orion Press.

Le Corbusier, 2008, *Toward an Architecture*, London: Frances Lincoln Ltd.

Leach, W., 1993, *Land of Desire: merchants, power, and the rise of a new American culture*, New York: Vintage Books.

Lella, J. W. and Pawluch, D., 1988, "Medical students and the cadaver in social and cultural context," in M. Lock and D. Gordon (eds), *Biomedicine Examined*, Norwell, MA: Kluwer Academic Publishers.

Leslie, C. and Young, A. (eds), 1992, *Paths to Asian Medical Knowledge*, Berkeley, CA: University of California Press.

Levin, D. M., 1993, *Modernity and the Hegemony of Vision*, Berkeley, CA: University of California Press.

Levy, M., 2002, *Why Buildings Fall Down: how structures fail*, London: W. W. Norton & Company.

Lichtenstein, N., 2009, *The Retail Revolution: how Wal-Mart created a brave new world of business*, New York: Metropolitan Books.

Lindqvist, S., 2001, *A History of Bombing*, London: The New Press.

Little, K., 1991, "On safari: the visual politics of a tourist representation," in D. Howes (ed.) *The Varieties of Sensory Experience*, Toronto: University of Toronto Press.

Lock, M., 1995, *Encounters with Aging: mythologies of menopause in Japan and North America*, Berkeley, CA: University of California Press.

Lock, M. and Gordon, D. (eds), 1988, *Biomedicine Examined*, Norwell, MA: Kluwer Academic Publishers.

Lofton, K. E., 2006, "The preacher paradigm: promotional biographies and the modern-made evangelist," *Religion and American Culture*, 16(1), 95–123.

Longstreth, R., 1997, *City Center to Regional Mall: architecture, the automobile, and retailing in Los Angeles, 1920–1950*, Cambridge, MA: MIT Press.

Longstreth, R., 2010, *The American Department Store Transformed*, New Haven, CT: Yale University Press.

Loos, A., 2006, *Ornament and Crime*, Riverside, CA: Ariadne Press.

Loviglio, J., 2005, *Radio's Intimate Public. Network broadcasting and mass mediated democracy*, Minneapolis, MN: University of Minnesota Press.

Lund, K., 2005, "Seeing in motion and the touching eye: walking over Scotland's mountains," *Etnofoor*, 181, 27–42.

Lyon, D., 2007, *Surveillance Studies: An Overview*, Cambridge: Polity Press.

MacCannell, D., 1976, *The Tourist*, London: Macmillan.

Mack, A., 2010, "'Speaking of tomatoes': supermarkets, the senses, and sexual fantasy in modern America," *Journal of Social History*, 43, 815–42.

Macnaghten, P. and Urry, J., 1998, *Contested Natures*, London: Sage.

Macnaughton, J., 2009, "Flesh revealed: medicine, art and anatomy," in C. Saunders, U. Maude, and J. Macnaughton (eds), *The Body and the Arts*, New York: Palgrave Macmillan.

Macpherson, F. (ed.), 2011, *The Senses: classic and contemporary philosophical perspectives*, Oxford: Oxford University Press.

Maines, D. R., 1977, "Tactile relationships in the subway as affected by racial, sexual, and crowded seating situations," *Journal of Nonverbal Behavior*, 2(2), 100–8.

Mall of America, 2012, *The Place for Fun: Media Info*, http://www.mallofamerica.com/content/doc/2011_MediaInfo_LoRes.pdf.

Malnig, J., 2009, *Ballroom, Boogie, Shimmy Sham, Shake: a social and popular dance reader*, Chicago, IL: University of Illinois Press.

Manalansan, M., 2006, "Immigrant lives and the politics of olfaction in the global city," in J. Drobnick (ed.), *The Smell Culture Reader*, London: Berg.

Maoz, D., 2006, "The mutual gaze," *Annals of Tourism Research*, 33(1), 221–39.

Marinetti, F. T., [1909] 1972, *Marinetti: selected writings*, ed. R.W. Flint and A. Coppotelli, London: Secker & Warburg.

Marinetti, F. T., [1919] 2002, *Selected Poems and Related Prose*, New Haven, CT: Yale University Press.

Marinetti, F. T., 1991, *The Futurist Cookbook*, San Francisco, CA: Chronicle Books.

Marinetti, F. T., 2006, *Critical Writings: new edition*, ed. G. Berghaus, New York: Farrar, Straus & Giroux.

Marr, D., 1982, *Vision*, New York: W. H. Freeman & Co. Ltd.

Marsden, G. M., 2006, *Fundamentalism and American Culture*, 2nd edn, New York: Oxford University Press.

Martin, E., 1987, *The Woman in the Body: a cultural analysis of reproduction*, Boston, MA: Beacon Press.

Martin, L. and Seagrave, K., 1988, *Anti-rock: the opposition to rock 'n' roll*, Hamden, CT: Archon Books.

Marx, K., [1844] 1987, *Economic and Philosophic Manuscripts of 1844*, trans. M. Milligan, Buffalo, NY: Prometheus Books.

Masco, J., 2010, "Atomic health, or how the bomb altered American notions of death," in J. M. Metzl and A. Kirkland (eds), *Against Health: how health became the new morality*, New York: New York University Press.

Massumi, B., 2002, *Parables for the Virtual: movement, affect, sensation*, Durham, NC: Duke University Press.

Maude, U., 2009, *Beckett, Technology and the Body*, Cambridge: Cambridge University Press.

Mauss, M., [1934] 1979, "Techniques of the body," in *Sociology and Psychology Essays*, trans. B. Brewster, London: Routledge & Kegan Paul.

May, E. T., 2008, *Homeward Bound: American families in the Cold War era*, 20th anniversary edn, New York: Basic Books.

McClelland, J. *et al.*, 1986, *Parallel Distributed Processing*, Vol. II, Cambridge, MA: MIT Press.

McClymond, K., 2006, "You are where you eat: negotiating Hindu utopias in Atlanta," in E. M. Madden and M. L. Finch (eds), *Eating in Eden: food & American utopias*, Lincoln, NE: University of Nebraska Press.

McKibbin, R., 1998, *Classes and Cultures: England 1918–1951*, Oxford: Oxford University Press.

McLuhan, M., 1962, *The Gutenburg Galaxy*, Toronto: University of Toronto Press.

McLuhan, M., 1964, *Understanding Media*, New York: New American Library.

McLuhan, M., 1967, *The Medium is the Message*, New York: Bantam Books.

McQuire, S., 2008, *The Media City: media, architecture and urban spaces*, London: Sage.

Meikle, J. L., 1995, *American Plastic: a cultural history*, New Brunswick. NJ: Rutgers University Press.

Mentor, S., 1998, "Witches, nurses, midwives, and cyborgs: IVF, ART and complex agency in the world of technobirth," in R. Davis-Floyd and J. Dumit (eds), *Cyborg Babies: from techno-sex to techno-tots*, New York: Routledge.

Merchant, S., 2011, "Negotiating underwater space: the sensorium, the body and the practice of scuba-diving," *Tourist Studies*, 11(3), 215–34.

Merleau-Ponty, M., 1992, *Phenomenology of Perception*, trans. C. Smith, London: Routledge.

Meyer, B., 2009, "Introduction: from imagined communities to aesthetic formations: religious mediations, sensational forms, and styles of binding," in B. Meyer (ed.), *Aesthetic Formations: media, religion, and the senses*, New York: Palgrave Macmillan.

Meyrowitz, J., 1985, *No Sense of Place: the impact of electronic media on social behaviour*, Oxford: Oxford University Press.

Mintz, S., 1985, *Sweetness and Power: the place of sugar in modern history*, New York: Penguin.

Mitchell, D., 1995, "The end of public space?: People's Park, definitions of the public, and democracy," *Annals of the Association of American Geographers*, 85, 108–33.

Mitchell, L. M. and Georges, E., 1998, "Baby's first picture: the cyborg fetus of ultrasound imaging," in R. Davis-Floyd and J. Dumit (eds), *Cyborg Babies: from techno-sex to techno-tots*, New York: Routledge.

Mitchell, W. J. T., 1986, *Iconology: image, text, ideology*, Chicago, IL: University of Chicago Press.

Montagu, A., [1971] 1986, *Touching: the human significance of the skin*, New York: Harper & Row.

Moore, G. E., 1922, "Some judgments of perception," in *Philosophical Studies*, London: Routledge & Kegan Paul.

Moore, G. E., 1959, "Visual sense-data," in C. Mace (ed.), *British Philosophy in Mid-Century*, London: George Allen & Unwin.

Moreton, B., 2009, *To Serve God and Wal-Mart: the making of Christian free enterprise*, Cambridge, MA: Harvard University Press.

Morgan, D. (ed.), 1996, *Icons of American Protestantism: the art of Warner Sallman*, New Haven, CT: Yale University Press.

Morgan, D., 2007, *The Lure of Images: a history of religion and visual media in America*, New York: Routledge.

Morley, D., 2000, *Home Territories: media, mobility and identity*, London: Routledge.

Morse, M., 1998, *Virtualities: television, media art, and cyberculture*, Bloomington, IN: Indiana University Press.

Mould, O., 2009, "Parkout, the city, the event," *Environment and Planning D: Society and Space*, 27(4), 738–50.

Mumford, L., 2010, *Technics and Civilization*, Chicago: University of Chicago Press.

Murphy, D. M., 2005, *WW2 People's War—A Cockney in the Blitz*, BBC, July 29, http://www.bbc.co.uk/history/ww2peopleswar/stories/23/a4611223.shtml.

Nasaw, D., 1999, *Going Out: the rise and fall of public amusements*, Boston, MA: Harvard University Press.

Ndalianis, A., 2012, *The Horror Sensorium: media and the senses*, Jefferson, NC: McFarland & Company.

Neal, S. and Walters, S., 2007, "'You can get away with loads because there's no one here': discourses of regulation and non-regulation in English rural spaces," *Geoforum*, 38(2), 252–63.

Norman, L. G., 1962, *Road Traffic Accidents, Epidemeology, Control and Prevention*, Geneva: World Health Organisation.

Obrador-Pons, P., 2007, "A haptic geography of the beach: naked bodies, vision and touch," *Social and Cultural Geography*, 8(1), 123–41.

Ogbar, J. O. G., 2004, *Black Power: radical politics and African American identity*, Baltimore, MD: The Johns Hopkins University Press.

Ong, W. J., 1967, *The Presence of the Word*, New Haven, CT: Yale University Press.

Ong, W. J., 1982, *Orality and Literacy: the technologization of the word*, New York: Methuen.

Orwell, G., 1958, *The Road to Wigan Pier*, New York: Houghton Mifflin Harcourt.

Otter, C., 2008, *The Victorian Eye: a political history of light and vision in Britain, 1800–1910*, Chicago: University of Chicago Press.

Pallasmaa, J., 2005, *The Eyes of the Skin: architecture and the senses*, London: John Wiley & Sons.

Palmer, B., 2000, *Cultures of Darkness: night travels in the histories of transgression (from medieval to modern)*, New York: Monthly Review Press.

Palmer, D. A., 2007, *Qigong Fever: body, science and utopia in China*, New York: Columbia University Press.

Palmer, S. E., 1999, *Vision Science: photons to phenomenology*, Cambridge, MA: MIT Press.

Paris, M., 1992, *Winged Warfare: the literature and theory of aerial warfare in Britain, 1859–1917*, Manchester: Manchester University Press.

Parr, J., 2010, *Sensing Changes: technologies, environments, and the everyday, 1953–2003*, Vancouver: University of British Columbia Press.

Paterson, M., 2009, "Haptic geographies: ethnography, haptic knowledges and sensuous dispositions," *Progress in Human Geography*, 33(6), 766–88.

Paterson, M., 2005, "Digital touch," in C. Classen (ed.), *The Book of Touch*, Oxford: Berg.

Peacocke, C., 1983, *Sense and Content*, Oxford: Oxford University Press.

Pells, R., 2011, *Modernist America: art, music, movies, and the globalization of American culture*, New Haven, CT: Yale University Press.

Peters, J. D., 1999, *Speaking to the Air: a history of communication*, Chicago, IL: University of Chicago Press.

Pine, J. B. II and Gilmore, J. H., 2011, *The Experience Economy*, Boston, MA: Harvard Business Review Press.

Pink, S., 2007, "Sensing Cittàslow: slow living and the constitution of the sensory city," *The Senses and Society*, 2(1), 59–78.

Pink, S., 2009, *Doing Sensory Ethnography*, London: Sage

Plate, S. B., 2008, *Religion and Film: cinema and the re-creation of the world*, New York: Wallflower.

Poggi, C., 2008, *Inventing Futurism: the art and politics of artificial optimism*, Princeton, NJ: Princeton University Press.

Postman, N., 1985, *Amusing Ourselves to Death: public discourse in the age of show business*, New York: Penguin.

Potter, E., 2006, *Feminism and the Philosophy of Science*, London: Routledge.

Price, H. H., 1932, *Perception*, London: Methuen.

Price, S. and Price, L., 1999, *Aromatherapy for Health Professionals*, 2nd edn, London: Churchill Livingstone.

Promey, S. M., 2006, "Taste cultures: the visual practice of liberal Protestantism, 1940–1965," in L. F. Maffly-Kipp, L. E. Schmidt, and M. Valeri (eds), *Practicing Protestants: histories of Christian life in America, 1630–1965*, Baltimore, MD: Johns Hopkins University Press.

Promey, S. M. and Brisman, S., 2010, "Sensory cultures: material and visual religion reconsidered," in P. Goff (ed.), *The Blackwell Companion to Religion in America*, Malden, MA: Wiley-Blackwell.

Proust, M., 1984, *Marcel Proust on Art and Literature*, New York: Carroll & Graf.

Rabinovitz, L., 2012, *Electric Dreamland: amusement parks, movies and American modernity*, New York: Columbia University Press.

Rancière, J., 2006, *The Politics of Aesthetics: the distribution of the sensible*, London: Continuum.

Reiser, S. J., 1993, "Technology and the use of the senses in twentieth-century medicine," in W. F. Bynum and R. Porter (eds), *Medicine and the Five Senses*, Cambridge: Cambridge University Press.

"Retailer Right on Target," 2012, *Chicago Tribune*, July 26.

Reynolds, S., 1998, *Energy Flash: a journey through rave culture and dance music*, London: Macmillan.

Rheingold, H., 1993, *Virtual Reality: exploring the brave new technologies of artificial intelligence and interactive world*, New York: Summit Books.

Richards, J., 2010, *The Age of the Dream Palace: cinema and society in 1930s Britain*, London: I. B. Tauris & Co.

Richter, H., 1965, *Dada and Anti-Art*, New York: McGraw-Hill.

Rickli, C., 2009, "An event 'like a movie'? Hollywood and 9/11," *Current Objectives of Postgraduate American Studies*, 110, 1.

Robbins, T. and Anthony, D., 1982, "Deprogramming, brainwashing and the medicalization of deviant religious groups," *Social Problems*, 29(3), 283–97.

Roberts, J. B. and Briand, P. L. (eds), 1957, *The Sound of Wings: readings for the air age*, New York: Henry Holt.

Robertson, J. E., 2005, *A Companion to the Anthropology of Japan*, London: Blackwell.

Rodriguez, R., 1983, *Hunger of Memory: the education of Richard Rodriguez*, New York: Bantam Books.

Rojek, C., 1995, *Decentring Leisure*, London: Sage.

Roseman, M., 1993, *Healing Sounds from the Malaysian Rainforest: Temiar music and medicine*, Berkeley, CA: University of California Press.

Rosenfeld, S., 2011, "On being heard: a case for paying attention to the historical ear," *American Historical Review*, 116(2), 316–34.

Ross, A. I., 2012, *The Anthropology of Alternative Medicine*, Oxford: Berg.

Rowley, L., 2003, *On Target: how the world's hottest retailer hit a bull's eye*, Hoboken, NJ: Wiley.

Rumelhart, D. *et al.*, 1986, *Parallel Distributed Processing*, Vol. I, Cambridge, MA: MIT Press.

Rushdie, S., 1981, *Midnight's Children*, London: Picador.

Russell, B., 1912, *The Problems of Philosophy*, Oxford: Oxford University Press.

Russell, B., 1927, *An Outline of Philosophy*, London: George Allen & Unwin.

Saia v. New York [1948], 334, US 558.

Saldanha, A., 2002, "Music tourism and factions of bodies in Goa," *Tourist Studies*, 2(1), 43–62.

Salimpoor, V. N., Benovoy, M., Larcher, K., Dagher, A., and Zatorre, R. J., 2011, "Anatomically distinct dopamine release during anticipation and experience of peak emotion to music," *Nature Neuroscience*, 14(2), 257–62.

Sally, L., 2006, "Fantasy lands and kinesthetic thrills: sensorial consumption, the shock of modernity and spectacle as total-body experience at Coney Island," *The Senses and Society*, 3(1), 293–310.

Sandburg, C., 2003, *The Complete Poems of Carl Sandburg*, New York: Harcourt.

Sarna, J. D., 2003, "The debate over mixed seating in the American synagogue," in D. G. Hackett (ed.), *Religion and American Culture: a reader*, New York: Routledge.

Sassoon, S., 1931, *Memoirs of an Infantry Officer*, London: Faber & Faber.

Schafer, R. M., 1994, *The Soundscape: our sonic environment and the tuning of the world*, Rochester, VT: Destiny Books.

Schultz, K. M., 2011, *Tri-Faith America: how Catholics and Jews held postwar America to its Protestant promise*, New York: Oxford University Press.

Schwartz, H., 2003, "The indefensible ear: a history," in M. Bull and L. Back (eds), *The Auditory Culture Reader*, Oxford: Berg.

Scruton, R., 1995, *The Classical Vernacular: architectural principles in an age of nihilism*, London: Palgrave Macmillan.

Searle, J. R., 1983, *Intentionality: an essay in the philosophy of mind*, Cambridge: Cambridge University Press.

Sennett, R., 1994, *Flesh and Stone: the body and the city in western civilization*, London: Faber.

Serematakis, C. N. (ed.), 1994, *The Senses Still: perception and memory as material culture in modernity*, Boulder, CO: Westview Press.

Sharpe, W., 2008, *New York Nocturne: the city after dark in literature, painting and photography, 1850–1950*, Princeton, NJ: Princeton University Press.

Sherrington, C. S., 1907, "On the proprioceptive system, especially in its reflex aspect," *Brain*, 29(4), 467–85.

Shields, R., 1991, *Places on the Margin*, London: Routledge.

Shove, E., 2004, *Comfort, Cleanliness and Convenience: the social organization of normality*, Oxford: Berg

Sibley, D., 1988, "Survey 13: purification of space," *Environment and Planning D: Society and Space*, 6, 409–21.

Simmel, G., 1995, "The metropolis and mental life," in P. Kasinitz (ed.) *Metropolis: centre and symbol of our times*, London: Macmillan.

Skeates, R., 2010, *An Archaeology of the Senses: prehistoric Malta*, Oxford: Oxford University Press.

Skinner, B. F., 1938, *The Behavior of Organisms*, New York: Appleton-Century-Crofts.

Skinner B. F., 1957, *Verbal Behavior*, Cambridge, MA: Prentice-Hall.

Slabbekoorn, H. and Ripmeester, E., 2008, "Birdsong and anthropogenic noise: implications and applications for conservation," *Molecular Ecology*, 17(1), 72–83.

Smith, D. W., 2011, "Phenomenology," in E. N. Zalta (ed.), *The Stanford Encyclopedia of Philosophy*, http://plato.stanford.edu/archives/fall2011/entries/phenomenology.

Smith, M. M., 2006, *How Race Is Made: slavery, segregation, and the senses*, Chapel Hill, NC: University of North Carolina Press.

Smith, M. M., 2007, *Sensing the Past: seeing, hearing, smelling, tasting and touching history*, Berkeley, CA: University of California Press.

Smith, S. M., 2010, "Nursing the nation: the 1930s public health nurse as image and icon," in D. Serlin (ed.), *Imagining Illness: public health and visual culture*, Minneapolis, MN: University of Minnesota Press.

Snow, J., 2004, "The civilization of white men: the race of the Hindu in *United States v. Bhagat Singh Thind*," in H. Goldschmidt and E. McAlister (eds), *Race, Nation, and Religion in the Americas*, New York: Oxford University Press.

Sobchack, V., 1998, "Beating the meat/surviving the text, or how to get out of this century alive," in P. Treichler, L. Cartwright, and C. Penley (eds), *The Visible Woman: imaging technologies, gender, and science*, New York: New York University Press.

Sontag, S., 1973, *On Photography*, New York: Picador.

Sontag, S., 2004, *Regarding the Pain of Others*, New York: Farrar, Straus & Giroux.

Spigel, L., 1992, *Make Room for TV: television and the family ideal in postwar America*, Chicago: University of Chicago Press.

Spock, B., [1946] 2012, *Dr. Spock's Baby and Child Care*, 9th edn, New York: Pocket Books.

Spock, B. and Parker, S., 1998, *Dr Spock's Baby and Child Care*, New York: Pocket Books.

Staples, W. G., 2000, *Everyday Surveillance: vigilance and visible in postmodern life*, Lanham, MD: Rowman & Littlefield.

Stein, B. (ed.), 2012, *The New Handbook of Multisensory Processing*, Cambridge, MA: MIT Press.

Sterne, J., 1997, "Sounds like the mall of America: programmed music and the architectonics of commercial space," *Ethnomusicology*, 41(1), 22–50.

Sterne, J., 2003, *The Audible Past: cultural origins of sound reproduction*, Durham, NC: Duke University Press.

Stodola, S., 2011, "Art meets leisure in Arkansas," *New York Times*, December 1.

Strasser, S., 1989, *Satisfaction Guaranteed: the making of the American mass market*, Washington, DC: Smithsonian Institution Press.

Sutton, D., 2001, *Remembrance of Repasts: an anthropology of food and memory*, Oxford: Berg.

Syman, S., 2010, *The Subtle Body: the story of yoga in America*, New York: Farrar, Straus & Giroux.

Synnott, A., 2005, "Handling children," in C. Classen (ed.), *The Book of Touch*, Oxford: Berg.

Taussig, M., 1993, *Mimesis and Alterity: a particular history of the senses*, London: Routledge.

Taylor, W. R., 1988, "New York and the origin of the skyline: the visual city as text," *Prospects*, 13, 225–48.

Tedlow, R. S., 1990, *New and Improved: the story of mass marketing in America*, New York: Basic Books.

Thomas, P., 2012, *Listen, Whitey: the sights and sounds of black power, 1965–1975*, Seattle, WA: Fantagraphics Books.

Tichi, C., 1987, *Shifting Gears: technology, literature, culture in modernist literature*, Durham, NC: University of North Carolina Press.

Tillich, P. and Green, T., 1954, "Authentic religious art," *Masterpieces of Religious Art exhibition held in connection with the Second Assembly of the World Council of Churches*, Chicago: Art Institute of Chicago.

Tiravanija, R., 2010, *Cook Book*, Bangkok, MA: River Books Press.

Tolbert, L. C., 2009, "The aristocracy of the market basket: self-service food shopping," in W. Belasco and R. Horowitz (eds), *Food Chains: from farm yard to shopping cart*, Philadelphia, PA: University of Pennsylvania Press.

Tonnies, F., 1955, *Community and Association*, London: Routledge & Kegan Paul.

Turing, L., 2006, *The Secret of Scent*, London: HarperCollins.

Turkle, S., 1995, *Life on the Screen: identity in the age of the internet*, New York: Simon & Schuster.

Turkle, S., 2011, *Alone Together: why we expect more from technology and less from each other*, New York: Basic Books.

Turner, V. W., 1968, *The Drums of Affliction*, Oxford: Clarendon Press.

United States v. *Thind* [1923], 261, US 204.

Urry, J., 2002, *The Tourist Gaze*, 2nd edn, London: Sage.

Vannini, P., Waskul, D., and Gottschalk, S., 2012, *The Senses in Self, Society and Culture: a sociology of the senses*, London: Routledge.

Virilio, P., 1989, *War and Cinema: the logistics of perception*, London: Verso.

Wacker, G., 2001, *Heaven Below: early Pentecostals and American culture*, Cambridge, MA: Harvard University Press.

Wacquant, L., 2007, "French working-class banlieues and Black American ghetto: from conflation to comparison," *Qui Parle*, 16(2), 5–38.

Walt Disney Company, 2011, *Fact Book: 2011*, http://thewaltdisneycompany.com/investors/fact-books.

Walt Disney Company, 2012, Disneyland Park website, http://disneyland.disney. go.com/disneyland.

Ware, V. and Back, L., 2002, *Out of Whiteness: color, politics, and culture*, Chicago, IL: University of Chicago Press.

Warner, M., 2006, "Wal-Mart extending its dominance of the grocery business," *New York Times*, March 3.

Watson, J. B., 1924, *Behaviorism*, New York: Norton.

Watts, S., 1995, "Walt Disney: art and politics in the American century," *Journal of American History*, 82, 84–110.

Waugh, P., 2009, "Writing the body: modernism and postmodernism," in C. Saunders *et al.* (eds), *The Body and the Arts*, Basingstoke: Palgrave Macmillan.

Weiner, I., 2014, *Religion Out Loud: religious sound, public space, and American pluralism*, New York: New York University Press.

Wenger, T., 2009, *We Have a Religion: the 1920s Pueblo Indian dance controversy and American religious freedom*, Chapel Hill, NC: University of North Carolina Press.

White, F., 1998, *The Overview Effect: space exploration and human evolution*, Reston, VA: American Institute of Aeronautics and Astronautics.

White, M., 2001, "Johannes Baader's Plasto-Dio-Dada-Drama: the mysticism of the mass-media," *Modernism/Modernity*, 8(4), 583–602.

Wilkerson, M., 2006, *Amazing Journey: the life of Peter Townshend*, Louisville, KY: Bad News Press.

Williamson, H., 1930, *The Patriot's Progress*, London: Geoffrey Bles.

Winterson, J., 2000, *The PowerBook*, London: Jonathan Cape.

Woolf, V., 1978, "Letter to Ethel Smyth, Thursday 28 August 1930," in N. Nicolson (ed.), *A Reflection of the Other Person: the letters of Virginia Woolf*, Vol. 4, London: Hogarth.

Woolf, V., 2000, *The Wave*, Ware: Wordsworth Editions.

Woolf, V., 2008a, "Modern fiction," in *Selected Essays*, ed. D. Bradshaw, Oxford: Oxford University Press.

Woolf, V., 2008b, "On being ill," in *Selected Essays*, ed. D. Bradshaw, Oxford: Oxford University Press.

Yoshimi, S., 2001, "America in Japan/Japan in Disneyfication: the Disney image and the transformation of 'America' in contemporary Japan," in J. Wasko, M. Philips, and E. R. Meehan (eds), *Dazzled by Disney? The global Disney audiences project*, London: Leicester University Press.

Young, M. and Willmott, P., 1992, *Family and Kinship in East London*, Berkeley, CA: University of California Press.

Zelizer, B., 2001, *About to Die. How news images move the public*, Oxford: Oxford University Press.

Zeller, B. E., 2012, "Food practices, culture, and social dynamics in the Hare Krishna movement," in C. M. Cusack and A. Norman (eds), *Handbook of New Religions and Cultural Production*, Leiden: Brill.

Zeller, B. E., 2014, "Quasi-religious American foodways: the cases of vegetarianism and locavorism," in B. E. Zeller, M. W. Dallam, R. L. Neilson, and N. L. Rubel (eds), *The Way of Food: religion, food, and eating in North America*, New York: Columbia University Press.

Zhdanov, A., [1934] 1992, "Speech to the Congress of Soviet Writers," in C. Harrison and P. Wood (eds), *Art in Theory: 1900–1990*, Oxford: Blackwell.

NOTES ON CONTRIBUTORS

Michael Bull is Reader in Media and Cultural Studies at the University of Sussex. His publications include *Sounding Out the City, Personal Stereos and the Management of Everyday Life* (2000) and *Sound Moves, iPod Culture and Urban Experience* (2007). He is the co-editor of *The Auditory Culture Reader* (2003) and editor of *Sound Studies* (Major Works) for Routledge (2013). He is a founding member of the European Association of Sound Studies and co-founder of the journal *The Senses and Society* (Bloomsbury).

Tim Edensor teaches cultural geography at Manchester Metropolitan University. He has authored *Tourists at the Taj* (1998), *National Identity, Popular Culture and Everyday Life* (2002), and *Industrial Ruins: Space, Aesthetics and Materiality*; edited *Geographies of Rhythm* (2010) and co-edited *Urban Theory Beyond the West: A World of Cities* (2011). He has written on national identity, tourism, industrial ruins, walking, driving, football cultures, and urban materiality and is currently investigating landscapes of illumination and darkness.

Ralf Hertel is Professor of English Literature at the University of Hamburg. His interests include the sensuousness of reading, early modern drama, and Anglo-Eastern encounters. He is the author of *Making Sense: Sense Perception in the British Novel of the 1980s and 1990s* (2005) and co-editor of *Performing National Identity: Anglo-Italian Cultural Transactions* (2008) as well as *Early Modern Encounters with the Islamic East* (2012). His most recent publication is *Staging England in the Elizabethan History Play* (2014).

Hannah B. Higgins is Professor of Art History at the University of Illinois, Chicago. Her publications include *Fluxus Experience* (2002) and *The Grid Book* (2009) as well as the anthology *Mainframe Experimentalism: Early Computing and the Foundations of Digital Art* (2012), co-edited with Douglas Kahn. She has received DAAD, Getty and Philips Collection Fellowships in support of her research, and is co-executor of the Estate of Dick Higgins and the Something Else Press.

David Howes is Professor of Anthropology and Director of the Centre for Sensory Studies at Concordia University, Montreal. He has conducted field research in Papua New Guinea, Northwestern Argentina, and the Southwestern United States. His research is in commerce, medicine, aesthetics, and law. He is the author or editor of numerous books, including *The Varieties of Sensory Experience* (1991), *Cross-Cultural Consumption* (1996), *Sensual Relations* (2003), and, most recently, *Ways of Sensing* (2014) with Constance Classen.

Adam Mack is Assistant Professor of History at the School of the Art Institute of Chicago. His research deals with sensory marketing, consumer culture, and urban studies. He is the author of *Sensing Chicago: The Rise of the Second City* (2014), and is currently working on a study of the sensory dimensions of the post-Second World War suburban marketplace.

Matthew Nudds is Professor of Philosophy and Head of the Philosophy Department at the University of Warwick. His research is in philosophy of mind and perception. In particular he is interested in what account should be given of the non-visual senses. He has published papers on the nature of the senses and on auditory perception and is editor—with Casey O'Callaghan—of *Sounds and Perception* (2010).

Alex Rhys-Taylor is Lecturer in Sociology and Deputy Director of the Centre for Urban and Community Research at Goldsmiths College, University of London. His research addresses questions around class, ethnicity, and gender in cities through the methods of multisensory ethnography and history. He has recently written on public space, olfaction, and multiculture for *Identities* (2013) and the relationship between class and disgust for *The Sociological Review* (2013). He is also the editor of *Street Signs* magazine.

Anamaria Iosif Ross is a Romanian-American anthropologist interested in preventive medicine, sensory dynamics of healing, human development, change, and revitalization movements. She has conducted fieldwork in Romania on healing and personhood after socialism. Her publications include *The Anthropology of Alternative Medicine* (2012) and articles in the *Journal of Religion and Society* and *Dilema Veche*. She currently explores environmental barriers to wellbeing in ethnically diverse communities.

Isaac A. Weiner is Assistant Professor of Religion and Culture in the Department of Comparative Studies at the Ohio State University. His research interests include American religious history, religious pluralism, religion and law, theory and method in the study of religion, and religion and the senses. He is the author of *Religion Out Loud: Religious Sound, Public Space, and American Pluralism* (2013).

INDEX

Degen, M. 43, 47, 69–70
Delvecchio Good, M. 151
democracy 110–11, 120, 123
Derrida, J. 183
Destination Moon ride 228
Die Hard 240
Diet for a Small Planet 23
Disneyland 1, 21, 77–80, 91, 94–5,
 228
Disneyworld 79, 235
Doors of Perception, The 25
Douglas, M. 67
"Downtown" 10
Dreamland 82–3
dress 117, 120–1, 156–7
drone aircraft 236–8
drugs 24–5, 42, 162–3
Duchamp, M. 199, 208
Dummett, D. 126

ear 13, 64, 99, 108, 196, 204
 see also hearing
Earth 5, 13, 18, 161
Eastern philosophies and religions 25,
 118, 164
Edible Woman, The 185
electric 17, 44, 64, 73, 82, 108
elevator 6–7 *see also* encapsulation
Eliot, T.S. 181
ELTA Universitate 167–9
Empire State Building 61
encapsulation 7, 62
Endgame 184, 186
England 9, 52, 59, 61, 69, 103
English Patient, The 189
environment 5, 16–17, 122, 180
environmentalism 19, 161
"Event" 210–12
everyday life 13, 111, 204, 210–11, 229,
 234
experience 79–80, 132–3, 134–6, 144–5,
 212, 219, 223, 234–5
 at a distance 224
 direct 221–2, 227
 economy 80

filmic 234
 mediated 221–2, 231
experimentation 135, 137, 161–2
expressway 62, 66
eye(s) 12, 13, 20, 63, 84, 104, 108, 196,
 204, 224 *see also* sight
Eye, The 184
Eyes of the Skin, The 58–9

faith 110, 114
family 10, 14, 15, 79, 80, 88, 91, 93, 97
 photo album 12
fantasy 45, 207–8, 211
Fascism 204–5, 158, 223
fear 45, 60, 66, 169
Febvre, L. 28
Feelies, The 219–20
Feminine Mystique, The 11
feminist 19
 concerns 183
 philosophy 126
Filliou, R. 213
film 106, 220–1, 223, 224–5, 227,
 239–40
 technique 224–5, 227, 239
"Flädlesoup" installation 215
flight 5, 64, 227–8
food 17, 42, 43, 49, 67–8, 69–71, 78, 87,
 91, 167–8
 culinary creolization 71
 in art 204–7, 213, 215–17
 natural 22–3
 slow 42
 raw 167–8
 retailing of 83–6, 89–91
Foucault, M. 28, 189
Foul and the Fragrant, The 28
Foxell, S. 57
fragmentation 102, 123
Frames 185
France 61, 129
Frau im Mond 227
Frege, G. 125
Freud, S. 174
Friedan, B. 11

www.ingramcontent.com/pod-product-compliance
Lightning Source LLC
Chambersburg PA
CBHW081430270326
41932CB00019B/3151